Atlas of Human Anatomy

Sobotta

**Volume 2 Trunk, Viscera,
Lower Limb**

Atlas of Human Anatomy
Sobotta

Edited by: R. Putz and R. Pabst
with assistance of Renate Putz

Volume 2 Trunk, Viscera, Lower Limb

13th English Edition
Nomenclature in English
21st German edition

755 colored figure tables
40 tables

Translated and edited by:

Andreas H. Weiglein, M.D.
Associate Professor
Institute of Anatomy
Medical School
Karl-Franzens-University Graz
Graz, Austria, Europe

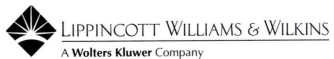

LIPPINCOTT WILLIAMS & WILKINS
A **Wolters Kluwer** Company
Philadelphia · Baltimore · New York · London
Buenos Aires · Hong Kong · Sydney · Tokyo

Correspondence and criticism to:
Urban & Fischer, lecturer for medical students, Dr. D. Hennesseen, Karlstrasse 45, 80333 Munich

Editors:

Professor R. Putz, M.D., Chairman
Institute of Anatomy
Ludwig-Maximillian-University
Pettenkofferstrasse 11, 80336 Munich

Professor R. Pabst, M.D., Chairman
Department of Functional and Applied Anatomy
Medical School
Carl-Neuberg-Strasse 8, 30625 Hannover

The atlas consists of two separate volumes:

Vol. 1: Head, Neck, Upper Limb

Vol. 2: Trunk, Viscera, Lower Limb

Program Director: Dorothea Hennessen, M.D.
Lecturer: Alexander Gattnarzik
Production: Renate Hausdorf
Graphics Design: Carsten Tschirner, Munich
Cover Design: prepress, Ulm
Cover Illustration: Michael Budowick

German Library Cataloging-in-Publication Data

Sobotta, Johannes:
Atlas der Anatomie des Menschen/ Sobotta [Hrsg. Von R. Putz und R. Pabst unter Mitarb. Von Renate Putz]. - München: Jena: Urban und Fischer
    Further editions in non-European languages.- until 20th edition by Urban und Schwarzenberg, Munich, Vienna, Baltimore
    Engl. Edition titled: Sobotta, Johannes: Atlas of human anatomy. -
    French edition titled: Sobotta, Johannes: Atlas d'anatomie humaine. -
    Turkish edition titled: Insan anatomisi atlasi

Vol. 2 Trunk, Viscera, Lower Limb: 40 tables. - 21st revised edition - 2000
ISBN 3-437-41950-1

00 01 02 03   5 4 3 2 1

Setting: Typodata, Munich
(Set in type in 9 Point Corporate in Quark Xpress in Apple Macintosh)
Reproduction: Typodata, Munich
Printing and Binding: Appl, Wemding
(Printed on Nopacoat 115 g)
Printed in Germany

The founder of this atlas, Johannes Sobotta; M.D. †, was the former Professor of Anatomy and Director of the Anatomical Institute of the University of Bonn.

German Editions and year of publication:
1st Edition: 1904-1907 J.F. Lehmanns Verlag, Munich
2nd - 11th Editions: 1913-1944 J.F. Lehmanns Verlag, Munich
12th Edition: 1948 and following editions Urban & Schwarzenberg, Munich
13th Edition: 1953
14th Edition: 1956
15th Edition: 1957
16th Edition: 1967 (ISBN 3-541-02826-2)
17th Edition: 1972 (ISBN 3-541-02827-0)
18th Edition: 1982 (ISBN 3-541-02828-9)
19th Edition: 1988 (ISBN 3-541-02829-7)
20th Edition: 1993 (ISBN 3-541-17370-X)
21st Edition: 2000 (ISBN 3-437-41950-1)

Licensed Editions:

Arabic Edition
Modern Technical Center, Damascus

Chinese Edition
Ho-Chi Book Publishing, Taiwan

Croatian Edition
Naklada Slap, Jastrebarsko

Dutch Edition
Bohn Stafleu van Loghum, Houten

English Edition (English Nomenclature)
Atlas of Human Anatomy
Lippincott Williams & Wilkins

English Edition (English Nomenclature)
Atlas of Human Anatomy
Urban & Fischer

French Edition
Atlas d'Anatomie Humaine
Tec & Doc Lavoisier, Paris

Greek Edition (Greek Nomenclature)
Maria G. Parissianos, Athens

Greek Edition (Latin Nomenclature)
Maria G. Parissianos, Athens

Hungarian Edition
az ember anatómiájának atlasza
Semmelweis Kiadó

Indonesian Edition
Atlas Anatomi Manusia
Penerbit Buku Kedokteran EGC, Jakarta

Italian Edition
Atlante di Anatomia Umana
UTET, Torino

Japanese Edition
Igaku Shoin Ltd., Tokyo

Korean Edition
Panmun Book Company, Seoul

Polish Edition
Atlas anatomia cztowieka
Urban & Partner

Portuguese Edition (Portuguese Nomenclature)
Atlas de Anatomia Humana
Editora Guanbara Koogan, Rio de Janeiro

Portuguese Edition (Latin Nomenclature)
Atlas de Anatomia Humana
Editora Guanbara Koogan, Rio de Janeiro

Spanish Edition
Atlas de Anatomia Humana
Editrial Medica Panamericana, Buenos Aires/ Madrid

Turkish Edition
Insan Anatomisi Atlasi
Bera Basim Yayim Dagitim, Istanbul

Contents

Preface

After the excellent acceptance of the 20th edition of the Atlas, that was founded in 1903 by J. Sobotta, the editors and the publishers considered what could be improved in a standard book like this. From many letters and from many discussions with both students and colleagues it became obvious that the concept still fits into the "study landscape," due to the fact that gross anatomy—besides the other basic sciences—unquestionably is one of the pillars of medicine, particularly with a practical point of view. Although this atlas primarily focuses on the pre-clinical student, it—as a "book for a life as a physician"—nevertheless meets all requirements to accompany the student throughout the clinical years and also as a reference book for the later professional activity. Following the most important wishes of the users, the 21st edition presents a number of innovations:

In the new edition we have

- drawn 133 new figures based on original prosections, e.g. the serial sections of the brain and the thorax,
- replaced the black and white figures,
- updated the figures according to technical development, e.g. endoscopic views or X-rays,
- introduced diagrams on joint load,
- completely redone the diagrams on the muscles.

As a second important goal we improved the readability by:
- the introduction of signal colors for the chapters,
- a color code of the labels of topographical figures,
- consistent introduction of orientation sketches for slice direction and visual angle,
- revision and renewal of the well accepted tables,
- the introduction of small "wind roses" referring to adjacent figures in different directions and sections.

Of course, the new nomenclature (Terminologia Anatomica) valid since October 1998 has been used consistently. The glossary builds a bridge of understanding for those interested in the background of our terminology.

With the exception of discussion about general concepts and mutual correction, the editors have maintained the division for the revision of the chapters as follows:

R. Putz:　general anatomy, upper limb, brain, eye, ear, back, lower limb;

R. Pabst:　head, neck, thoracic and abdominal walls, thorax, abdomen, pelvis

For the large number of new figures the following medical illustrators deserve our acknowledgment: Mrs. Ulrike Brugger, Mr. Ruediger Himmelhan, Mrs. Sonja Klebe, and Mr. Horst Russ. It is owing to them that the familiar and successful "Sobotta style" has essentially been maintained. The electronic processing of photographs and the production of graphs have been accomplished by Mr. Michael Budowick. We also owe a debt of gratitude to our clinical colleagues, who again made several figures available for this edition (see acknowledgements). We also would like to thank the involved members of the institutes and departments for their insight and their suggestions. Mr. Dr. N. Sokolov and Mr. A. Buchhorn have done the delicate dissections to serve as the basis for many new illustrations; Mrs. S. Fryk and Mrs. G. Hoppmann supported us in text processing. The glossary was critically reviewed by Mr. cand. phil. T. Lederer.

The editors would also like to express their gratitude to the lecturers, particularly to Mrs. Dr. D. Hennessen and Mr. A. Gattnarzik, who despite some external turbulence helped us to consistently pursue the accomplishment of this new edition. In the beginning the production was assisted in the proved way by Mr. P. Mazzetti and later on by Mrs. R. Hausdorf with great effort. Mrs. Renate Putz was responsible for both the realization of the Nomina Anatomica and for the standardization of references and text. We would like to express our special thanks to all ladies and gentlemen who devoted themselves to the nerve-wracking job of the correction and the assembly of the index. It is only possible that the "SOBOTTA" now is published with lots of new contents and in new brilliance with the constructive collaboration of all people involved. We also wish to thank our families for their understanding for this time-consuming project.

Many innovations of this atlas are based upon the critiques and the suggestions of both students and colleagues. This is highly appreciated by the editors, and we would like to ask the users of this edition not to hesitate to send us their comments.

Munich and Hannover, September 1999
R. Putz and R. Pabst

General Terms

The following terms indicate opposite positions of organs and parts of the body, partially regardless of the position of the body, as well as the position and direction in the extremities. These terms are not only used in human anatomy, but also in practical medicine and comparative anatomy.

General terms

anterior-posterior = in front of-in back of (e.g. anterior and posterior tibial arteries)

ventral-dorsal = closer to the belly-closer to the back

superior-inferior = higher-lower (e.g. superior and inferior nasal conchae)

cranial-caudal = closer to the cranium-closer to the tail

internal-external = inward-outward

superficial-deep = close to the surface-in the depth

middle, intermediate = between two other structures (e.g. the middle nasal concha lies between the superior and inferior nasal conchae)

median = in the median plane (anterior median fissure of the spinal cord). A "median section" divides the body into two symmetrical parts.

medial-lateral = closer to the middle of the body, closer to the side of the body (e.g. medial and lateral inguinal fossae)

Terms for directions and positions in the extremities

proximal-distal = closer to the root of the extremity-closer to the end of the extremity (e.g. proximal and distal radio-ulnar joints)

for the upper limb:
radial-ulnar = on the side of the radius-on the side of the ulna (e.g. radial and ulnar arteries)

for the hand:
palmar [volar]-dorsal = on the palm of the hand-on the back of the hand (e.g. palmar aponeurosis, dorsal interossei)

for the lower limb:
tibial-fibular [peroneal] = on the side of the tibia-on the side of the fibula (e.g. anterior tibial artery)

for the foot:
plantar-dorsal = on the sole-on the dorsum of foot (e.g. lateral and medial plantar arteries, dorsalis pedis artery [dorsal artery of foot])

Instructions for colored figures

The multicolored figures of this book are based on didactic considerations: contrasts should be enhanced, structures that are difficult to distinguish should be more obvious. The colors used for different tissues (such as tendons, cartilage, bone, muscles) and pathways (such as arteries, veins, lymph vessels, nerves) differ from those in the living or dead body or the embalmed cadaver. Arteries are colored in red, veins in blue, nerves in yellow, lymph vessels and nodes generally in green.

In addition to the artists (K. Hajek, Professor E. Lepier, F. Bathe, H. von Eickstedt, K. Endtresser, J. Kosanke, J. von Marchtaler, J. Dimes, U. Brugger, N. Lechenbauer, I. Schnellbaecher, and K. Schuhmacher) that produced the base for the entire figure set together with Professor Sobotta and the later editors Professor Becher, Professor Ferner, and Professor Staubesand, the following artists worked for this present issue: Mrs. Ulrike Brugger, Mr. Ruediger Himmelhan, Mrs. Sonja Klebe, and Mr. Horst Russ. A series of original photographs were processed electronically by Mr. Michael Budowick. Some CT-scan diagrams were produced by Mrs. Henriette Rintelen.

The following figure numbers indicate both newly developed figures and new drawings due to main corrections:
U. Brugger
707, 923, 924, 927-932, 934, 936, 937, 1266,1378
R. Himmelhan
1367, 1368, 1370, 1372, 1374, 1375
S. Klebe
1162, 1174, 1175, 1218, 1222, 1223, 1250, 1349
H. Russ
788, 798, 1281-1284, 1302-1304

Acknowledgements

The authors are greatly obliged to the following clinical colleagues for their contribution of ultrasound, computer-tomographic, and magnetic resonance images as well as endoscopic photographs and color photographs of surgical procedures:

Prof. Altaras, Center of Radiology, University of Giessen (Figs. 964, 979, 980)

Dr. Baumeister, Department of Radiology, University of Freiburg (Fig. 1095)

Prof. Daniel, Department of Cardiology, Hannover Medical School (Figs. 862–864, 935)

Prof. Galanski, Dr. Kirchhoff, Department of Diagnostic Radiology I, Hannover Medical School (Figs 924, 1144 a, b, 1154, 1155)

Prof. Galanski, Dr. Schäfer, Department of Diagnostic Radiology I, Hannover Medical School (Figs. 838 a, b, 888, 933, 958, 1139, 1147, 1150, 1152)

Prof. Gebel, Department of Gastro-enterology and Hepatology, Hannover Medical School (Figs. 253 a, b, 966, 975, 976, 981, 990, 991, 1026, 1043)

Dr. Goel, Radiology, Heerlen, Netherlands (Figs. 1010, 1011) (with permission: Radiology 173: 137–141, 1989)

Dr. Greeven, St. Elisabeth Hospital, Neuwied (Figs. 166, 1182)

Prof. Von der Hardt, Clinic of Pediatrics, Hannover Medical School (Fig. 893)

Dr. Hennig, Department of Radiology, University of Freiburg (Fig. 529)

Prof. Jonas, Urology, Hannover Medical School (Figs. 1050 a, b, 1051)

Prof. Kremers, Policlinic of Preservative Dentistry and Parodontology, Munich University (Fig. 182)

Prof. Kunze, Clinic of Pediatrics, Munich University (Figs. 15–18)

Dr. Meyer, Department of Gastro-enterology and Hepatology, Hannover Medical School (Figs. 906, 949 a, b, 959, 1086)

Prof. Pfeifer, Division of Radiology, Clinic of Surgery, Munich University (Figs. 306, 319, 321, 748–751, 789–792, 1199, 1230, 1231, 1260, 1261)

Priv.-Doz. Rau, Department of Radiology, University of Freiburg (Figs. 875, 886, 887)

Prof. Ravelli, Institute of Anatomy, Innsbruck University (Fig. 746)

Prof. Reich, Clinic of Orofacial Surgery, Bonn University (Figs. 133, 134)

Prof. Reiser, Dr. Glaser, Institute of Clinical Radiology, Munich University (Figs. 307, 578–582, 705 a, b, 771, 1369, 1371, 1373, 1377)

Prof. Rudzki-Janson, Policlinic of Pediatric Orthopedics, Munich University (Figs 80, 81)

Dr. Scheibe, Department of Surgery, Rosman Hospital, Breisach (Figs. 1233 a–c)

Prof. Schillinger, Women's Clinic, Freiburg University (Figs. 1072–1074)

Dr. Dr. Schliephake, Orofacial Surgery, Hannover Medical School (Figs. 167, 212, 213)

Prof. Schloesser, Center of Gynecology, Hannover Medical School (Figs. 1071 a, b, 1080, 1082, 1083, 1130)

Prof. Schumacher, Neuroradiology, Department of Radiology, Freiburg University – (Figs. 448 a, b)

Dr. Sommer and Priv.-Doz. Bauer, Radiologists, Munich (Figs. 650, 1234–1236)

Prof. Stotz, Policlinic of Orthopedics, Munich University (Fig. 1193)

Prof. Vogl, Policlinic of Radiology, Munich University (Figs. 440, 442, 631, 632)

Prof. Vollrath, Clinic of ENT Surgery, Moenchengladbach (Figs. 246–248)

Prof. Wagner †, Department of Diagnostic Radiology II, Hannover Medical School (Figs. 914, 1014, 1017, 1020, 1023, 1090)

Prof. Wenz, Department of Radiology, Freiburg University (Fig. 747)

Dr. Willfuehr, Abdominal and Transplant Surgery, Hannover Medical School (Fig. 1001)

Priv.-Doz. Wimmer, Department of Radiology, Freiburg University (Fig. 778)

Additional illustrations were taken from the following books:

Birkner, R.: Das typische Roentgenbild des Skeletts. (The Typical Radiograph of the Skeleton.) Urban & Schwarzenberg, Munich-Vienna-Baltimore, 1990 (Fig. 1200)

Welsch, U. (ed.): Sobotta-Histologie (Sobotta-Histology), 5th edition, Urban & Schwarzenberg, Munich-Vienna-Baltimore, 1997 (Figs. 635, 646)

Wicke, L.: Atlas der Roentgenanatomie (Atlas of Radiological Anatomy), 3rd edition, Urban & Schwarzenberg, Munich-Vienna-Baltimore, 1985 (Figs. 905 a, b, 1076)

Wilhelm, K.R., R. Putz, R. Hierner, R.E. Giunta: Lappenplastiken in der Handchirurgie (Flaps in Handsurgery). Urban & Schwarzenberg, Munich-Vienna-Baltimore, 1997 (Fig. 58)

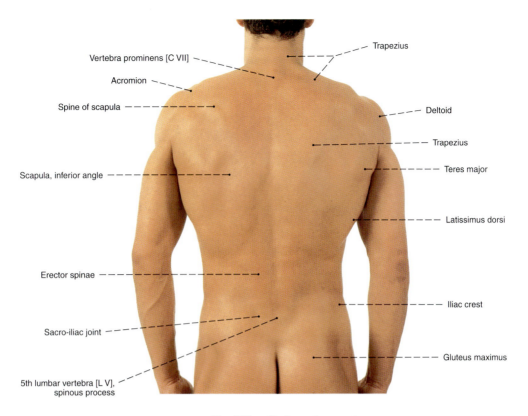

Vertebra prominens [C VII]
Acromion
Spine of scapula
Scapula, inferior angle
Erector spinae
Sacro-iliac joint
5th lumbar vertebra [L V], spinous process

Trapezius
Deltoid
Trapezius
Teres major
Latissimus dorsi
Iliac crest
Gluteus maximus

Fig. 706 Back, surface anatomy.

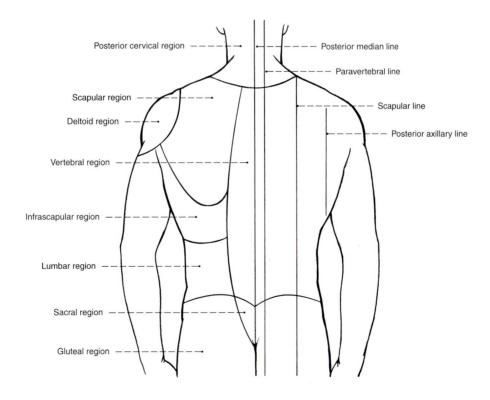

Posterior cervical region
Scapular region
Deltoid region
Vertebral region
Infrascapular region
Lumbar region
Sacral region
Gluteal region

Posterior median line
Paravertebral line
Scapular line
Posterior axillary line

Fig. 707 Posterior planes and axes of the human body.

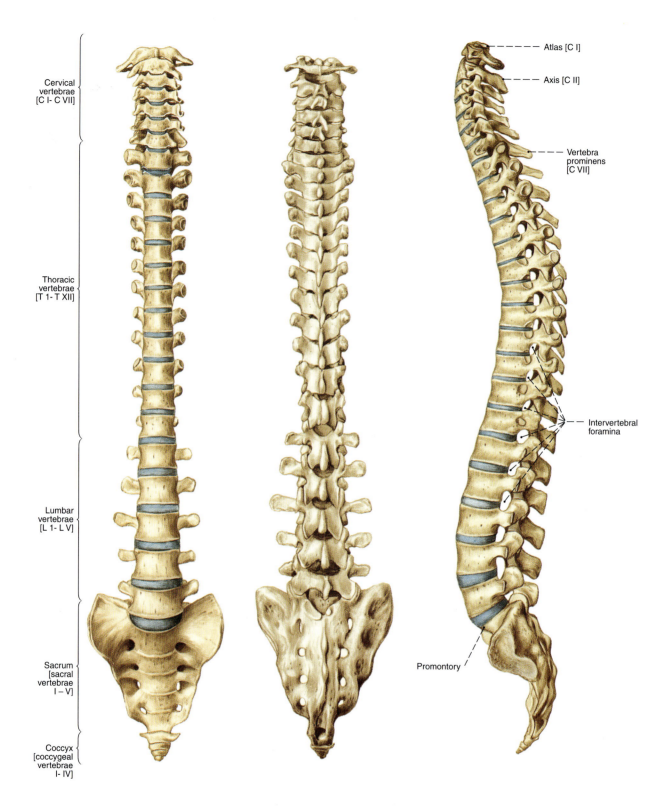

Cervical
vertebrae
[C I- C VII]

Thoracic
vertebrae
[T 1- T XII]

Lumbar
vertebrae
[L 1- L V]

Sacrum
[sacral
vertebrae
I – V]

Coccyx
[coccygeal
vertebrae
I- IV]

Atlas [C I]

Axis [C II]

Vertebra
prominens
[C VII]

Intervertebral
foramina

Promontory

Fig. 708 Vertebral column, intervertebral discs in blue color; ventral aspect (30%).

Fig. 709 Vertebral column, dorsal aspect (30%).

Fig. 710 Vertebral column; intervertebral discs in blue color; left lateral aspect (30%).

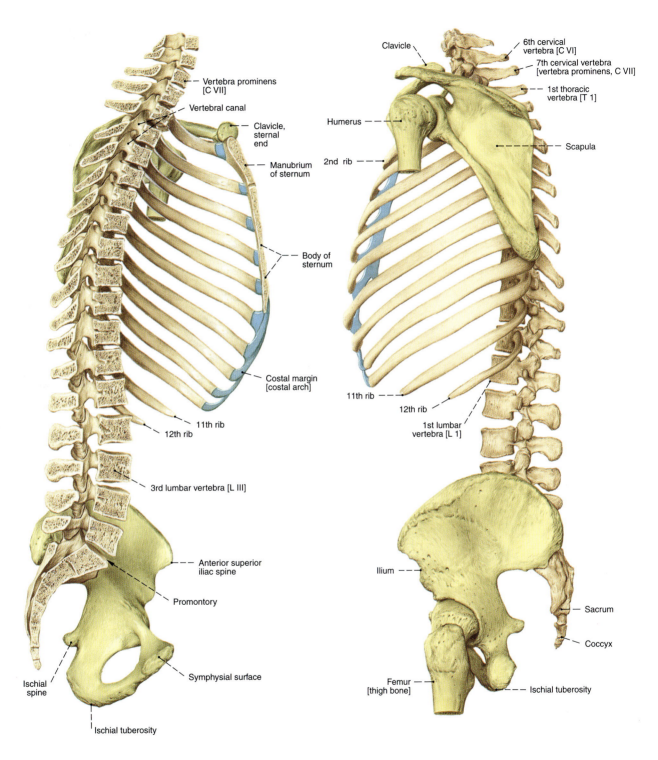

Vertebra prominens [C VII]

Vertebral canal

Clavicle, sternal end

Manubrium of sternum

Body of sternum

Costal margin [costal arch]

11th rib

12th rib

3rd lumbar vertebra [L III]

Anterior superior iliac spine

Promontory

Symphysial surface

Ischial spine

Ischial tuberosity

Clavicle

6th cervical vertebra [C VI]

7th cervical vertebra [vertebra prominens, C VII]

1st thoracic vertebra [T 1]

Humerus

Scapula

2nd rib

11th rib

12th rib

1st lumbar vertebra [L 1]

Ilium

Sacrum

Coccyx

Femur [thigh bone]

Ischial tuberosity

Fig. 711 Vertebral column; pectoral girdle [shoulder girdle]; pelvic girdle; vertebral column sectioned in the median plane; left medial aspect (25%).

Fig. 712 Vertebral column; pectoral girdle [shoulder girdle]; pelvic girdle; vertebral column sectioned in the median plane; left lateral aspect (25%).

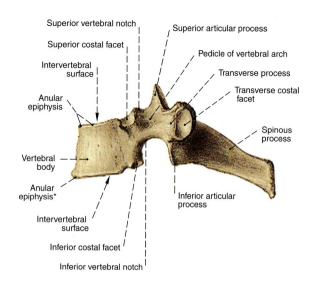

Fig. 713   Vertebra; typical features for example in the 5th thoracic vertebra [T V]; lateral aspect (80%).

* Also: rim of vertebral body.

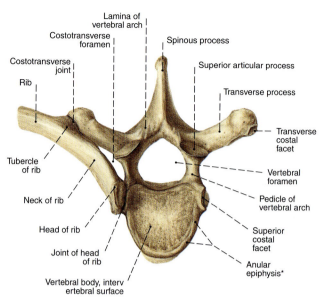

Fig. 714   Vertebra; typical features, for example, in the 5th thoracic vertebra [T V]; cranial aspect (80%).

* Also: rim of vertebral body.

Features of typical vertebrae (excluding atlas and axis)

	7 cervical vertebrae [CI–C VII]	12 thoracic vertebrae [TI–TXII]	5 lumbar vertebrae [LI–LV]	Sacrum [sacral vertebrae I–V]
Intervertebral surfaces of vertebral bodies	Rectangular, small with uncus of body [uncinate process] on cranial surface	Basically triangular, caudal vertebrae rounded	Bean-shaped, large	
Vertebral foramen	Large, triangular	Round	Small, triangular	Sacral canal, oval
Articular processes	Oblique dorsal inclination	Frontal, dorsal inclination	Lateral part : sagittal ; medial part : frontal	Fused to intermediate sacral crest
Transverse processes	Comprise an anterior and a posterior tubercle, a groove for spinal nerve and a foramen transversarium	Club-shaped with costal facets	Mammillary and accessory processes	Fused to lateral sacral crest
Spinous processes	Horizontal, short, bifurcated	Different steep downward direction	Horizontal, laterally flattened, massive	Fused to median sacral crest
Costal elements	Ventral part of transverse process and dorsal tubercle	None, because there are ribs	Costal processes	Lateral parts
Characteristic feature	Foramen transversarium	Superior and inferior costal facets	Mammillary and accessory processes	Synostotic fusion of vertebrae

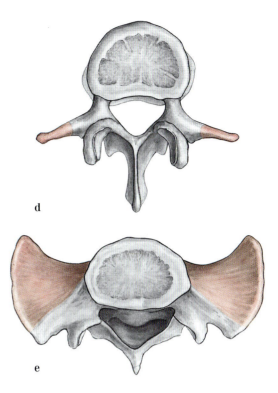

a

b

c

d

e

Fig. 715 a-e Regional characteristic features of vertebrae. The material derived from the embryonic costal processes (pink) form ribs only in the thoracic region.

a 1st cervical vertebra [atlas, C I]
b 4th cervical vertebra [C IV]
c 1st thoracic vertebra [T I], respective ribs and sternum
d 3rd lumbar vertebra [L III]
e Sacrum [sacral vertebrae I- V]

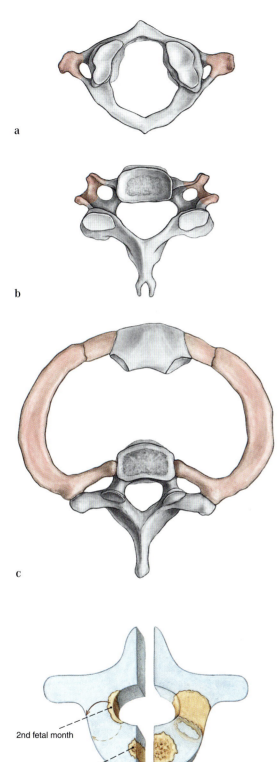

2nd fetal month

3rd – 6th fetal months

Fig. 716 Vertebral development.
Appearance of primary ossification centers (pedicle, 2nd fetal month; body, 3rd-6th fetal months) in a lumbar vertebra. Synostosis of ossification centers of vertebral arch with those of vertebral body occurs between 3rd and 6th year of life.

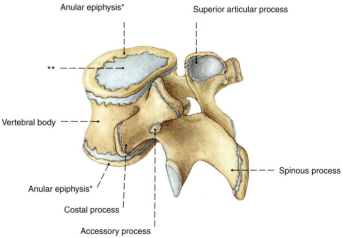

Anular epiphysis*

Superior articular process

**

Vertebral body

Spinous process

Anular epiphysis*

Costal process

Accessory process

Fig. 717 Vertebral development.
In the epiphyses of vertebral bodies ring-shaped ossification centers (rims*) appear during the 8th year of life and fuse with the vertebral bodies until the 18th year of life. The central parts of epiphyses remain as hyaline cartilaginous plates (**) throughout life. Secondary ossification centers (apophyses) form on the processes.

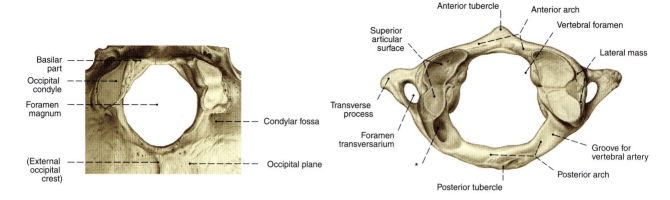

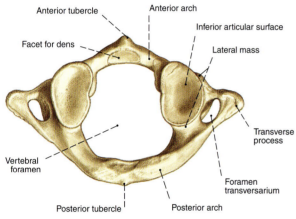

Fig. 718 Occipital bone; part showing foramen magnum and articular processes of atlanto-occipital joint; caudal aspect (80%).

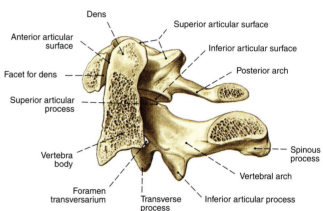

Fig. 719 1st cervical vertebra [atlas, C I]; cranial aspect (85%).
The superior articular surfaces of atlas are frequently divided.

* Variation: canal for vertebral artery.

Fig. 720 1st cervical vertebra [atlas, C I]; caudal aspect (85%).

Fig. 721 1st and 2nd cervical vertebrae [atlas and axis, C I, C II]; median section, medial aspect (90%).

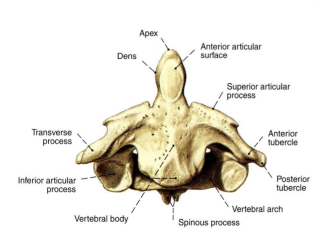

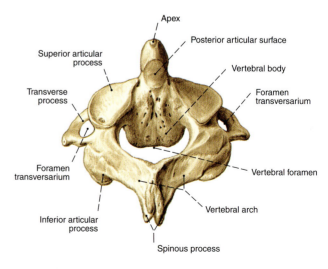

Fig. 722 2nd cervical vertebra [axis, C II]; ventral aspect (90%).

Fig. 723 2nd cervical vertebra [axis, C II]; dorsocranial aspect (90%).

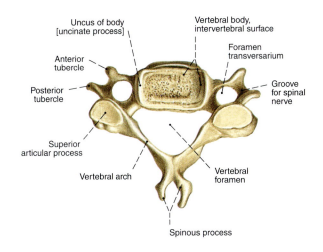

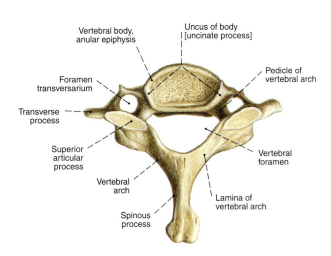

Fig. 724   5th cervical vertebra [C V];
cranial aspect (100%).
The spinous processes of the 2nd–6th
cervical vertebrae are usually bifurcated.

Fig. 725   7th cervical vertebra [C VII];
cranial aspect (100%).
The 7th cervical vertebra, also called vertebra
prominens, is usually easy to identify due to its
prominent spinous process. However, the spinous
process of the 1st thoracic vertebra is usually
even longer.

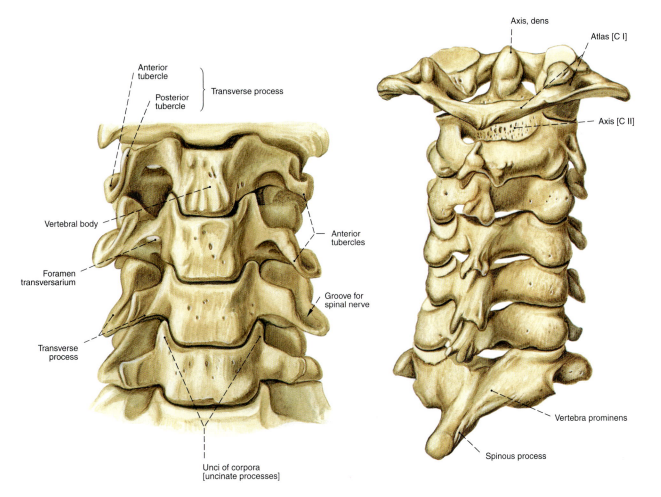

Fig. 726   2nd–7th cervical vertebrae [C II–C VII];
ventral aspect (120%).

Fig. 727   1st–7th cervical vertebrae [C I–C VII];
dorsolateral aspect (110%).

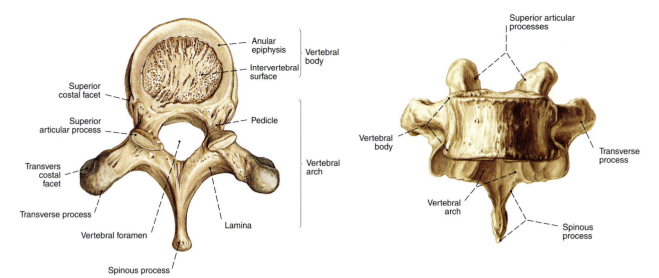

Superior
costal facet

Superior
articular process

Transvers
costal
facet

Transverse process

Vertebral foramen

Spinous process

Anular
epiphysis

Intervertebral
surface

⎫
⎬ Vertebral
⎭ body

Pedicle

⎫
⎪
⎬ Vertebral
⎪ arch
⎭

Lamina

Fig. 728   10th thoracic vertebra [T X];
cranial aspect (90%).

Superior articular
processes

Vertebral
body

Vertebral
arch

Transverse
process

Spinous
process

Fig. 729   10th thoracic vertebra [T X];
ventral aspect (90%).

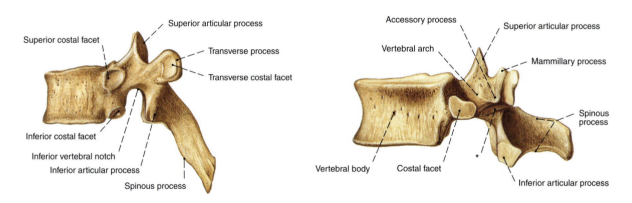

Superior costal facet

Superior articular process

Transverse process

Transverse costal facet

Inferior costal facet

Inferior vertebral notch

Inferior articular process

Spinous process

Fig. 730   6th thoracic vertebra [T VI];
left lateral aspect (90%).

Accessory process

Vertebral arch

Vertebral body

Costal facet

Superior articular process

Mammillary process

Spinous
process

Inferior articular process

Fig. 731 12th thoracic vertebra [T XII];
left lateral aspect (80%).

* Region of vertebral arch between superior and inferior
   articular processes (so-called "isthmus" = intra-articular portion).

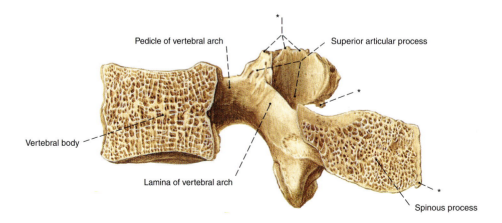

Pedicle of vertebral arch

Superior articular process

Vertebral body

Lamina of vertebral arch

Spinous process

Fig. 732   3rd lumbar vertebra [L III]; median section;
specimen of older person; medial aspect (110%).

* Ossified ligamentous insertions.

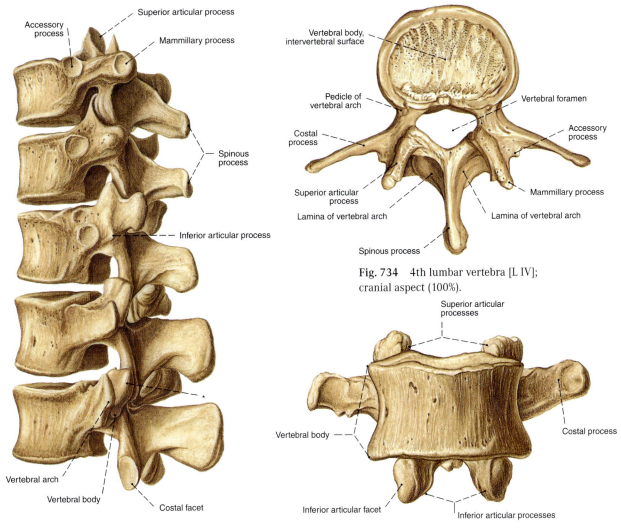

Fig. 733   10th–12th thoracic vertebrae
[T X–T XII] and 1st–2nd lumbar vertebrae
[L I–L II]; dorsolateral aspect (70%).

Fig. 734   4th lumbar vertebra [L IV];
cranial aspect (100%).

Fig. 735   4th lumbar vertebra [L IV];
ventral aspect (100%).

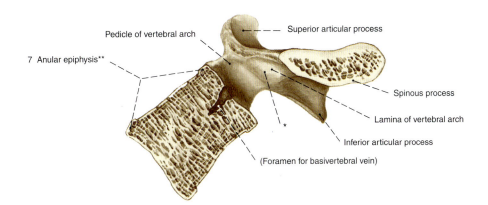

Fig. 736   5th lumbar vertebra [L V];
median section; medial aspect (100%).
**Note the characteristic wedge shape
of the body of the 5th lumbar vertebra.**

* Region of vertebral arch between superior and inferior articular processes.
  Here, in the 5th, rarely also in the 4th lumbar vertebrae, a cleft bridged
  by connective tissue (spondylolysis) may occur, probably due to excessive
  local flexion stress. Subsequently the cranial vertebra may slide (olisthesis)
  from the top of the caudal vertebra (spondylolisthesis).

** In this specimen the anterior border is pathologically oblique.

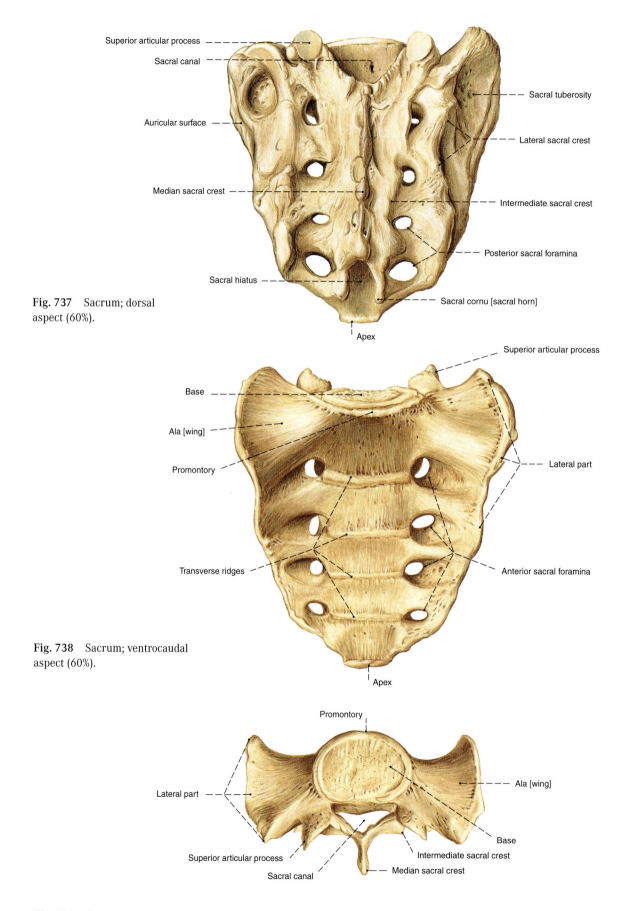

Superior articular process

Sacral canal

Auricular surface

Median sacral crest

Sacral hiatus

Sacral tuberosity

Lateral sacral crest

Intermediate sacral crest

Posterior sacral foramina

Sacral cornu [sacral horn]

Apex

Fig. 737 Sacrum; dorsal aspect (60%).

Superior articular process

Base

Ala [wing]

Promontory

Transverse ridges

Lateral part

Anterior sacral foramina

Apex

Fig. 738 Sacrum; ventrocaudal aspect (60%).

Promontory

Lateral part

Ala [wing]

Superior articular process

Base

Intermediate sacral crest

Sacral canal

Median sacral crest

Fig. 739 Sacrum; cranial aspect (55%).

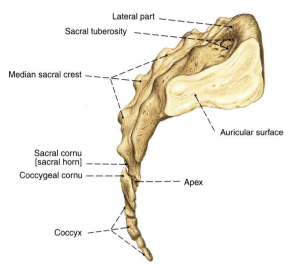

Lateral part
Sacral tuberosity
Median sacral crest
Auricular surface
Sacral cornu [sacral horn]
Coccygeal cornu
Apex
Coccyx

Fig. 740   Sacrum; right lateral aspect (45%).

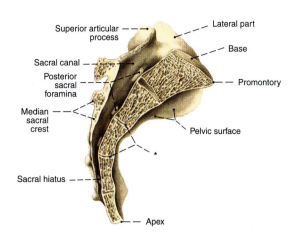

Superior articular process
Sacral canal
Posterior sacral foramina
Median sacral crest
Sacral hiatus
Lateral part
Base
Promontory
Pelvic surface
*
Apex

Fig. 741   Sacrum, median section; medial aspect (45%).

* Remnants of the intervertebral discs also remain in the adult.

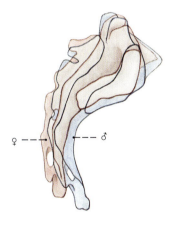

♀   ♂

Fig. 742   Sacrum; sex differences; lateral aspect.

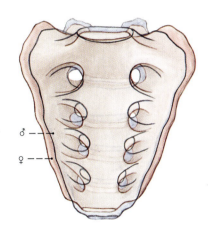

♂
♀

Fig. 743   Sacrum; sex differences; ventral aspect.

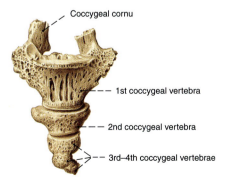

Coccygeal cornu
1st coccygeal vertebra
2nd coccygeal vertebra
3rd–4th coccygeal vertebrae

Fig. 744   Coccyx; ventrocranial aspect (105%). Despite variations in the development of intervertebral discs, the entire postsacral vertebral rudiments are called coccyx.

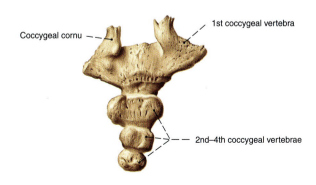

Coccygeal cornu
1st coccygeal vertebra
2nd–4th coccygeal vertebrae

Fig. 745   Coccyx; dorsocaudal aspect (105%).

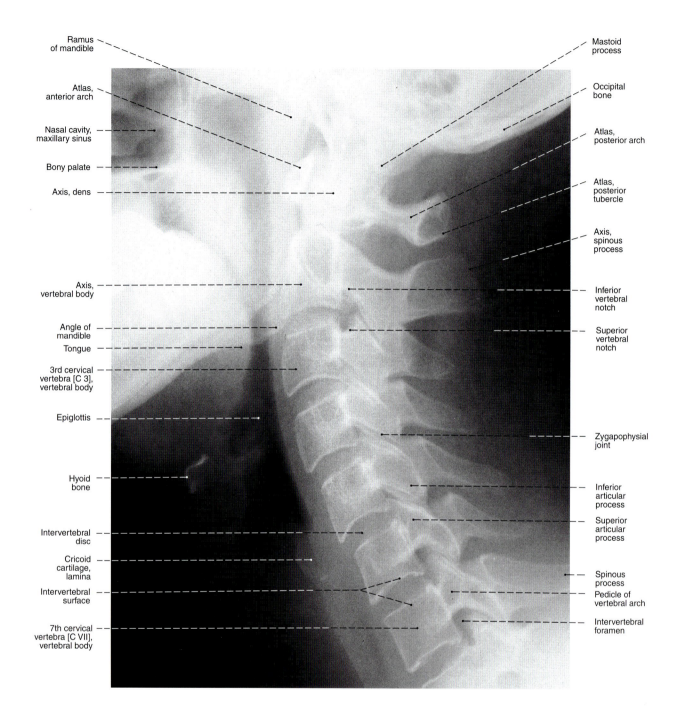

Ramus of mandible

Atlas, anterior arch

Nasal cavity, maxillary sinus

Bony palate

Axis, dens

Axis, vertebral body

Angle of mandible

Tongue

3rd cervical vertebra [C 3], vertebral body

Epiglottis

Hyoid bone

Intervertebral disc

Cricoid cartilage, lamina

Intervertebral surface

7th cervical vertebra [C VII], vertebral body

Mastoid process

Occipital bone

Atlas, posterior arch

Atlas, posterior tubercle

Axis, spinous process

Inferior vertebral notch

Superior vertebral notch

Zygapophysial joint

Inferior articular process

Superior articular process

Spinous process

Pedicle of vertebral arch

Intervertebral foramen

Fig. 746 Cervical vertebrae; lateral radiograph of cervical vertebral column in upright position; central beam directed toward 3rd cervical vertebra; shoulders depressed.

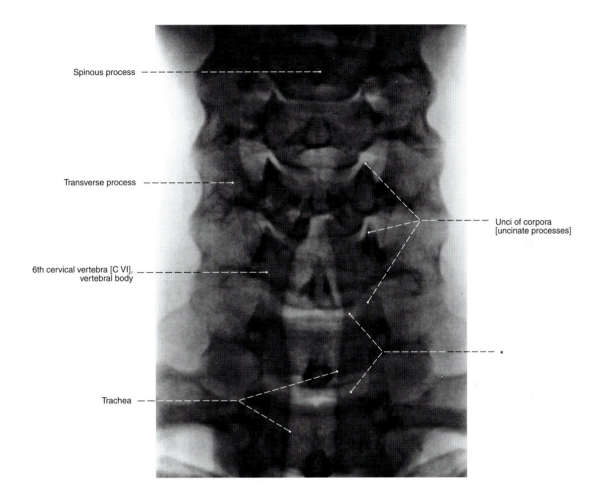

Spinous process

Transverse process

Unci of corpora
[uncinate processes]

6th cervical vertebra [C VI],
vertebral body

*

Trachea

Fig. 747 Cervical vertebrae; AP radiograph of cervical
vertebral column in upright position; central beam
directed toward 3rd cervical vertebra.

* Spaces of intervertebral discs.

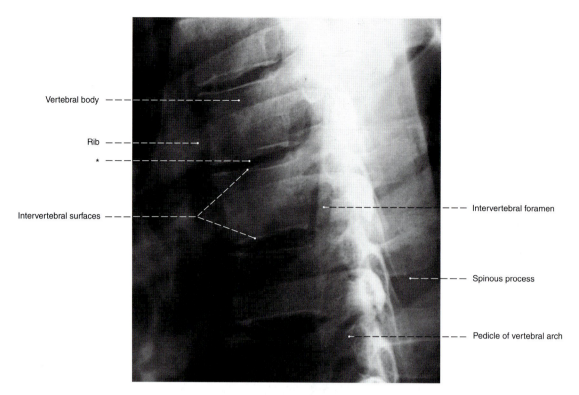

Vertebral body
Rib
*
Intervertebral surfaces

Intervertebral foramen
Spinous process
Pedicle of vertebral arch

Fig. 748   Thoracic vertebrae; lateral radiograph of thoracic vertebral column in upright position; thorax in inspiration; central beam directed toward 6th thoracic vertebra.

* Space of intervertebral discs.

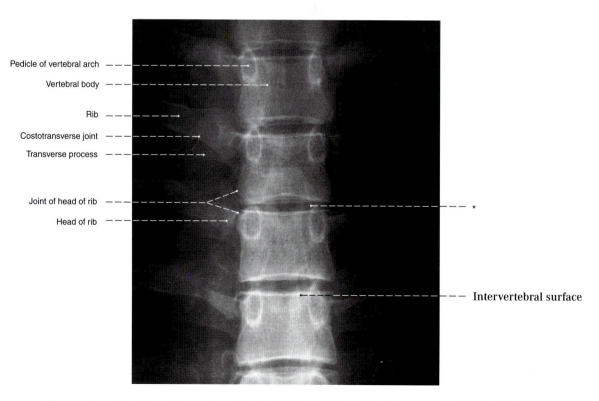

Pedicle of vertebral arch
Vertebral body
Rib
Costotransverse joint
Transverse process
Joint of head of rib
Head of rib

*

Intervertebral surface

Fig. 749   Thoracic vertebrae; AP radiograph of thoracic vertebral column in upright position; thorax in inspiration; central beam directed toward 6th thoracic vertebra.

* Space of intervertebral discs.

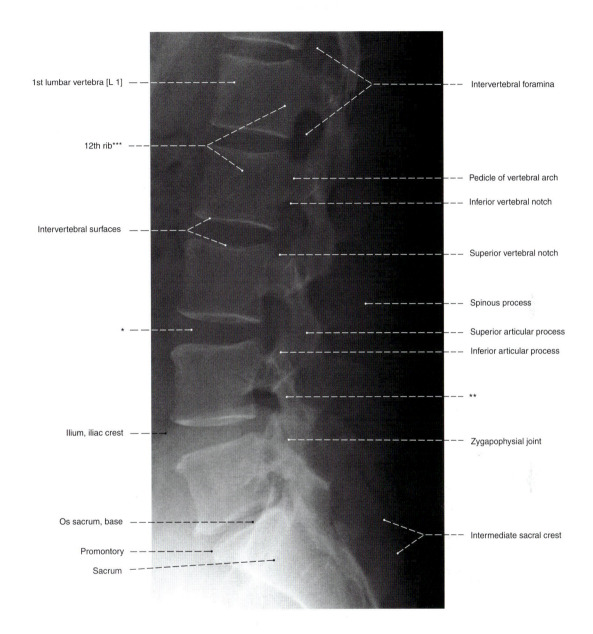

1st lumbar vertebra [L 1] —— Intervertebral foramina

12th rib*** —— Pedicle of vertebral arch

—— Inferior vertebral notch

Intervertebral surfaces —— Superior vertebral notch

—— Spinous process

* —— Superior articular process

—— Inferior articular process

**

Ilium, iliac crest —— Zygapophysial joint

Os sacrum, base —— Intermediate sacral crest

Promontory

Sacrum

Fig. 750   Lumbar vertebrae; lateral radiograph of lumbar vertebral column in upright position; central beam directed toward 2nd lumbar vertebra.

The oblique anterior borders of the lower lumbar vertebrae are pathological alterations.

*   Space of intervertebral disc.

**   Region of vertebral arch between superior and inferior articular processes (so-called "isthmus" = intra-articular portion).

***   Ends of lines indicate the course of the hardly visible 12th rib.

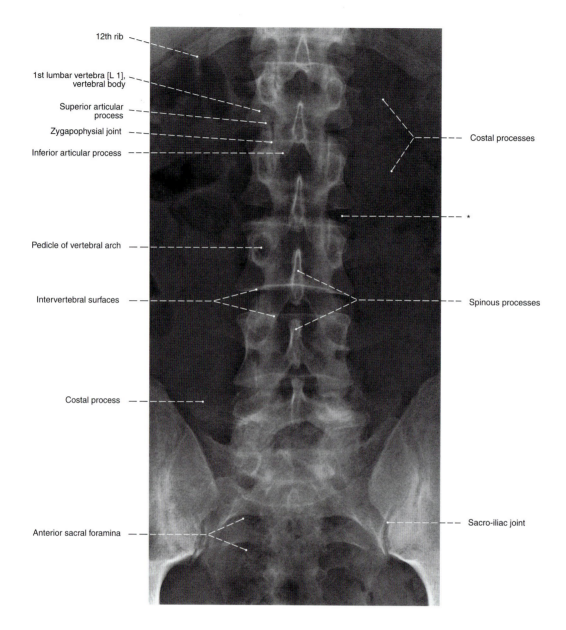

12th rib

1st lumbar vertebra [L 1], vertebral body

Superior articular process

Zygapophysial joint

Inferior articular process

Costal processes

*

Pedicle of vertebral arch

Intervertebral surfaces

Spinous processes

Costal process

Sacro-iliac joint

Anterior sacral foramina

Fig. 751   Lumbar vertebrae; AP radiograph of lumbar vertebral
column and sacrum in upright position; central beam directed
toward 2nd lumbar vertebra. The oblique anterior borders of
the lower lumbar vertebrae are pathological alterations.

*   Space of intervertebral disc.

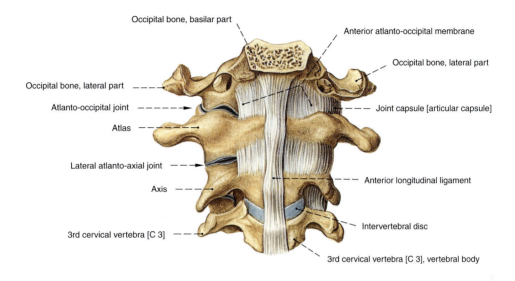

Occipital bone, basilar part

Anterior atlanto-occipital membrane

Occipital bone, lateral part

Occipital bone, lateral part

Atlanto-occipital joint

Atlas

Lateral atlanto-axial joint

Axis

3rd cervical vertebra [C 3]

Joint capsule [articular capsule]

Anterior longitudinal ligament

Intervertebral disc

3rd cervical vertebra [C 3], vertebral body

Fig. 752   Craniocervical joints and upper cervical vertebral column; joint capsules removed on the left; ventral aspect.

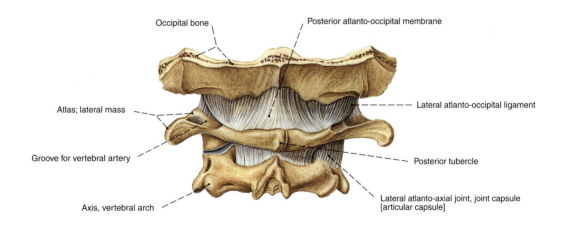

Occipital bone

Posterior atlanto-occipital membrane

Atlas; lateral mass

Groove for vertebral artery

Axis, vertebral arch

Lateral atlanto-occipital ligament

Posterior tubercle

Lateral atlanto-axial joint, joint capsule [articular capsule]

Fig. 753   Craniovertebral joints; joint capsules of lateral atlanto-axial joint removed on the left; dorsal aspect.

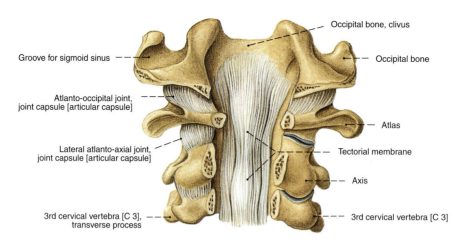

Fig. 754   Craniocervical joints, deep ligaments exposed after opening foramen magnum and vertebral canal; joint capsules partially removed on the right; dorsal aspect.

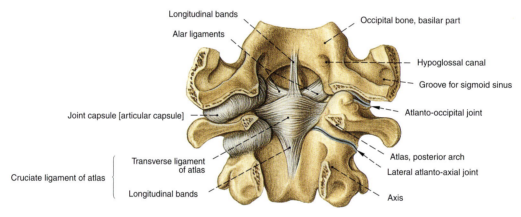

Fig. 755   Craniocervical joints, deep ligaments exposed after opening foramen magnum and vertebral canal; joint capsules partially removed on the right; dorsal aspect.

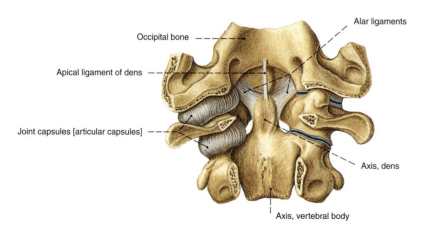

Fig. 756   Craniocervical joints, deep ligaments exposed after opening foramen magnum and vertebral canal; joint capsules removed on the right; dorsal aspect.

The alar ligaments frequently insert also at the lateral masses of atlas.

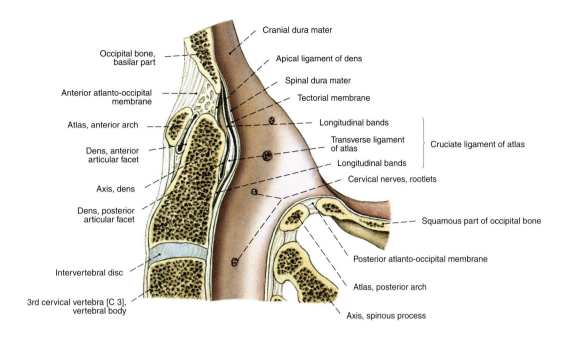

Occipital bone, basilar part

Anterior atlanto-occipital membrane

Atlas, anterior arch

Dens, anterior articular facet

Axis, dens

Dens, posterior articular facet

Intervertebral disc

3rd cervical vertebra [C 3], vertebral body

Cranial dura mater

Apical ligament of dens

Spinal dura mater

Tectorial membrane

Longitudinal bands

Transverse ligament of atlas

Longitudinal bands

Cruciate ligament of atlas

Cervical nerves, rootlets

Squamous part of occipital bone

Posterior atlanto-occipital membrane

Atlas, posterior arch

Axis, spinous process

Fig. 757   Craniocervical joints; median section; medial aspect.

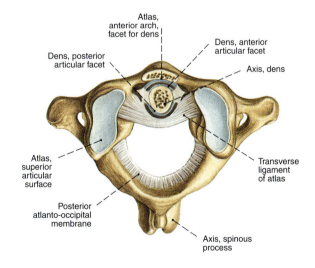

Atlas, anterior arch, facet for dens

Dens, posterior articular facet

Dens, anterior articular facet

Axis, dens

Atlas, superior articular surface

Transverse ligament of atlas

Posterior atlanto-occipital membrane

Axis, spinous process

Fig. 758   Craniocervical joints; occipital bone removed; cranial aspect.

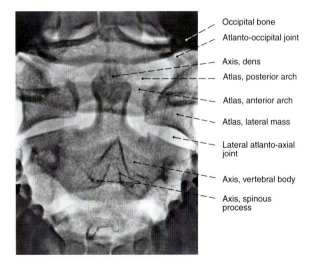

Occipital bone

Atlanto-occipital joint

Axis, dens

Atlas, posterior arch

Atlas, anterior arch

Atlas, lateral mass

Lateral atlanto-axial joint

Axis, vertebral body

Axis, spinous process

Fig. 759   Craniocervical joints, AP radiograph; open mouth view.

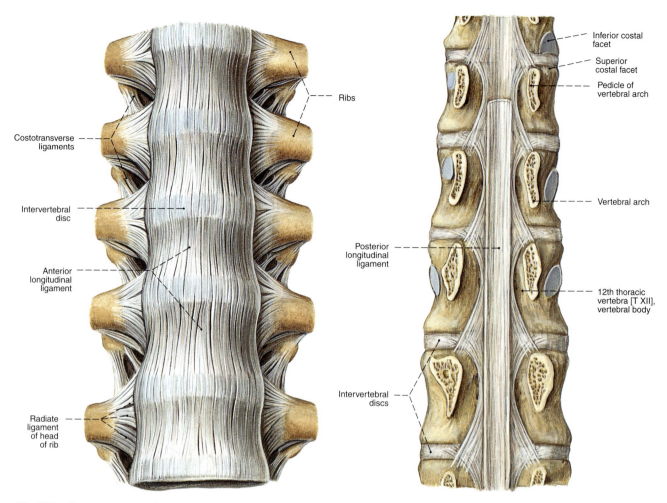

Ribs

Costotransverse ligaments

Intervertebral disc

Anterior longitudinal ligament

Radiate ligament of head of rib

Inferior costal facet

Superior costal facet

Pedicle of vertebral arch

Vertebral arch

Posterior longitudinal ligament

12th thoracic vertebra [T XII], vertebral body

Intervertebral discs

Fig. 760 Ligaments of vertebral column; e.g. in the lower thoracic vertebral column; ventral aspect.

Fig. 761 Ligaments of vertebral column; e.g. in the lower thoracic and the upper lumbar vertebral column; vertebral canal opened by a frontal section through pedicles; dorsal aspect.

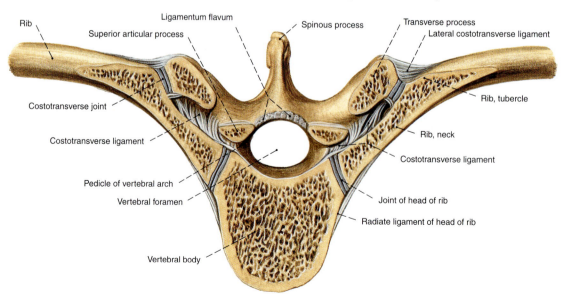

Rib

Superior articular process

Ligamentum flavum

Spinous process

Transverse process

Lateral costotransverse ligament

Costotransverse joint

Costotransverse ligament

Pedicle of vertebral arch

Vertebral foramen

Rib, tubercle

Rib, neck

Costotransverse ligament

Joint of head of rib

Radiate ligament of head of rib

Vertebral body

Fig. 762 Costovertebral joints; horizontal section at level of lower part of joint of head of rib; cranial aspect.

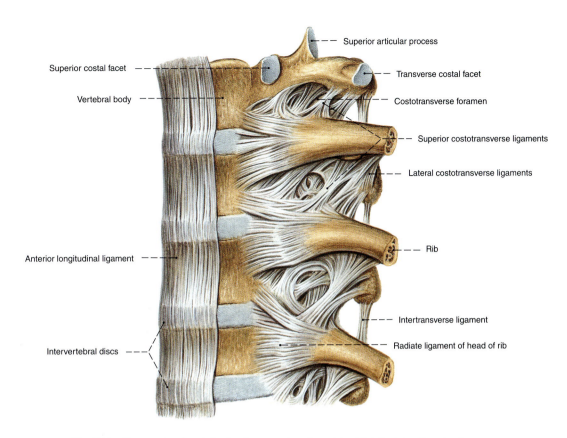

Superior articular process

Superior costal facet

Transverse costal facet

Vertebral body

Costotransverse foramen

Superior costotransverse ligaments

Lateral costotransverse ligaments

Rib

Anterior longitudinal ligament

Intertransverse ligament

Radiate ligament of head of rib

Intervertebral discs

Fig. 763   Ligaments of vertebral column and costovertebral joints; lateral parts of anterior longitudinal ligament removed; left lateral aspect.

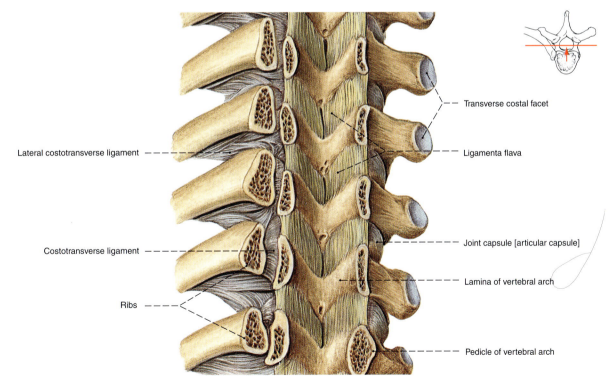

Transverse costal facet

Lateral costotransverse ligament

Ligamenta flava

Costotransverse ligament

Joint capsule [articular capsule]

Lamina of vertebral arch

Ribs

Pedicle of vertebral arch

Fig. 764   Ligaments of vertebral arches; vertebral canal opened by a frontal section through pedicles; ventral aspect.

The ligamenta flava of the lumbar vertebra lie ventral to the zygapophysial joints, thus forming the posterior wall of the intervertebral foramina.

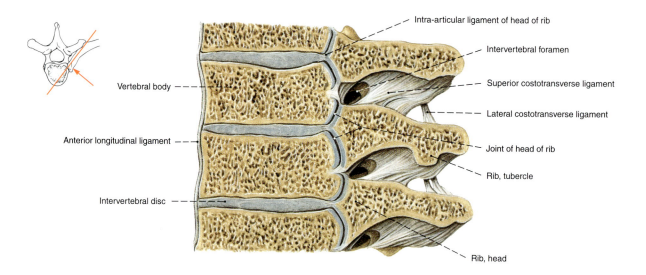

Intra-articular ligament of head of rib

Intervertebral foramen

Superior costotransverse ligament

Lateral costotransverse ligament

Joint of head of rib

Rib, tubercle

Vertebral body

Anterior longitudinal ligament

Intervertebral disc

Rib, head

Fig. 765   Costovertebral joints; oblique vertical section through joints of heads of ribs; left lateral aspect.

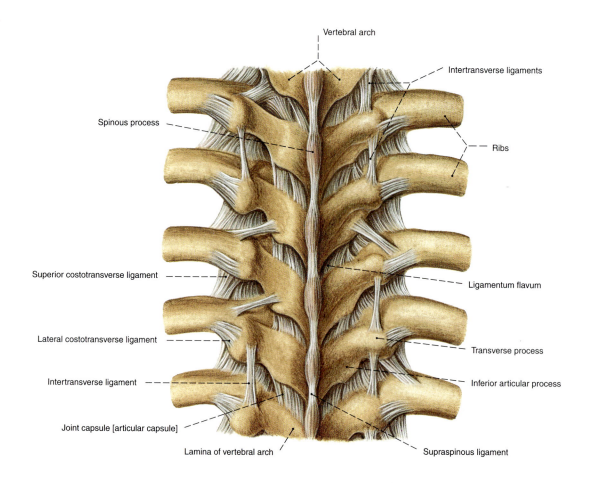

Vertebral arch

Intertransverse ligaments

Spinous process

Ribs

Superior costotransverse ligament

Ligamentum flavum

Lateral costotransverse ligament

Transverse process

Intertransverse ligament

Inferior articular process

Joint capsule [articular capsule]

Lamina of vertebral arch

Supraspinous ligament

Fig. 766   Ligaments of vertebral arches and costovertebral joints; dorsal aspect.

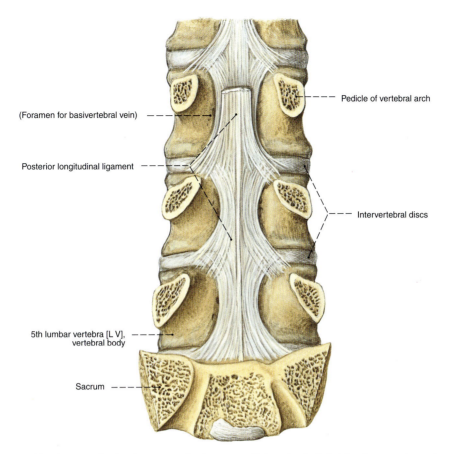

(Foramen for basivertebral vein)

Posterior longitudinal ligament

5th lumbar vertebra [L V], vertebral body

Sacrum

Pedicle of vertebral arch

Intervertebral discs

Fig. 767 Ligaments of lumbar vertebral column; vertebral canal opened; dorsal aspect.

Below the 2nd–3rd lumbar vertebrae the superficial layer of the posterior longitudinal ligament becomes a thin band, whereas the deep layer merges into the anulus fibrosus.

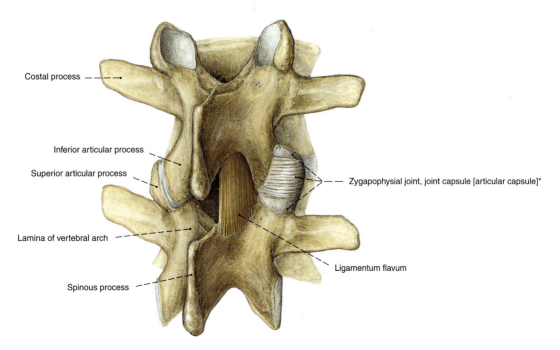

Costal process

Inferior articular process

Superior articular process

Lamina of vertebral arch

Spinous process

Zygapophysial joint, joint capsule [articular capsule]*

Ligamentum flavum

Fig. 768 Lumbar zygapophysial joints; ligamentum flavum removed on the left; right dorsal aspect.

* Only in the lumbar vertebral column are the zygapophysial joints strengthened by transverse running fibers ("transverse ligaments").

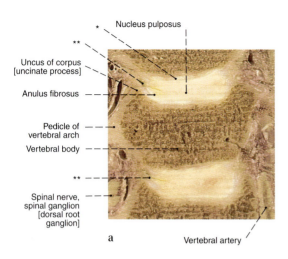

Nucleus pulposus

*

**

Uncus of corpus [uncinate process]

Anulus fibrosus

Pedicle of vertebral arch

Vertebral body

**

Spinal nerve, spinal ganglion [dorsal root ganglion]

a

Vertebral artery

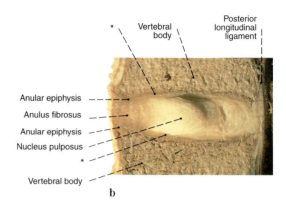

*

Vertebral body

Posterior longitudinal ligament

Anular epiphysis

Anulus fibrosus

Anular epiphysis

Nucleus pulposus

*

Vertebral body

b

Fig. 769 a, b   Intervertebral discs.

a   Cervical intervertebral disc; frontal section at level of middle of vertebral body; ventral aspect (115%).

b   Lumbar intervertebral disc; median section (115%).

*   Hyaline cartilaginous covers of end plates of vertebral bodies as non-ossified part of the epiphyses.

**   Already in the first decade of life, clefts—the so-called "uncovertebral clefts"—develop in the lateral parts of the intervertebral discs. These clefts individually progress further medially in the following decades.

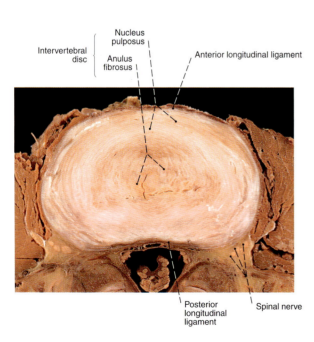

Intervertebral disc

Nucleus pulposus

Anulus fibrosus

Anterior longitudinal ligament

Posterior longitudinal ligament

Spinal nerve

Fig. 770   Lumbar intervertebral disc; ventrocranial aspect (115%).

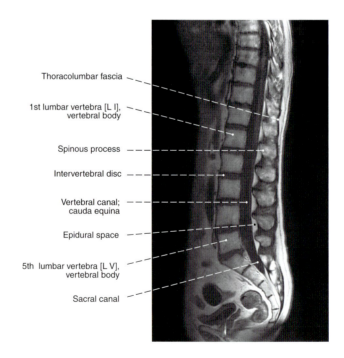

Thoracolumbar fascia

1st lumbar vertebra [L I], vertebral body

Spinous process

Intervertebral disc

Vertebral canal; cauda equina

Epidural space

5th lumbar vertebra [L V], vertebral body

Sacral canal

Fig. 771   Lumbar vertebral column; MRI; median section.

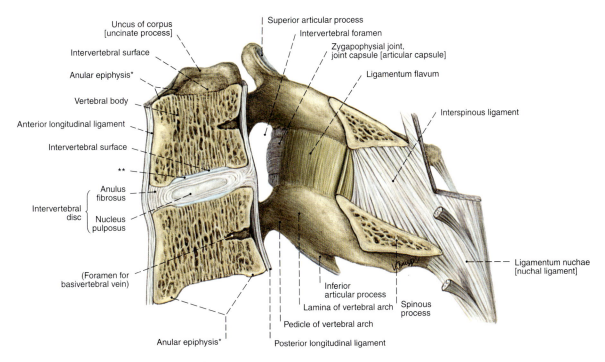

Uncus of corpus [uncinate process]

Intervertebral surface

Anular epiphysis*

Vertebral body

Anterior longitudinal ligament

Intervertebral surface

**

Intervertebral disc { Anulus fibrosus

Nucleus pulposus

(Foramen for basivertebral vein)

Anular epiphysis*

Superior articular process

Intervertebral foramen

Zygapophysial joint, joint capsule [articular capsule]

Ligamentum flavum

Interspinous ligament

Ligamentum nuchae [nuchal ligament]

Inferior articular process

Lamina of vertebral arch   Spinous process

Pedicle of vertebral arch

Posterior longitudinal ligament

Fig. 772   Cervical intervertebral joints; diagram, median section (160%).

*   Also: rim of vertebral body.
** Hyaline cartilaginous covers of end plates of vertebral bodies as non-ossified part of the epiphyses.

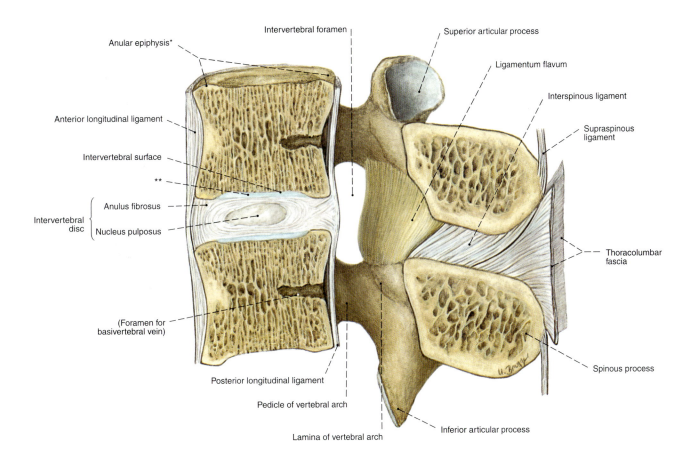

Anular epiphysis*

Anterior longitudinal ligament

Intervertebral surface

**

Intervertebral disc { Anulus fibrosus

Nucleus pulposus

(Foramen for basivertebral vein)

Intervertebral foramen

Superior articular process

Ligamentum flavum

Interspinous ligament

Supraspinous ligament

Thoracolumbar fascia

Spinous process

Posterior longitudinal ligament

Pedicle of vertebral arch

Lamina of vertebral arch

Inferior articular process

Fig. 773   Lumbar intervertebral joints; diagram, median section (120%).

*   Also: rim of vertebral body.
** Hyaline cartilaginous covers of end plates of vertebral bodies as non-ossified part of the epiphyses.

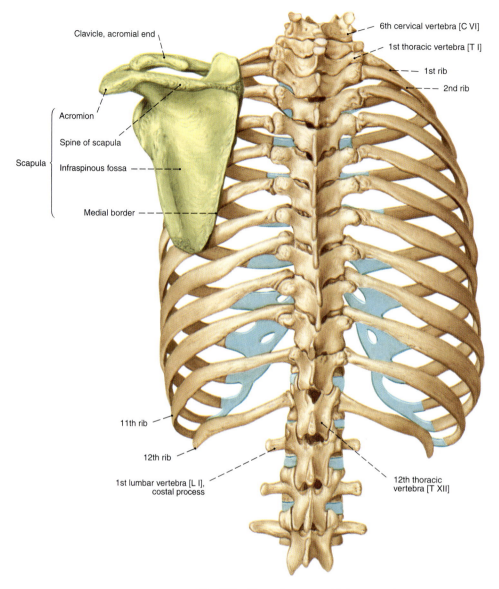

Clavicle, acromial end

6th cervical vertebra [C VI]

1st thoracic vertebra [T I]

1st rib

2nd rib

Acromion

Spine of scapula

Scapula

Infraspinous fossa

Medial border

11th rib

12th rib

1st lumbar vertebra [L I], costal process

12th thoracic vertebra [T XII]

Fig. 774   Thoracic cage and left pectoral girdle [shoulder girdle]; dorsal aspect.

Trunk–pectoral girdle muscles (Figs. 775, 776)

The dorsal muscles of this group, trapezius, levator scapulae, rhomboid major, and rhomboid minor belong to the superficial muscles of the back according to their position; according to their development and innervation they are called immigrated muscles of the back. Serratus anterior muscle is located on the lateral thoracic wall and is hidden under the scapula when it courses dorsally.
The pectoralis minor and subclavius originate from the anterior thoracic wall. Both muscles are dealt with in the ventral muscles group of the shoulder.

Muscle *Innervation*	Origin	Insertion	Functions
1. Trapezius *Accessory nerve [XI] and direct branches from cervical plexus* In the area of origin between the middle and lower thoracic vertebrae a characteristic aponeurosis is developed.	**Descending part [superior part]:** squamous part of occipital bone (between highest and superior nuchal lines), spinous processes of upper cervical vertebrae (above ligamentum nuchae [nuchal ligament]) **Transverse part [middle part]:** spinous processes of lower cervical and upper thoracic vertebrae **Ascending part [inferior part]:** spinous processes of middle and lower thoracic vertebrae	**Descending part [superior part]:** clavicle (acromial third) **Transverse part [middle part]:** acromion **Ascending part [inferior part]:** spine of scapula	**Pectoral girdle [shoulder girdle]:** Descending part [superior part]: carry weight of shoulder girdle and arm (e.g. carrying a suitcase), elevation (e.g. inspiration) and upward rotation of scapula (for raising the arm above 90° - serratus anterior); when shoulder is fixed, rotation of head to contralateral side, both muscles together extend the cervical vertebral column Transverse part [middle part]: retraction of scapula Ascending part [inferior part]: depression of scapula and medial rotation Vertebral column: Transverse and ascending part of both sides together decrease thoracic kyphosis

Continued → S. 28

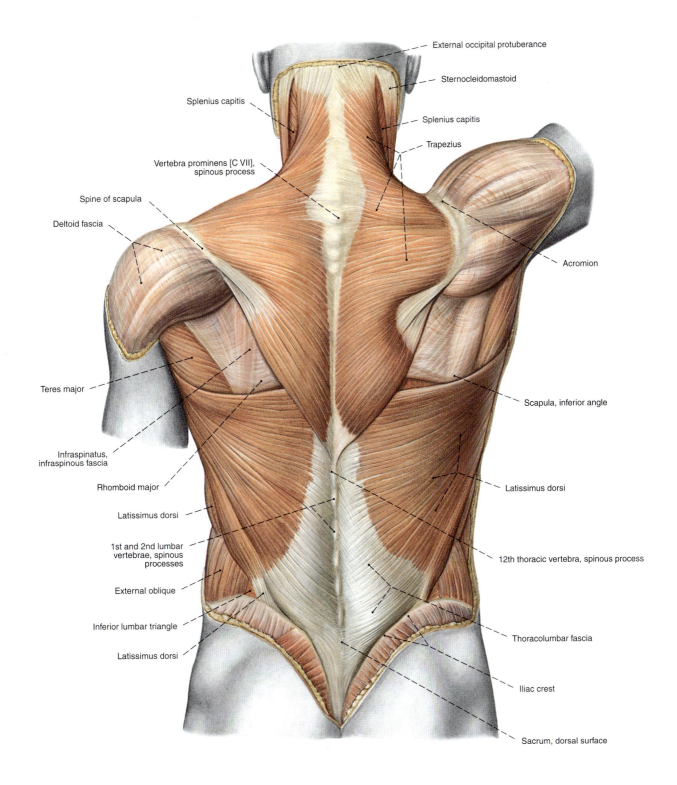

External occipital protuberance

Sternocleidomastoid

Splenius capitis

Splenius capitis

Trapezius

Vertebra prominens [C VII], spinous process

Spine of scapula

Deltoid fascia

Acromion

Teres major

Scapula, inferior angle

Infraspinatus, infraspinous fascia

Latissimus dorsi

Rhomboid major

Latissimus dorsi

1st and 2nd lumbar vertebrae, spinous processes

12th thoracic vertebra, spinous process

External oblique

Inferior lumbar triangle

Thoracolumbar fascia

Latissimus dorsi

Iliac crest

Sacrum, dorsal surface

Fig. 775 Muscles of back; superficial layer of trunk-arm and trunk-pectoral girdle muscles; dorsal aspect.

Trunk – pectoral girdle muscles (continued)

Muscle *Innervation*	Origin	Insertion	Function
2. **Levator scapulae** *Direct branches from cervical plexus and dorsal scapular nerve (brachial plexus, supraclavicular part)*	Posterior tubercles of transverse processes of 1st–4th cervical vertebrae [C I–C IV]	Superior angle and immediate adjacent borders of scapula	**Pectoral girdle [shoulder girdle]:** elevation and medial rotation of scapula
3. **Rhomboid major** *Dorsal scapular nerve (brachial plexus, supraclavicular part)*	Spinous process of four upper thoracic vertebrae	Medial border of scapula (caudal to spine of scapula)	**Pectoral girdle [shoulder girdle]:** together with rhomboid minor retraction and elevation of scapula; together with serratus anterior fixation of scapula to trunk
4. **Rhomboid minor** *Dorsal scapular nerve (brachial plexus, supraclavicular part)*	Spinous process of 6th and 7th thoracic vertebrae	Medial border of scapula (cranial to spine of scapula)	**Pectoral girdle [shoulder girdle]:** together with rhomboid major, retraction and elevation of scapula; together with serratus anterior, fixation of scapula to trunk
5. **Serratus anterior** *Long thoracic nerve (brachial plexus, supraclavicular part)*	**Superior part:** 1st and 2nd ribs (slightly convergent) **Middle part:** 2nd–4th ribs (divergent) **Inferior part:** 5th–8th (9th) ribs (much convergent)	**Superior part:** superior angle of scapula **Middle part:** medial border of scapula **Inferior part:** inferior angle of scapula	**Pectoral girdle [shoulder girdle]:** All parts: protraction of scapula; together with rhomboid fixation of scapula to trunk (scapula alata or winged scapula when one part is paralyzed) Superior part: elevation Middle part: depression Inferior part: depression, lateral rotation (for elevation of arm above 90°) **Thorax:** When scapula is fixed elevation of ribs (inspiration)

Trunk – arm muscles (Fig. 775)

This group comprises the latissimus dorsi and pectoralis major muscles. Both originate from the trunk and course to the arm. Because of the position of its muscle belly, the latissimus dorsi belongs to the superficial muscles of back; like them it has immigrated from ventral.

The pectoralis major originates from the thoracic wall and is dealt with among the other ventral muscles of the shoulder.

Muscle *Innervation*	Origin	Insertion	Function
Latissimus dorsi *Thoracodorsal nerve (brachial plexus, supraclavicular part)*	Spinous processes of six lower thoracic vertebrae, all lumbar vertebrae (via thoracolumbar fascia), dorsal surface of sacrum, outer lip of iliac crest (dorsal third), (9th) 10th–12th rib; frequently from inferior angle of scapula	Crest of lesser tubercle [medial lip] (with a flat tendon spiraling around the teres major tendon; the two tendons separated by the subtendinous bursa of latissimus dorsi)	**Glenohumeral joint [shoulder joint]:** Adduction, medial rotation, extension **Pectoral girdle [shoulder girdle]:** Retraction and depression of scapula

Spinocostal muscles (Fig. 776)

The spinocostal muscles, serratus posterior superior and serratus posterior inferior lie superficial to the deep muscles of back.

Muscle *Innervation*	Origin	Insertion	Function
1. **Serratus posterior superior** *Ventral rami of cervical nerves [C 6] to thoracic nerve [T 2]*	Spinous process of 6th and 7th cervical and 1st and 2nd thoracic vertebrae	2nd–5th rib (lateral to angle of rib)	Elevation of 2nd–5th ribs (inspiration)
2. **Serratus posterior inferior** *Ventral rami of thoracic nerves [T 11] to lumbar nerve [L 2]*	Spinous process of 11th and 12th thoracic and 1st and 2nd lumbar vertebrae	9th–12th rib (caudal border)	Depression of 9th–12th rib (expiration); counteracts the diaphragm also in forced inspiration

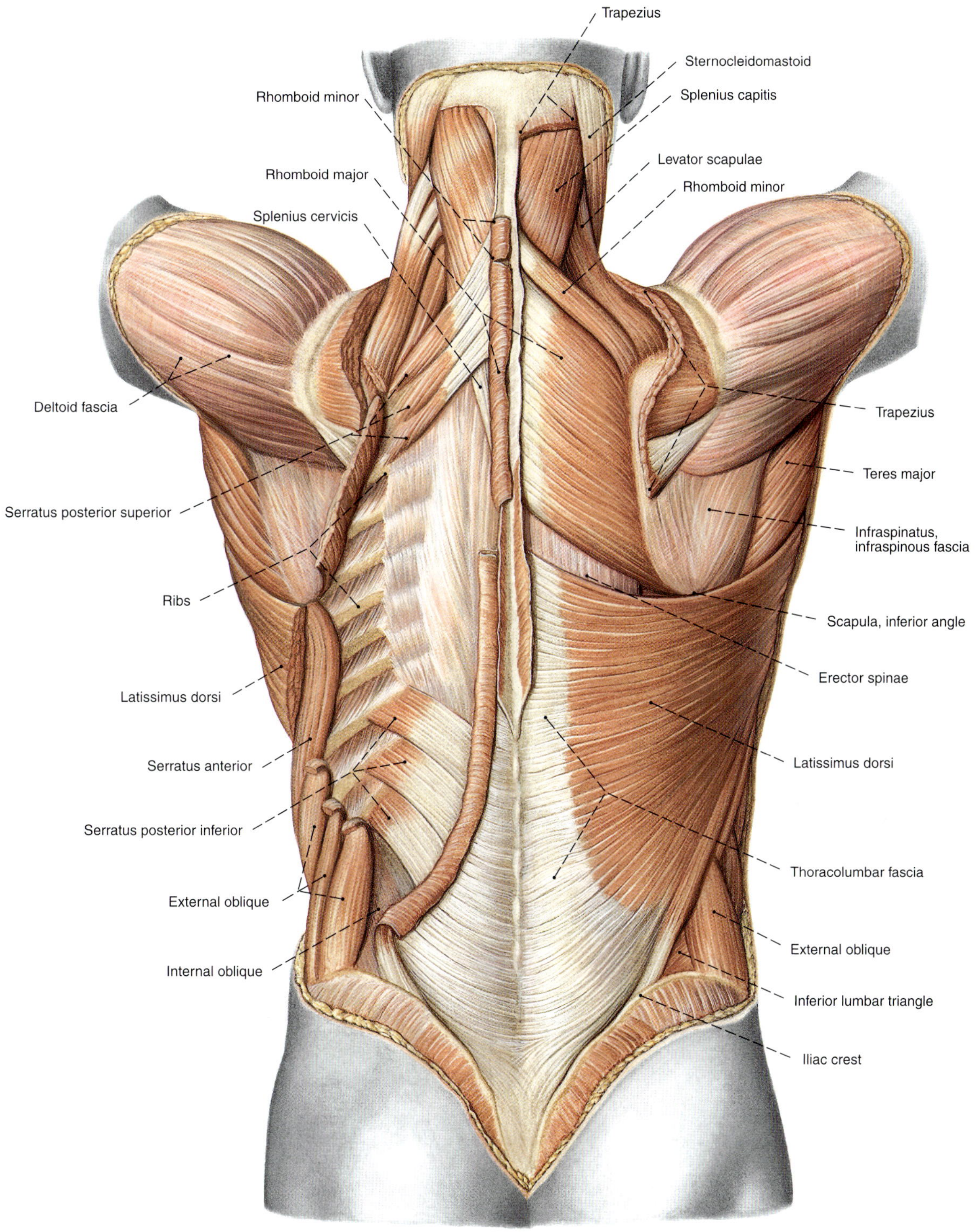

Fig. 776   Muscles of back; deep layer of trunk-arm and trunk-pectoral girdle muscles after extensive removal of superficial muscles on the left; dorsal aspect.

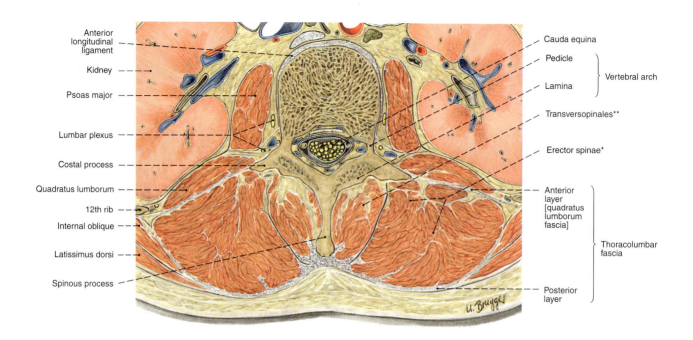

Anterior longitudinal ligament

Kidney

Psoas major

Lumbar plexus

Costal process

Quadratus lumborum

12th rib

Internal oblique

Latissimus dorsi

Spinous process

Cauda equina

Pedicle

Lamina
} Vertebral arch

Transversopinales**

Erector spinae*

Anterior layer [quadratus lumborum fascia]
} Thoracolumbar fascia

Posterior layer

Fig. 777 Muscles of back; horizontal section at level of 2nd lumbar vertebra; caudal aspect.

The muscles of back proper lie in an osseofibrous tube, which is formed by dorsal parts of the vertebrae and by the thoracolumbar fascia. The muscles are grouped into a lateral* and medial tract **.

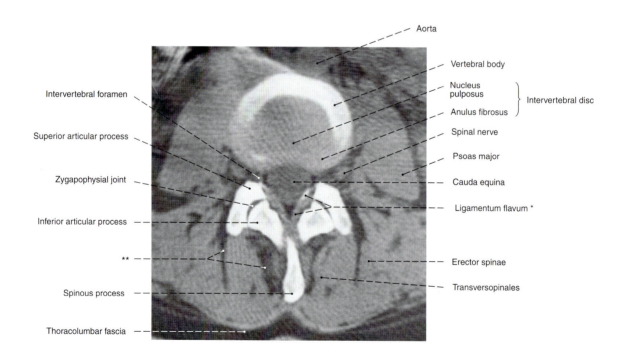

Intervertebral foramen

Superior articular process

Zygapophysial joint

Inferior articular process

**

Spinous process

Thoracolumbar fascia

Aorta

Vertebral body

Nucleus pulposus

Anulus fibrosus
} Intervertebral disc

Spinal nerve

Psoas major

Cauda equina

Ligamentum flavum *

Erector spinae

Transversopinales

Fig. 778 Muscles of back; horizontal CT section at level of intervertebral disc between 3rd and 4th lumbar vertebrae; caudal aspect.

* Calcification or ossification at the sites of attachment of the ligamenta flava frequently occurs even in younger individuals.
** Fatty deposits.

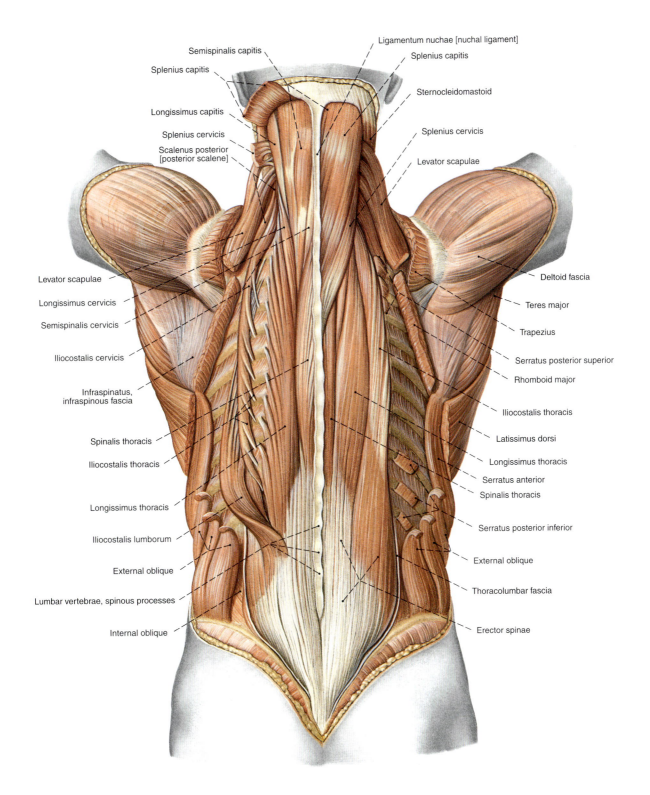

Semispinalis capitis

Splenius capitis

Longissimus capitis

Splenius cervicis

Scalenus posterior
[posterior scalene]

Levator scapulae

Longissimus cervicis

Semispinalis cervicis

Iliocostalis cervicis

Infraspinatus,
infraspinous fascia

Spinalis thoracis

Iliocostalis thoracis

Longissimus thoracis

Iliocostalis lumborum

External oblique

Lumbar vertebrae, spinous processes

Internal oblique

Ligamentum nuchae [nuchal ligament]

Splenius capitis

Sternocleidomastoid

Splenius cervicis

Levator scapulae

Deltoid fascia

Teres major

Trapezius

Serratus posterior superior

Rhomboid major

Iliocostalis thoracis

Latissimus dorsi

Longissimus thoracis

Serratus anterior

Spinalis thoracis

Serratus posterior inferior

External oblique

Thoracolumbar fascia

Erector spinae

Fig. 779 Muscles of back; superficial layer of muscles of back proper after removal of posterior layer of thoracolumbar fascia and overlying trunk-arm and trunk-pectoral girdle muscles; dorsal aspect.

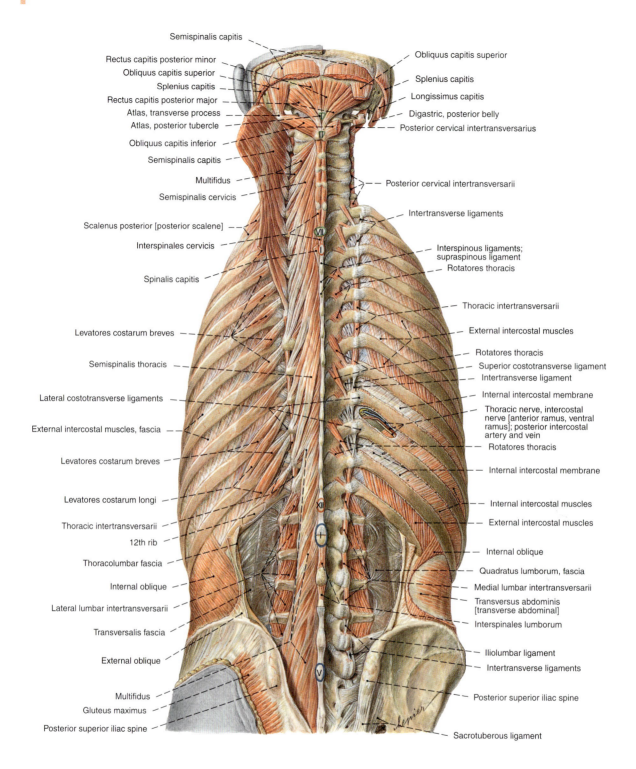

Semispinalis capitis

Rectus capitis posterior minor

Obliquus capitis superior

Splenius capitis

Rectus capitis posterior major

Atlas, transverse process

Atlas, posterior tubercle

Obliquus capitis inferior

Semispinalis capitis

Multifidus

Semispinalis cervicis

Scalenus posterior [posterior scalene]

Interspinales cervicis

Spinalis capitis

Levatores costarum breves

Semispinalis thoracis

Lateral costotransverse ligaments

External intercostal muscles, fascia

Levatores costarum breves

Levatores costarum longi

Thoracic intertransversarii

12th rib

Thoracolumbar fascia

Internal oblique

Lateral lumbar intertransversarii

Transversalis fascia

External oblique

Multifidus

Gluteus maximus

Posterior superior iliac spine

Obliquus capitis superior

Splenius capitis

Longissimus capitis

Digastric, posterior belly

Posterior cervical intertransversarius

Posterior cervical intertransversarii

Intertransverse ligaments

Interspinous ligaments;
supraspinous ligament

Rotatores thoracis

Thoracic intertransversarii

External intercostal muscles

Rotatores thoracis

Superior costotransverse ligament

Intertransverse ligament

Internal intercostal membrane

Thoracic nerve, intercostal
nerve [anterior ramus, ventral
ramus]; posterior intercostal
artery and vein

Rotatores thoracis

Internal intercostal membrane

Internal intercostal muscles

External intercostal muscles

Internal oblique

Quadratus lumborum, fascia

Medial lumbar intertransversarii

Transversus abdominis
[transverse abdominal]

Interspinales lumborum

Iliolumbar ligament

Intertransverse ligaments

Posterior superior iliac spine

Sacrotuberous ligament

Fig. 781 Muscles of back and suboccipital muscles; deep layer after removal of all superficial muscles and thoracolumbar fascia; 9th intercostal space partially opened; dorsal aspect. Roman numerals indicate spinous processes of respective vertebrae.

Muscles of back proper, medial tract (Figs. 780, 781)

The medial tract of muscles of back lies deep to the lateral tract and thus is also called the deep part of the muscles of back proper. These comprise the straight running interspinales and spinalis. The rotatores, multifidus, and semispinalis converge obliquely cranial (transversospinales).

Muscle *Innervation*	Origin	Insertion	Function
1. **Interspinales lumborum** *Posterior rami [dorsal rami] of spinal nerves*	Spinous processes of 5th–1st lumbar vertebrae	Median sacral crest (superior border), spinous process of 5th–2nd lumbar vertebrae	Segmental extension
2. **Interspinales thoracis** *Posterior rami [dorsal rami] of spinal nerves*	Spinous processes of (12th)11th–2nd (1st) thoracic vertebrae	Spinous process of (1st lumbar) 12th–3rd (2nd) thoracic vertebra	
3. **Interspinales cervicis** *Posterior rami [dorsal rami] of spinal nerves*	Spinous processes of 7th–2nd cervical vertebrae	Spinous process of 1st thoracic –3rd cervical vertebrae	
4. **Spinalis thoracis** *Posterior rami [dorsal rami] of spinal nerves*	Spinous processes of (3rd) 2nd, 1st lumbar and 112th–10th thoracic vertebrae (blends with longissimus thoracis)	Spinous process of (10th) 9th–2nd thoracic vertebrae (blends with multifidus)	
5. **Spinalis cervicis** *Posterior rami [dorsal rami] of spinal nerves*	Spinous processes of (4th)3rd–1st thoracic and 7th–6th cervical vertebrae	Spinous process of 6th (5th)–2nd cervical vertebrae	Acting unilateral: lateral flexion; Acting bilateral: extension
6. **Spinalis capitis** *Posterior rami [dorsal rami] of spinal nerves (inconstant muscle)*	Spinous processes of 3rd–1st thoracic and 7th–6th cervical vertebrae	Squamous part of occipital bone (between highest and superior nuchal lines near to external occipital protuberance)	
7. **Rotatores** *Posterior rami [dorsal rami] of spinal nerves* The rotatores comprise: rotatores cervicis, rotatores thoracis, and rotatores lumborum (inconstant)	Mammillary processes of lumbar vertebrae, transverse processes of thoracic vertebrae, inferior articular processes of cervical vertebrae (rotatores longi extend over two vertebrae, rotatores breves insert in the next cranial vertebra)	Spinous process (roots) of 3rd–1st lumbar, 12th–1st thoracic, and 7th–2nd cervical vertebrae	Acting unilateral: segmental lateral flexion, rotation Acting bilateral: extension
8. **Multifidus** *Posterior rami [dorsal rami] of spinal nerves*	Dorsal surface of sacrum, posterior sacroiliac ligament, iliac crest (dorsal part), mammillary processes of lumbar vertebrae, inferior articular processes of 7th–4th cervical vertebrae (fibers extend over two–four vertebrae)	Spinous process of 5th–1st lumbar, 12th–1st thoracic, and 7th–2nd cervical vertebrae	
9. **Semispinalis thoracis** *Posterior rami [dorsal rami] of spinal nerves*	Transverse processes of (12th) 11th–7th (6th) thoracic vertebrae	Spinous processes of 3rd thoracic–6th cervical vertebrae	
10. **Semispinalis cervicis** *Posterior rami [dorsal rami] of spinal nerves*	Transverse processes of (7th) 6th thoracic–7th cervical vertebrae	Spinous processes of 6th–2nd cervical vertebrae	Acting unilateral: rotation of vertebral column and head to contralateral side Acting bilateral: extension
11. **Semispinalis capitis** *Posterior rami [dorsal rami] of spinal nerves*	Transverse processes of (8th) 7th thoracic–3rd cervical vertebrae	Squamous part of occipital bone (between highest and superior nuchal lines, medial part)	

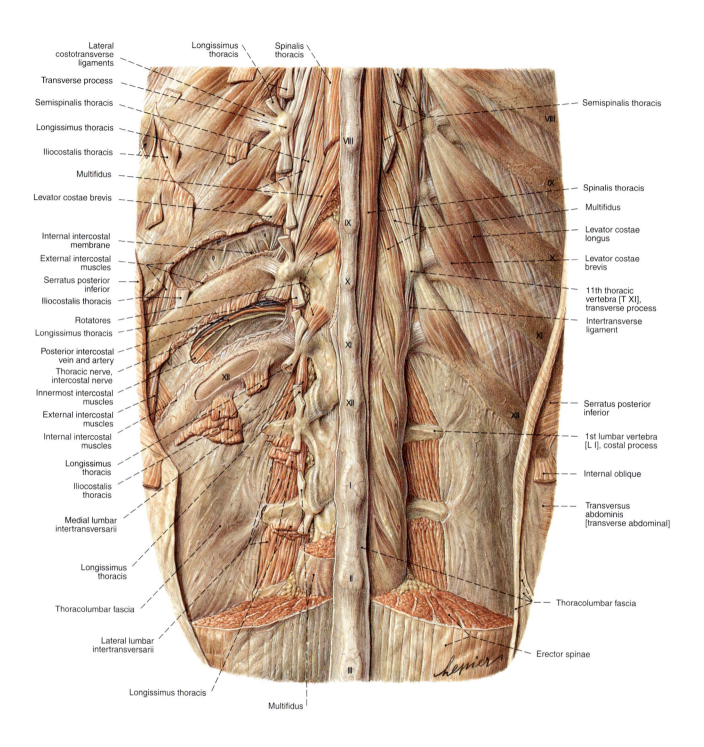

Lateral costotransverse ligaments

Transverse process

Semispinalis thoracis

Longissimus thoracis

Iliocostalis thoracis

Multifidus

Levator costae brevis

Internal intercostal membrane

External intercostal muscles

Serratus posterior inferior

Iliocostalis thoracis

Rotatores

Longissimus thoracis

Posterior intercostal vein and artery

Thoracic nerve, intercostal nerve

Innermost intercostal muscles

External intercostal muscles

Internal intercostal muscles

Longissimus thoracis

Iliocostalis thoracis

Medial lumbar intertransversarii

Longissimus thoracis

Thoracolumbar fascia

Lateral lumbar intertransversarii

Longissimus thoracis

Multifidus

Longissimus thoracis

Spinalis thoracis

Semispinalis thoracis

Spinalis thoracis

Multifidus

Levator costae longus

Levator costae brevis

11th thoracic vertebra [T XI], transverse process

Intertransverse ligament

Serratus posterior inferior

1st lumbar vertebra [L I], costal process

Internal oblique

Transversus abdominis [transverse abdominal]

Thoracolumbar fascia

Erector spinae

Fig. 782　Muscles of back; stepwise exposure of muscles of back proper and muscles of trunk between 8th and 12th thoracic vertebrae (VIII–XII) and 1st to 3rd lumbar vertebrae (I–III); 11th intercostal space partially opened; dorsal aspect.

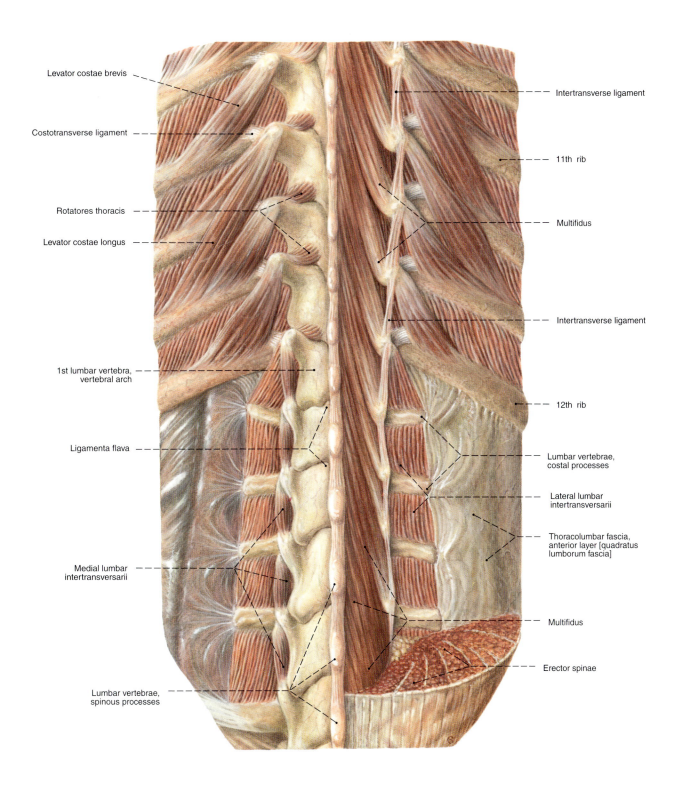

Levator costae brevis

Costotransverse ligament

Rotatores thoracis

Levator costae longus

1st lumbar vertebra, vertebral arch

Ligamenta flava

Medial lumbar intertransversarii

Lumbar vertebrae, spinous processes

Intertransverse ligament

11th rib

Multifidus

Intertransverse ligament

12th rib

Lumbar vertebrae, costal processes

Lateral lumbar intertransversarii

Thoracolumbar fascia, anterior layer [quadratus lumborum fascia]

Multifidus

Erector spinae

Fig. 783   Muscles of back; deepest layer in the region of lower thoracic and upper lumbar vertebrae after removal of thoracolumbar fascia; dorsal aspect.

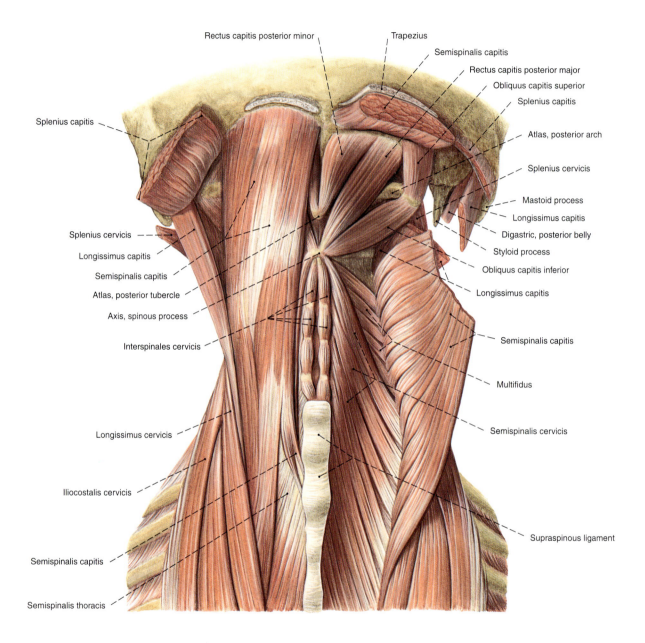

Rectus capitis posterior minor

Trapezius

Semispinalis capitis

Rectus capitis posterior major

Obliquus capitis superior

Splenius capitis

Splenius capitis

Atlas, posterior arch

Splenius cervicis

Mastoid process

Longissimus capitis

Digastric, posterior belly

Styloid process

Obliquus capitis inferior

Longissimus capitis

Splenius cervicis

Longissimus capitis

Semispinalis capitis

Atlas, posterior tubercle

Axis, spinous process

Interspinales cervicis

Semispinalis capitis

Multifidus

Semispinalis cervicis

Longissimus cervicis

Iliocostalis cervicis

Supraspinous ligament

Semispinalis capitis

Semispinalis thoracis

Fig. 784   Muscles of back and suboccipital muscles;
after removal of some superficial muscles; dorsal aspect.

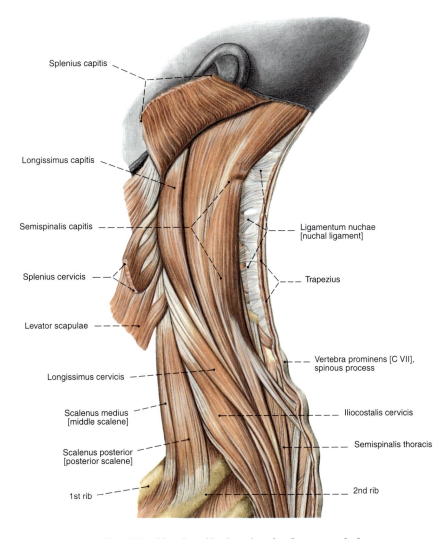

Splenius capitis

Longissimus capitis

Semispinalis capitis

Splenius cervicis

Levator scapulae

Longissimus cervicis

Scalenus medius
[middle scalene]

Scalenus posterior
[posterior scalene]

1st rib

Ligamentum nuchae
[nuchal ligament]

Trapezius

Vertebra prominens [C VII],
spinous process

Iliocostalis cervicis

Semispinalis thoracis

2nd rib

Fig. 785   Muscles of back and neck; after removal of
superficial muscles of back; left lateral aspect.

Suboccipital muscles (Figs. 784, 786)

The medial tract of the muscles of back proper comprise the rectus capitis posterior minor and major, and the obliquus capitis
superior and inferior, the rectus capitis lateralis belongs to the lateral tract.

Muscle/*Innervation*	Origin	Insertion	Function
1. Rectus capitis posterior major *Suboccipital nerve (dorsal ramus of 1st cervical nerve [C 1]*	Spinous process of axis	Inferior nuchal line (medial third)	
2. Rectus capitis posterior minor *Suboccipital nerve (see no. 1)*	Posterior tubercle of posterior arch of atlas	Inferior nuchal line (medial third)	They act together in fine control of position and kinematics of craniocervical joints
3. Obliquus capitis superior *Suboccipital nerve (see no. 1)*	Posterior tubercle of transverse process of atlas	Inferior nuchal line (lateral third)	
4. Obliquus capitis inferior *Suboccipital nerve (see no. 1)*	Spinous process of axis	Transverse process of atlas (posterior border)	
5. Rectus capitis lateralis *Cervical nerve (ventral ramus of 1st cervical nerve [C 1])*	Transverse process of atlas (anterior border)	Jugular process of occipital bone	

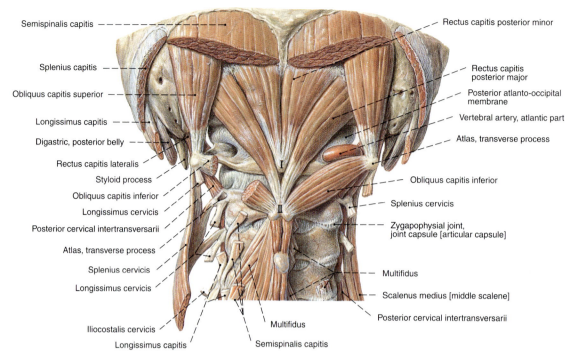

Semispinalis capitis

Splenius capitis

Obliquus capitis superior

Longissimus capitis

Digastric, posterior belly

Rectus capitis lateralis

Styloid process

Obliquus capitis inferior

Longissimus cervicis

Posterior cervical intertransversarii

Atlas, transverse process

Splenius cervicis

Longissimus cervicis

Iliocostalis cervicis

Longissimus capitis

Multifidus

Semispinalis capitis

Rectus capitis posterior minor

Rectus capitis posterior major

Posterior atlanto-occipital membrane

Vertebral artery, atlantic part

Atlas, transverse process

Obliquus capitis inferior

Splenius cervicis

Zygapophysial joint, joint capsule [articular capsule]

Multifidus

Scalenus medius [middle scalene]

Posterior cervical intertransversarii

Fig. 786 Suboccipital muscles; dorsal aspect.
I = Posterior tubercle of atlas
II = Spinous process of axis

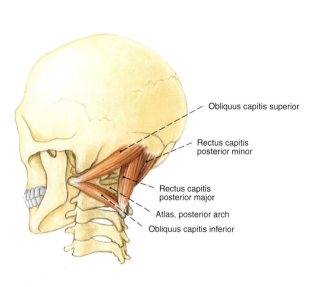

Obliquus capitis superior

Rectus capitis posterior minor

Rectus capitis posterior major

Atlas, posterior arch

Obliquus capitis inferior

Fig. 787 Suboccipital muscles; semischematic diagram; dorsolateral aspect.

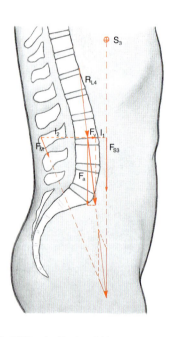

S_3 Center of gravity of 3/6 parts of body weight
F_{S3} Force of body weight effective in lumbar vertebral column
R_{L4} Resulting force effective in intervertebral joints L3/L4
F_M Force of muscles of back
F_V Ventral directed shear-stress effective in zygapophysial joints
F_a Axial pressure force effective in intervertebral disc and vertebral body
l_1 Lever arm of parts of body weight effective in lumbar vertebral column in upright position
l_2 Lever arm of muscles of back

Fig. 788 Load of lumbar vertebral column in upright position.

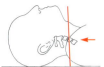

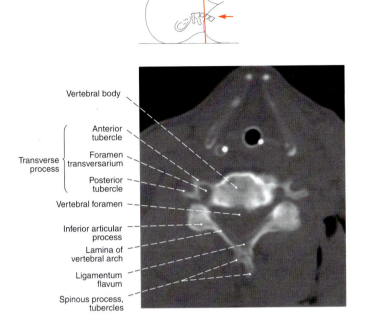

Vertebral body

Transverse process {
  Anterior tubercle
  Foramen transversarium
  Posterior tubercle
}

Vertebral foramen

Inferior articular process

Lamina of vertebral arch

Ligamentum flavum

Spinous process, tubercles

Fig. 789 Cervical vertebral column; computer tomographic horizontal section at level of intervertebral disc between 4th and 5th cervical vertebrae; caudal aspect.

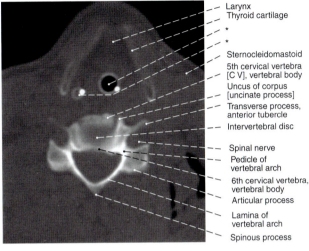

Larynx
Thyroid cartilage
*
*
Sternocleidomastoid
5th cervical vertebra [C V], vertebral body
Uncus of corpus [uncinate process]
Transverse process, anterior tubercle
Intervertebral disc
Spinal nerve
Pedicle of vertebral arch
6th cervical vertebra, vertebral body
Articular process
Lamina of vertebral arch
Spinous process

Fig. 790 Cervical vertebral column; computer tomographic horizontal section at level of 5th/6th cervical vertebrae; caudal aspect.

* Respiratory tube and endoscopic instrument.

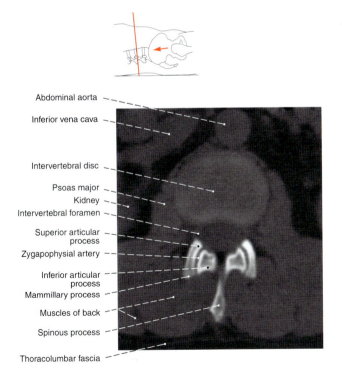

Abdominal aorta

Inferior vena cava

Intervertebral disc

Psoas major

Kidney

Intervertebral foramen

Superior articular process

Zygapophysial artery

Inferior articular process

Mammillary process

Muscles of back

Spinous process

Thoracolumbar fascia

Fig. 791 Lumbar vertebral column; computer tomographic horizontal section at level of intervertebral disc between 2nd and 3rd lumbar vertebrae; caudal aspect.

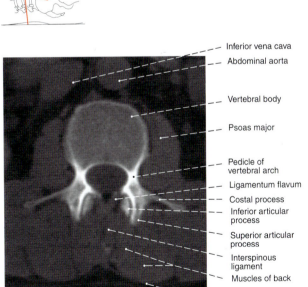

Inferior vena cava

Abdominal aorta

Vertebral body

Psoas major

Pedicle of vertebral arch

Ligamentum flavum

Costal process

Inferior articular process

Superior articular process

Interspinous ligament

Muscles of back

Thoracolumbar fascia

Fig. 792 Lumbar vertebral column; computer tomographic horizontal section at level of pedicles of 3rd lumbar vertebra; caudal aspect.

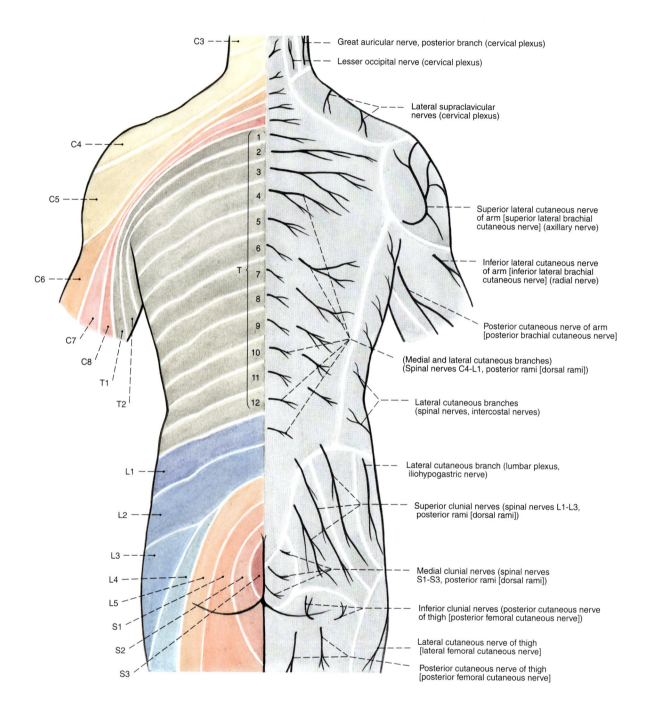

C3

Great auricular nerve, posterior branch (cervical plexus)

Lesser occipital nerve (cervical plexus)

Lateral supraclavicular nerves (cervical plexus)

C4

C5

C6

C7
C8
T1
T2

1
2
3
4
5
6
7
8
9
10
11
12

T

Superior lateral cutaneous nerve of arm [superior lateral brachial cutaneous nerve] (axillary nerve)

Inferior lateral cutaneous nerve of arm [inferior lateral brachial cutaneous nerve] (radial nerve)

Posterior cutaneous nerve of arm [posterior brachial cutaneous nerve]

(Medial and lateral cutaneous branches) (Spinal nerves C4-L1, posterior rami [dorsal rami])

Lateral cutaneous branches (spinal nerves, intercostal nerves)

Lateral cutaneous branch (lumbar plexus, iliohypogastric nerve)

L1

L2

L3

L4

L5

S1

S2

S3

Superior clunial nerves (spinal nerves L1-L3, posterior rami [dorsal rami])

Medial clunial nerves (spinal nerves S1-S3, posterior rami [dorsal rami])

Inferior clunial nerves (posterior cutaneous nerve of thigh [posterior femoral cutaneous nerve])

Lateral cutaneous nerve of thigh [lateral femoral cutaneous nerve]

Posterior cutaneous nerve of thigh [posterior femoral cutaneous nerve]

Fig. 793 Segmental innervation of skin (dermatomes) and cutaneous nerves of back; dorsal aspect.

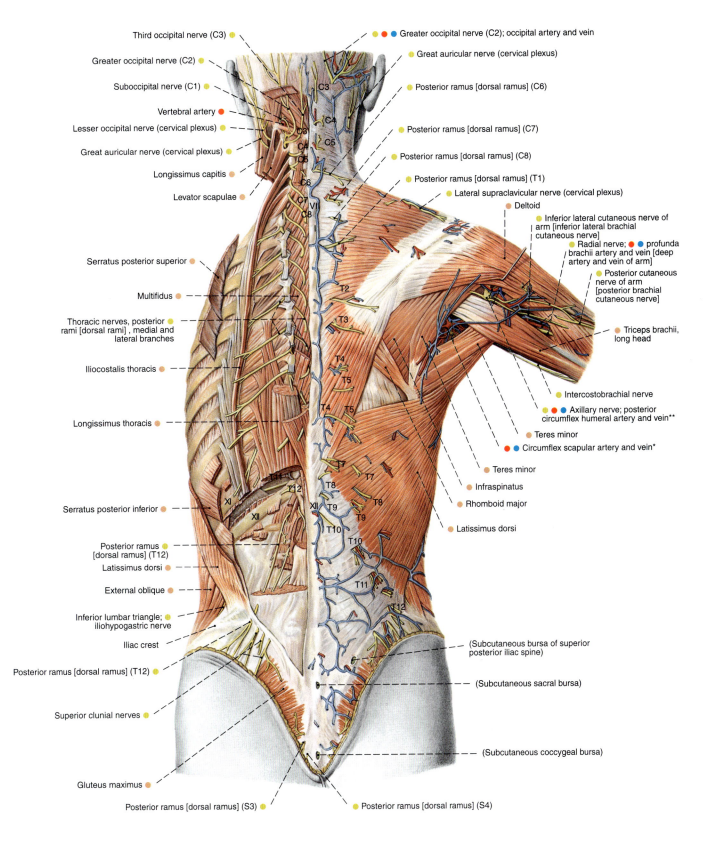

Third occipital nerve (C3)

Greater occipital nerve (C2)

Suboccipital nerve (C1)

Vertebral artery

Lesser occipital nerve (cervical plexus)

Great auricular nerve (cervical plexus)

Longissimus capitis

Levator scapulae

Serratus posterior superior

Multifidus

Thoracic nerves, posterior rami [dorsal rami] , medial and lateral branches

Iliocostalis thoracis

Longissimus thoracis

Serratus posterior inferior

Posterior ramus [dorsal ramus] (T12)

Latissimus dorsi

External oblique

Inferior lumbar triangle; iliohypogastric nerve

Iliac crest

Posterior ramus [dorsal ramus] (T12)

Superior clunial nerves

Gluteus maximus

Posterior ramus [dorsal ramus] (S3)

Greater occipital nerve (C2); occipital artery and vein

Great auricular nerve (cervical plexus)

Posterior ramus [dorsal ramus] (C6)

Posterior ramus [dorsal ramus] (C7)

Posterior ramus [dorsal ramus] (C8)

Posterior ramus [dorsal ramus] (T1)

Lateral supraclavicular nerve (cervical plexus)

Deltoid

Inferior lateral cutaneous nerve of arm [inferior lateral brachial cutaneous nerve]

Radial nerve; profunda brachii artery and vein [deep artery and vein of arm]

Posterior cutaneous nerve of arm [posterior brachial cutaneous nerve]

Triceps brachii, long head

Intercostobrachial nerve

Axillary nerve; posterior circumflex humeral artery and vein**

Teres minor

Circumflex scapular artery and vein*

Teres minor

Infraspinatus

Rhomboid major

Latissimus dorsi

(Subcutaneous bursa of superior posterior iliac spine)

(Subcutaneous sacral bursa)

(Subcutaneous coccygeal bursa)

Posterior ramus [dorsal ramus] (S4)

Fig. 794 Blood vessels and nerves of back; after removal of superficial muscles of shoulder girdle on the left; dorsal aspect.
* Blood vessels and nerves in triangular space.
** Blood vessels and nerves in quadrangular space.

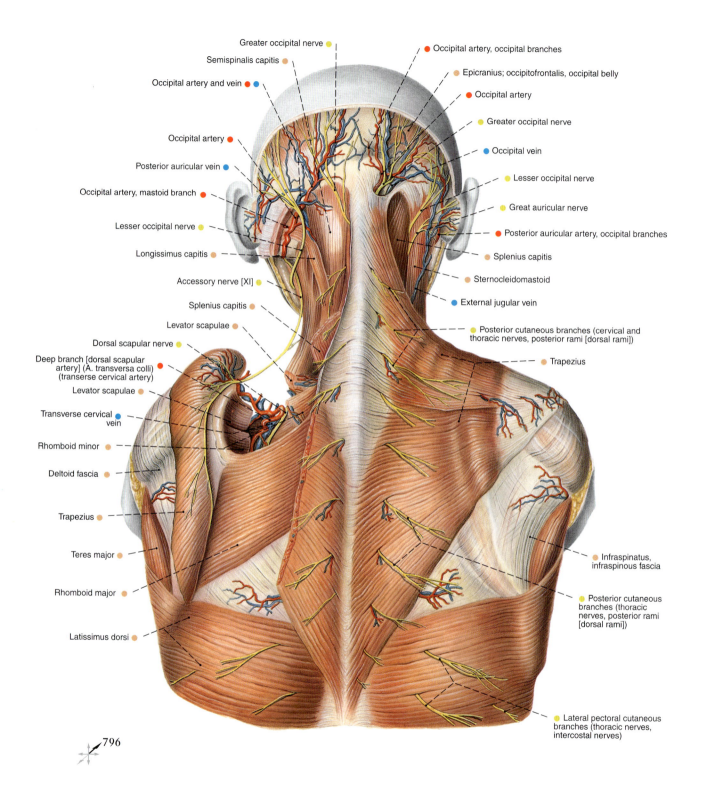

Greater occipital nerve
Semispinalis capitis
Occipital artery and vein
Occipital artery
Posterior auricular vein
Occipital artery, mastoid branch
Lesser occipital nerve
Longissimus capitis
Accessory nerve [XI]
Splenius capitis
Levator scapulae
Dorsal scapular nerve
Deep branch [dorsal scapular artery] (A. transversa colli) (transerse cervical artery)
Levator scapulae
Transverse cervical vein
Rhomboid minor
Deltoid fascia
Trapezius
Teres major
Rhomboid major
Latissimus dorsi

Occipital artery, occipital branches
Epicranius; occipitofrontalis, occipital belly
Occipital artery
Greater occipital nerve
Occipital vein
Lesser occipital nerve
Great auricular nerve
Posterior auricular artery, occipital branches
Splenius capitis
Sternocleidomastoid
External jugular vein
Posterior cutaneous branches (cervical and thoracic nerves, posterior rami [dorsal rami])
Trapezius
Infraspinatus, infraspinous fascia
Posterior cutaneous branches (thoracic nerves, posterior rami [dorsal rami])
Lateral pectoral cutaneous branches (thoracic nerves, intercostal nerves)

796

Fig. 795   Blood vessels and nerves of occipital and posterior cervical region and upper back; after partial removal of superficial muscles of back on the left; dorsal aspect.

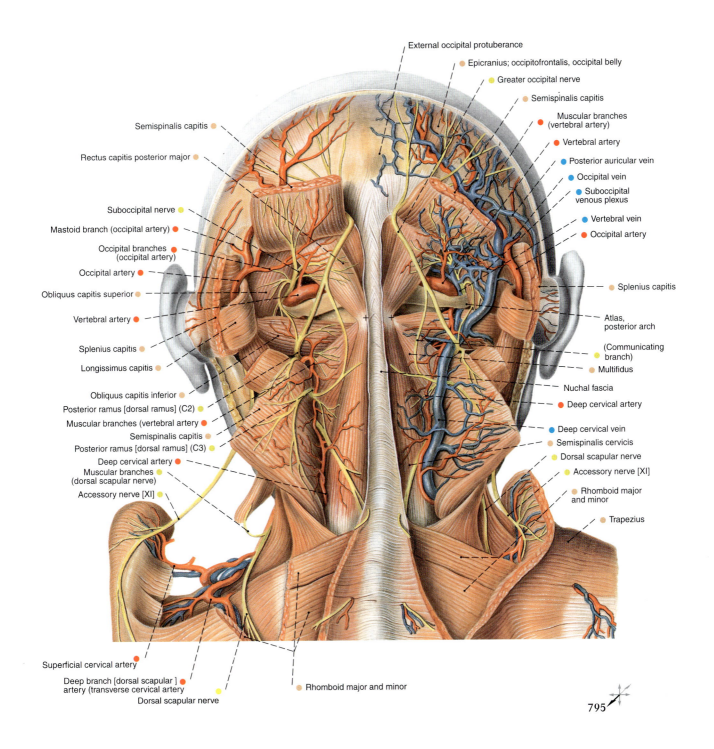

External occipital protuberance

Epicranius; occipitofrontalis, occipital belly

Greater occipital nerve

Semispinalis capitis

Muscular branches (vertebral artery)

Vertebral artery

Posterior auricular vein

Occipital vein

Suboccipital venous plexus

Vertebral vein

Occipital artery

Splenius capitis

Atlas, posterior arch

(Communicating branch)

Multifidus

Nuchal fascia

Deep cervical artery

Deep cervical vein

Semispinalis cervicis

Dorsal scapular nerve

Accessory nerve [XI]

Rhomboid major and minor

Trapezius

Semispinalis capitis

Rectus capitis posterior major

Suboccipital nerve

Mastoid branch (occipital artery)

Occipital branches (occipital artery)

Occipital artery

Obliquus capitis superior

Vertebral artery

Splenius capitis

Longissimus capitis

Obliquus capitis inferior

Posterior ramus [dorsal ramus] (C2)

Muscular branches (vertebral artery)

Semispinalis capitis

Posterior ramus [dorsal ramus] (C3)

Deep cervical artery

Muscular branches (dorsal scapular nerve)

Accessory nerve [XI]

Superficial cervical artery

Deep branch [dorsal scapular] artery (transverse cervical artery)

Dorsal scapular nerve

Rhomboid major and minor

795

Fig. 796   Blood vessels and nerves of occipital and posterior cervical region; dorsal aspect.

* Tubercles of spinous process of axis.

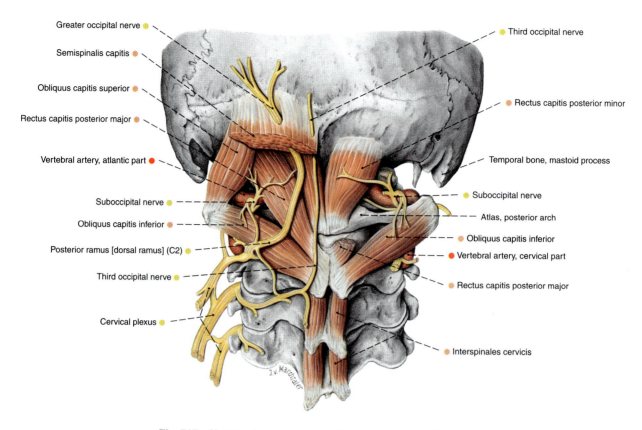

Greater occipital nerve

Semispinalis capitis

Obliquus capitis superior

Rectus capitis posterior major

Vertebral artery, atlantic part

Suboccipital nerve

Obliquus capitis inferior

Posterior ramus [dorsal ramus] (C2)

Third occipital nerve

Cervical plexus

Third occipital nerve

Rectus capitis posterior minor

Temporal bone, mastoid process

Suboccipital nerve

Atlas, posterior arch

Obliquus capitis inferior

Vertebral artery, cervical part

Rectus capitis posterior major

Interspinales cervicis

Fig. 797　Nerves of posterior cervical region and vertebral artery;
dorsal aspect.

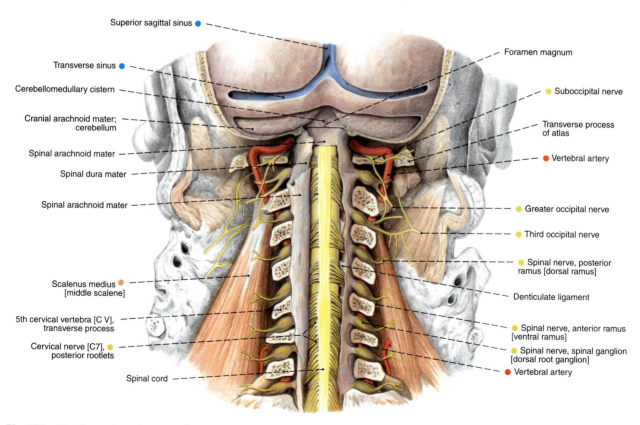

Superior sagittal sinus

Transverse sinus

Cerebellomedullary cistern

Cranial arachnoid mater;
cerebellum

Spinal arachnoid mater

Spinal dura mater

Spinal arachnoid mater

Scalenus medius
[middle scalene]

5th cervical vertebra [C V],
transverse process

Cervical nerve [C7],
posterior rootlets

Spinal cord

Foramen magnum

Suboccipital nerve

Transverse process
of atlas

Vertebral artery

Greater occipital nerve

Third occipital nerve

Spinal nerve, posterior
ramus [dorsal ramus]

Denticulate ligament

Spinal nerve, anterior ramus
[ventral ramus]

Spinal nerve, spinal ganglion
[dorsal root ganglion]

Vertebral artery

Fig. 798　Blood vessels and nerves of posterior cervical region
and contents of vertebral canal; occipital bone partially and
vertebral arches completely removed; stepwise exposure of
meninges; dorsal aspect.

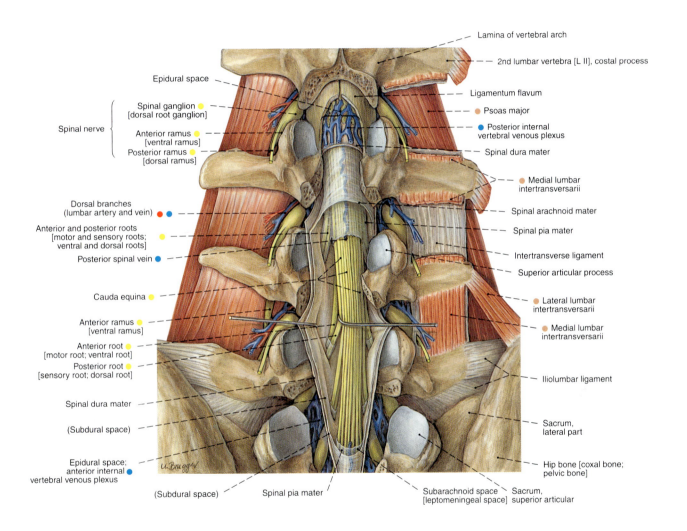

Lamina of vertebral arch

2nd lumbar vertebra [L II], costal process

Epidural space

Ligamentum flavum

Spinal ganglion ● [dorsal root ganglion]

● Psoas major

Anterior ramus ● [ventral ramus]

● Posterior internal vertebral venous plexus

Spinal nerve

Posterior ramus ● [dorsal ramus]

Spinal dura mater

● Medial lumbar intertransversarii

Dorsal branches (lumbar artery and vein) ● ●

Spinal arachnoid mater

Anterior and posterior roots [motor and sensory roots; ventral and dorsal roots] ●

Spinal pia mater

Posterior spinal vein ●

Intertransverse ligament

Superior articular process

Cauda equina ●

● Lateral lumbar intertransversarii

Anterior ramus ● [ventral ramus]

● Medial lumbar intertransversarii

Anterior root ● [motor root; ventral root]

Posterior root ● [sensory root; dorsal root]

Iliolumbar ligament

Spinal dura mater

(Subdural space)

Sacrum, lateral part

Epidural space; anterior internal ● vertebral venous plexus

Hip bone [coxal bone; pelvic bone]

(Subdural space)

Spinal pia mater

Subarachnoid space [leptomeningeal space]

Sacrum, superior articular

Fig. 799   Blood vessels and nerves of lumbar vertebral canal; vertebral arches removed; stepwise exposure of meninges; dorsal aspect.

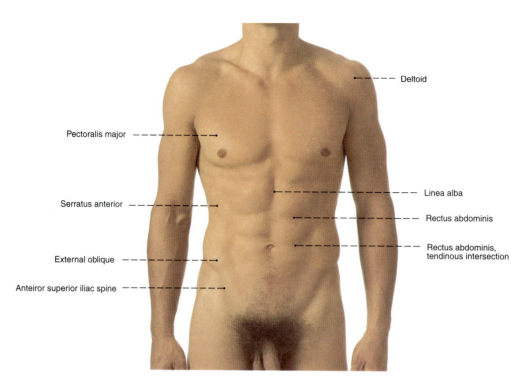

Fig. 800 Surface anatomy of thoracic and abdominal walls of a young male with prominent muscles indicated.
Note the upper border of pubic hair, which in the male extends triangularly to the umbilicus, whereas in the female it has a horizontal border (Fig. 801).
Regions of thoracic and abdominal walls are shown in Fig. 7.

Deltoid

Pectoralis major

Linea alba

Serratus anterior

Rectus abdominis

Rectus abdominis, tendinous intersection

External oblique

Anteiror superior iliac spine

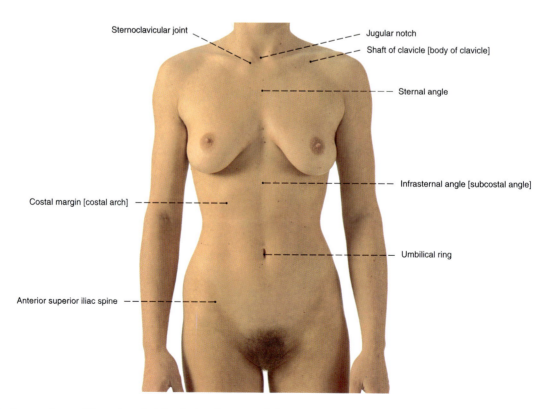

Sternoclavicular joint

Jugular notch

Shaft of clavicle [body of clavicle]

Sternal angle

Infrasternal angle [subcostal angle]

Costal margin [costal arch]

Umbilical ring

Anterior superior iliac spine

Fig. 801 Surface anatomy of thoracic and abdominal walls of a young female with prominent bones indicated.

Orientation lines of thoracic and abdominal walls are shown in Fig. 2.

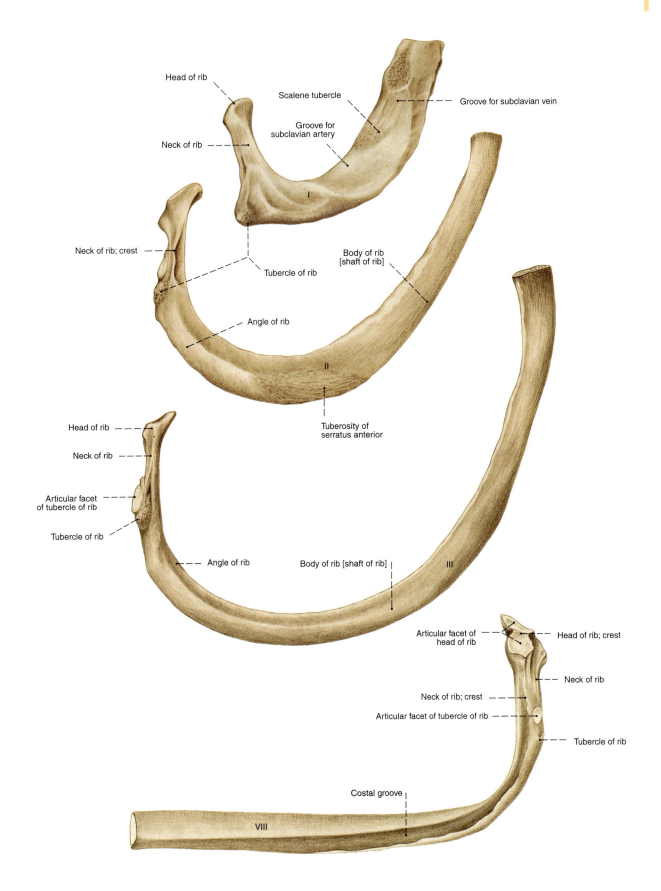

Head of rib

Scalene tubercle

Groove for subclavian vein

Neck of rib

Groove for subclavian artery

Neck of rib; crest

Tubercle of rib

Body of rib [shaft of rib]

Angle of rib

I

II

Tuberosity of serratus anterior

Head of rib

Neck of rib

Articular facet of tubercle of rib

Tubercle of rib

Angle of rib

Body of rib [shaft of rib]

III

Articular facet of head of rib

Head of rib; crest

Neck of rib

Neck of rib; crest

Articular facet of tubercle of rib

Tubercle of rib

Costal groove

VIII

Fig. 802   Ribs;
Ribs I–III; superior aspect.
Rib VIII; inferior aspect.

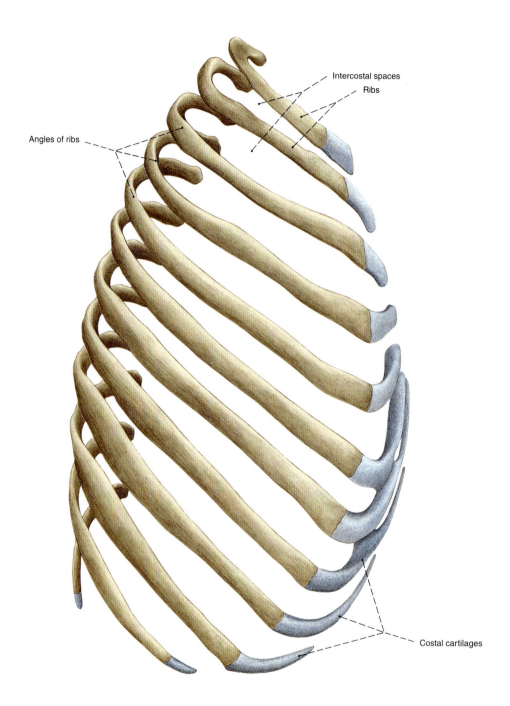

Fig. 803   Ribs; right aspect.
Ribs shown in their natural distance.

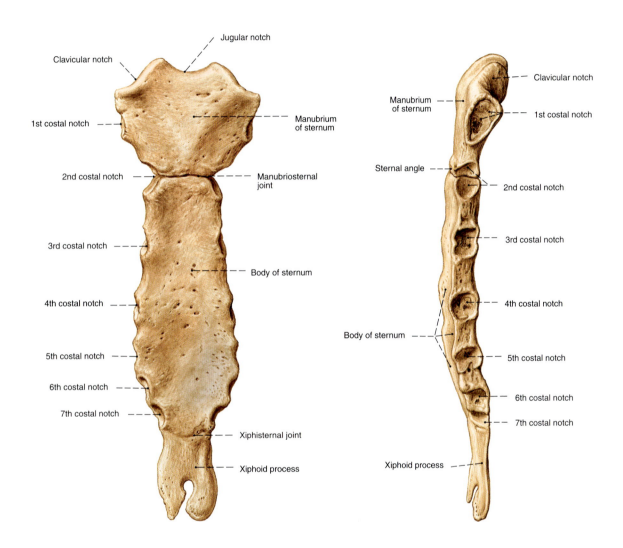

Fig. 804 Sternum; anterior aspect. Shape, length, and direction (dorsal or ventral) of xiphoid process vary considerably.

Fig. 805 Sternum; left lateral aspect. For counting ribs and intercostal spaces on the anterior thoracic wall the sternal angle, to which the 2nd rib is attached, is important

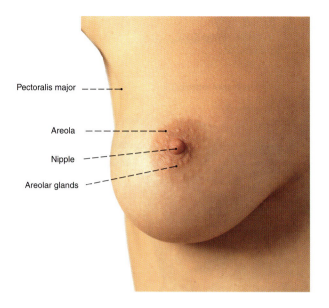

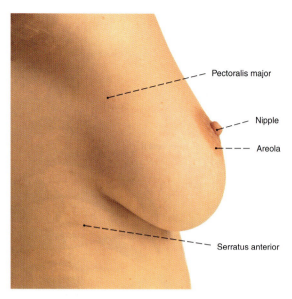

Fig. 809   Breast; anterior aspect.

Fig. 810   Breast; right lateral aspect.

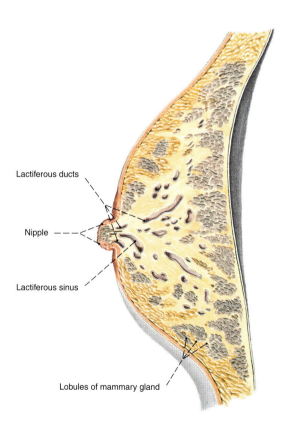

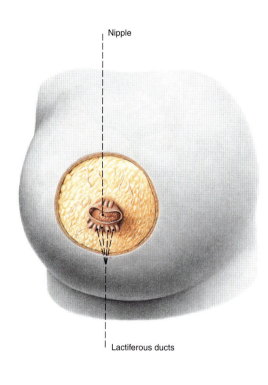

Fig. 811   Mammary gland of a pregnant woman; sectioned sagittally into halves; lateral aspect.

Fig. 812   Mammary gland of a pregnant woman; skin of areola removed and skin surrounding nipple reflected; anterior aspect.

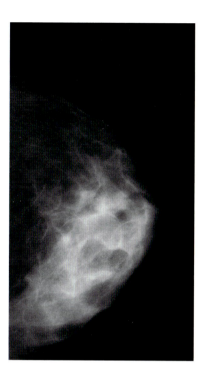

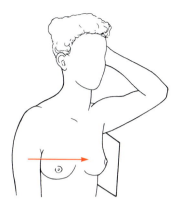

Fig. 813   Radiograph of mammary gland;
lateral mammography of a 47-year-old woman.

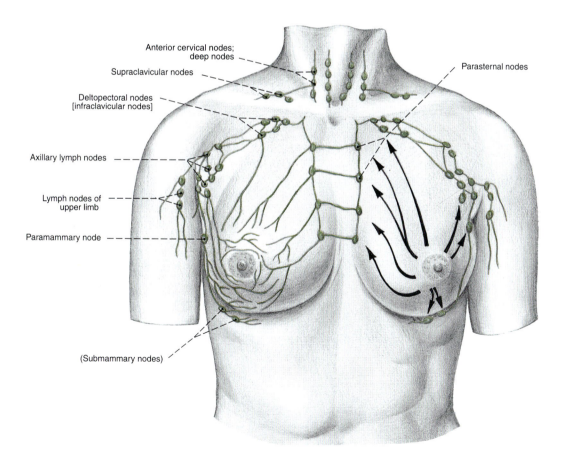

Anterior cervical nodes;
deep nodes

Supraclavicular nodes

Parasternal nodes

Deltopectoral nodes
[infraclavicular nodes]

Axillary lymph nodes

Lymph nodes of
upper limb

Paramammary node

(Submammary nodes)

Fig. 814   Lymphatic drainage of female mammary gland and
site of regional lymph nodes.
(From: BENNINGHOFF/ GOERTTLER: Lehrbuch der Anatomie
des Menschen, vol. 2, 12th ed., Urban & Schwarzenberg,
Munich 1979).

Note the communications of lymphatic vessels of both sides
and lymphatic drainage into intrathoracic lymph nodes.

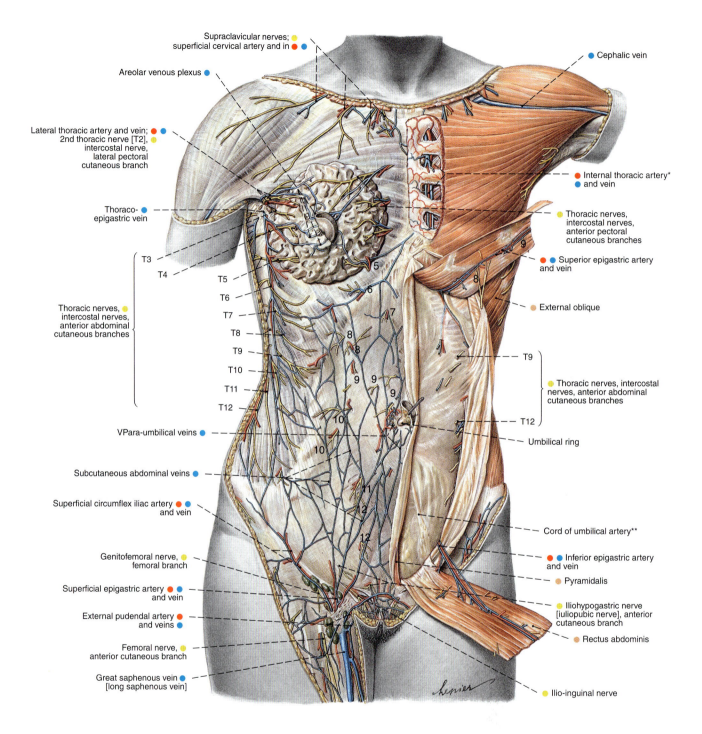

Fig. 815   Blood vessels and nerves of thoracic and abdominal walls; superficial layer shown on the right; anterior aspect. Arabic numerals indicate cutaneous branches of respective intercostal nerves.

*   Clinically: internal mammary artery.
**   The cord of umbilical artery causes the medial umbilical fold internally.

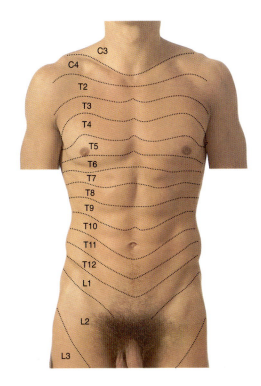

Fig. 816   Segmental sensory innervation of thoracic
and abdominal walls (dermatomes).
Letters and numerals indicate respective spinal cord segments.

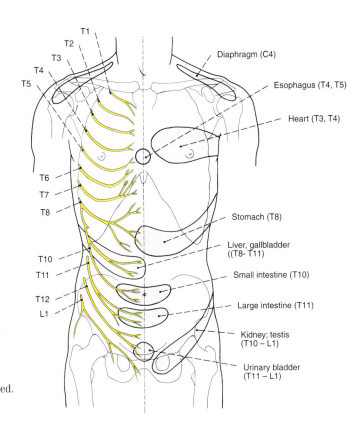

Fig. 817   Segmental sensory innervation of anterior thoracic
and abdominal walls (dermatomes).
On the left side of the body regions of pain projection due to
diseases of respective internal viscera (Head's zones) are indicated.

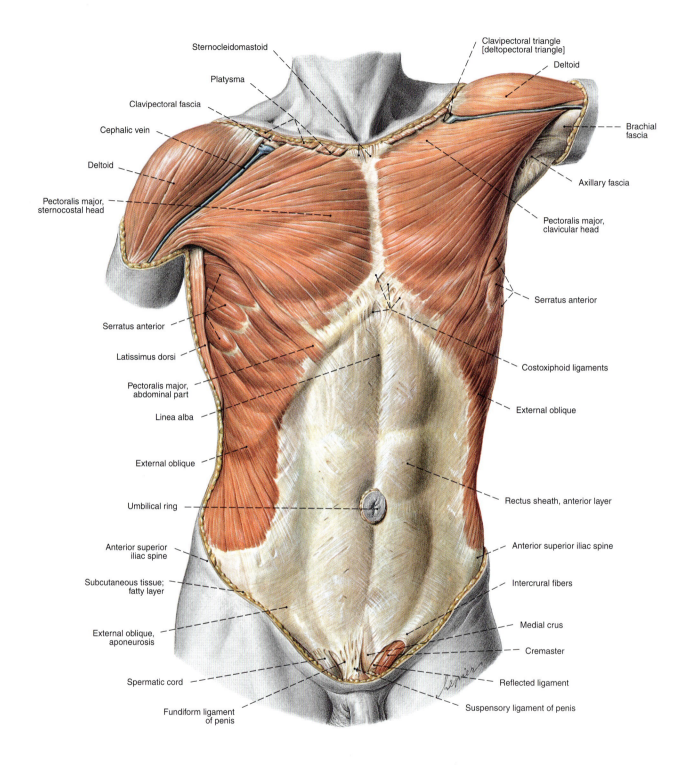

Fig. 818   Muscles of thoracic and abdominal walls;
superficial layer; anterior aspect.

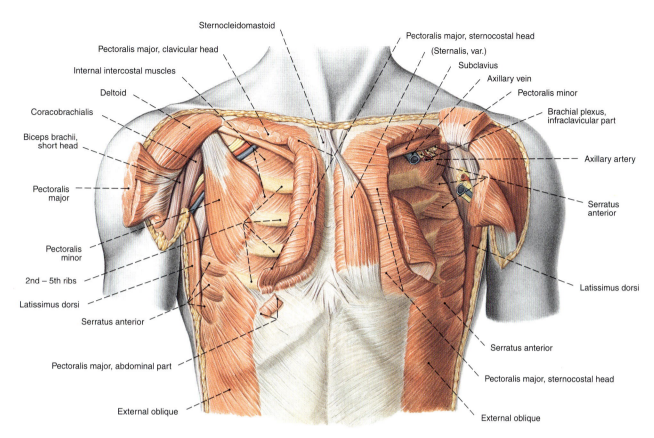

Sternocleidomastoid

Pectoralis major, clavicular head

Internal intercostal muscles

Deltoid

Coracobrachialis

Biceps brachii, short head

Pectoralis major

Pectoralis minor

2nd – 5th ribs

Latissimus dorsi

Serratus anterior

Pectoralis major, abdominal part

External oblique

Pectoralis major, sternocostal head
(Sternalis, var.)

Subclavius

Axillary vein

Pectoralis minor

Brachial plexus, infraclavicular part

Axillary artery

Serratus anterior

Latissimus dorsi

Serratus anterior

Pectoralis major, sternocostal head

External oblique

Fig. 819 Muscles of thorax; right pectoralis major partially removed, left pectoralis minor sectioned and reflected; external intercostal membrane removed; anterior aspect.

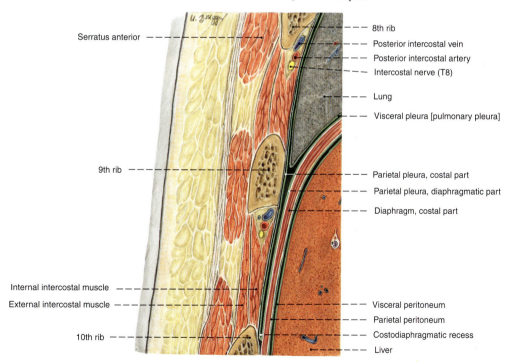

Serratus anterior

9th rib

Internal intercostal muscle

External intercostal muscle

10th rib

8th rib

Posterior intercostal vein

Posterior intercostal artery

Intercostal nerve (T8)

Lung

Visceral pleura [pulmonary pleura]

Parietal pleura, costal part

Parietal pleura, diaphragmatic part

Diaphragm, costal part

Visceral peritoneum

Parietal peritoneum

Costodiaphragmatic recess

Liver

Fig. 820 Muscles of thorax; frontal section exposing thoracic wall, thoracic and abdominal cavity; right ventral aspect. During puncture for aspiration of fluid in the pleural cavity or during puncture of the liver, the course of intercostal nerves and blood vessels, the position of the diaphragm, and the expansion of the lung into the costodiaphragmatic recess must be considered.

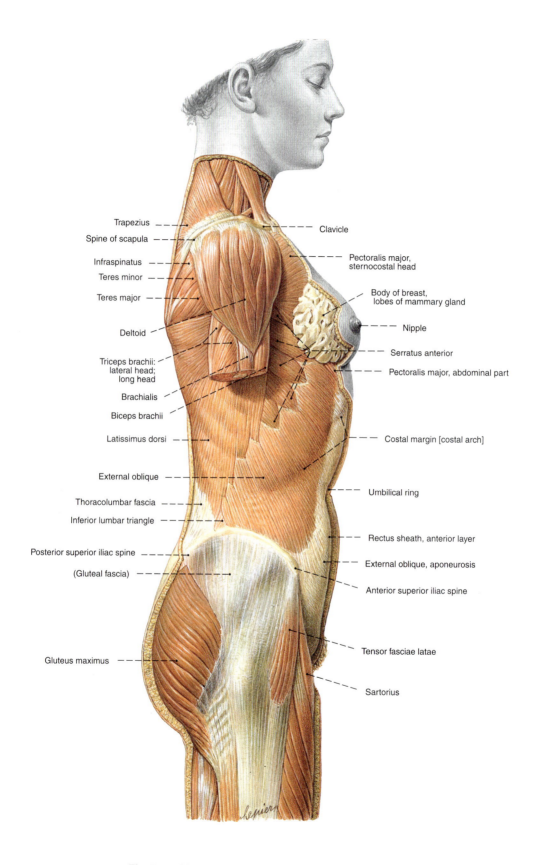

Trapezius

Spine of scapula

Infraspinatus

Teres minor

Teres major

Deltoid

Triceps brachii:
lateral head;
long head

Brachialis

Biceps brachii

Latissimus dorsi

External oblique

Thoracolumbar fascia

Inferior lumbar triangle

Posterior superior iliac spine

(Gluteal fascia)

Gluteus maximus

Clavicle

Pectoralis major,
sternocostal head

Body of breast,
lobes of mammary gland

Nipple

Serratus anterior

Pectoralis major, abdominal part

Costal margin [costal arch]

Umbilical ring

Rectus sheath, anterior layer

External oblique, aponeurosis

Anterior superior iliac spine

Tensor fasciae latae

Sartorius

Fig. 823 Muscles of thoracic and abdominal walls;
mammary gland dissected; lateral aspect.

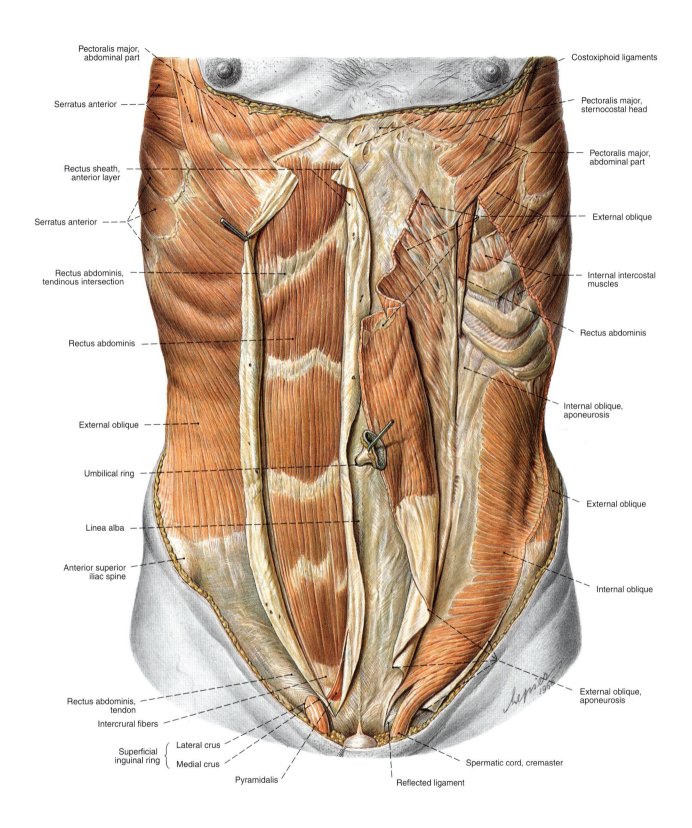

Pectoralis major, abdominal part

Serratus anterior

Rectus sheath, anterior layer

Serratus anterior

Rectus abdominis, tendinous intersection

Rectus abdominis

External oblique

Umbilical ring

Linea alba

Anterior superior iliac spine

Rectus abdominis, tendon

Intercrural fibers

Superficial inguinal ring { Lateral crus / Medial crus }

Pyramidalis

Costoxiphoid ligaments

Pectoralis major, sternocostal head

Pectoralis major, abdominal part

External oblique

Internal intercostal muscles

Rectus abdominis

Internal oblique, aponeurosis

External oblique

Internal oblique

External oblique, aponeurosis

Spermatic cord, cremaster

Reflected ligament

Fig. 824 Muscles of abdomen; anterior layer of rectus sheath split on the right to expose rectus abdominis and pyramidalis; external oblique sectioned on the left to expose internal oblique; anterior aspect.

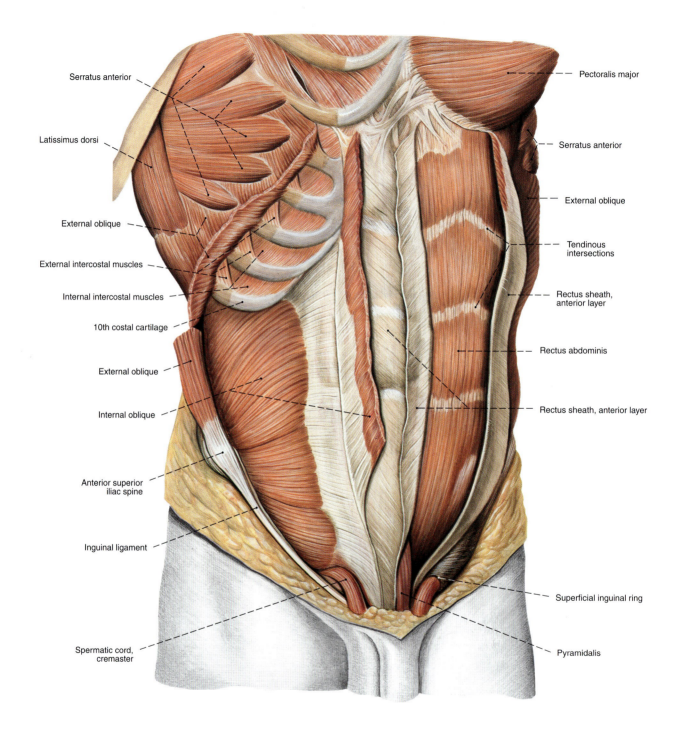

Fig. 825   Muscles of abdomen; anterior layer of rectus sheath opened on the right; external oblique sectioned on the left; external intercostal membrane removed; anterolateral aspect.

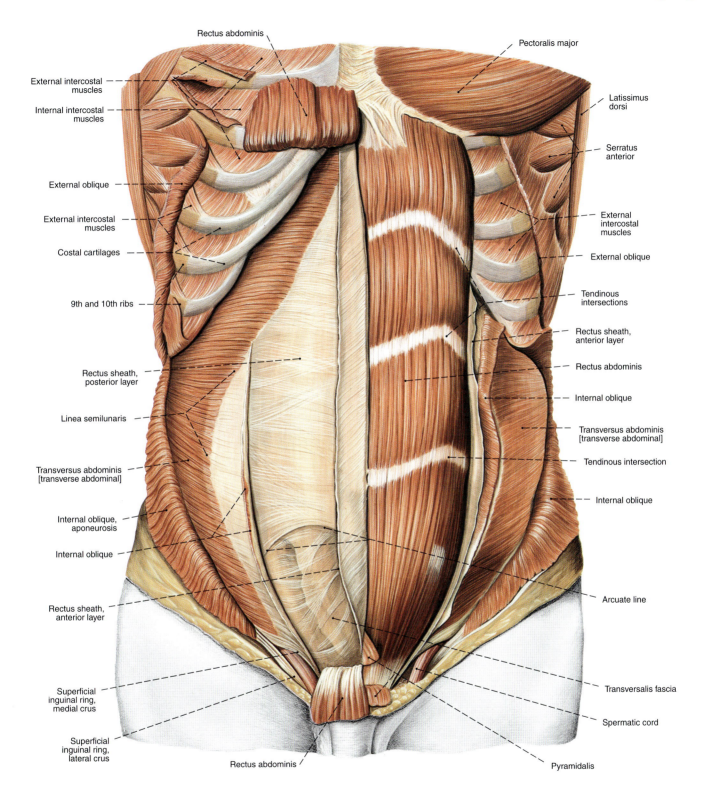

Rectus abdominis

External intercostal muscles

Internal intercostal muscles

External oblique

External intercostal muscles

Costal cartilages

9th and 10th ribs

Rectus sheath, posterior layer

Linea semilunaris

Transversus abdominis [transverse abdominal]

Internal oblique, aponeurosis

Internal oblique

Rectus sheath, anterior layer

Superficial inguinal ring, medial crus

Superficial inguinal ring, lateral crus

Rectus abdominis

Pectoralis major

Latissimus dorsi

Serratus anterior

External intercostal muscles

External oblique

Tendinous intersections

Rectus sheath, anterior layer

Rectus abdominis

Internal oblique

Transversus abdominis [transverse abdominal]

Tendinous intersection

Internal oblique

Arcuate line

Transversalis fascia

Spermatic cord

Pyramidalis

Fig. 826   Muscles of abdomen; pyramidalis sectioned on the left; rectus abdominis reflected upward and downward and external oblique opened on the right; anterior layer of rectus sheath reflected to the right over the midline; anterior aspect.

Ventral muscles of abdominal wall (Fig. 826)

Both the anterior muscles of the abdominal wall, rectus abdominis, and pyramidalis lie within the rectus sheath.

Muscle *Innervation*	Origin	Insertion	Function
1. **Rectus abdominis** *Intercostal nerves (thoracic nerves); occasionally ventral rami of upper lumbar nerves*	5th – 7th costal cartilages (external surface), xiphoid process, costoxiphoid ligaments	Pubic crest, pubic symphysis	Flexes trunk toward pelvis, increases abdominal pressure, compresses abdomen in expiration
2. **Pyramidalis** *Caudal intercostal nerves (thoracic nerves) (inconstant muscle)*	Pubic crest, pubic symphysis (ventral of rectus abdominis)	Linea alba	Tenses linea alba

Lateral muscles of abdominal wall (Figs. 824, 826)

The lateral muscles of the abdominal wall comprise the external and internal oblique, and the transversus abdominis [transverse abdominal].
In the male the cremaster separates from the internal oblique and the transversus abdominis [transverse abdominal].

Muscle *Innervation*	Origin	Insertion	Function
1. **External oblique** *Caudal intercostal nerves (thoracic nerves), iliohypogastric nerve [iliopubic nerve; ilio-inguinal nerve; (lumbar plexus)*	5th–12th ribs (outer surface, interdigitations with serratus anterior)	Outer lip of iliac crest, inguinal ligament, pubic tubercle, pubic crest, linea alba (contributes to anterior layer of rectus sheath)	Acting unilateral: rotation of thorax to contralateral side, lateral flexion of vertebral column Acting bilateral: flexes trunk toward pelvis, increases abdominal pressure, compresses abdomen in expiration
2. **Internal oblique** *Caudal intercostal nerves (thoracic nerves), iliohypogastric nerve [iliopubic nerve; ilio-inguinal nerve; (lumbar plexus)*	Thoracolumbar fascia (posterior layer), intermediate zone of iliac crest, inguinal ligament (lateral 2/3)	(9th) 10th- 12th costal cartilage (lower border), linea alba (contributes to anterior and posterior layer of rectus sheath above arcuate line; below arcuate line all tendon fibers blend with the anterior layer). In the male the lowest fibers separate to form the cremaster, that continues in the spermatic cord.	Acting unilateral: rotation of thorax to ipsilateral side, lateral flexion of vertebral column Acting bilateral: flexes trunk toward pelvis, increases abdominal pressure, compresses abdomen in expiration Cremaster draws testis and sheaths upward.
3. **Transversus abdominis [transverse abdominal]** *Caudal intercostal nerves (thoracic nerves), iliohypogastric nerve [iliopubic nerve; ilio-inguinal nerve; genitofemoral nerve (lumbar plexus)*	(5th, 6th) 7th-12th costal cartilages (inner surface), costal processes of lumbar vertebrae (via anterior layer of thoracolumbar fascia), inner lip of iliac crest, inguinal ligament (lateral third)	Linea alba (contributes to posterior layer of rectus sheath above arcuate line and to the anterior layer below arcuate line). In the male the lowest fibers separate to form the cremaster, that continues in the spermatic cord.	Increases abdominal pressure, compresses abdomen in expiration

Posterior muscles of abdominal wall (Fig. 829)

The muscular base of the posterior abdominal wall is represented by the lumbar part of diaphragm superiorly and the quadratus lumborum inferiorly. This muscle is joined by the psoas major medially.

Muscle *Innervation*	Origin	Insertion	Function
1. **Quadratus lumborum** *Muscular branches (lumbar plexus); intercostal nerve (12th thoracic nerve)*	Outer lip of iliac crest (posterior third), iliolumbar ligament	12th rib (medial part), costal processes of 4th-1st lumbar vertebrae	Lowers ribs (expiration), lateral flexion of vertebral column

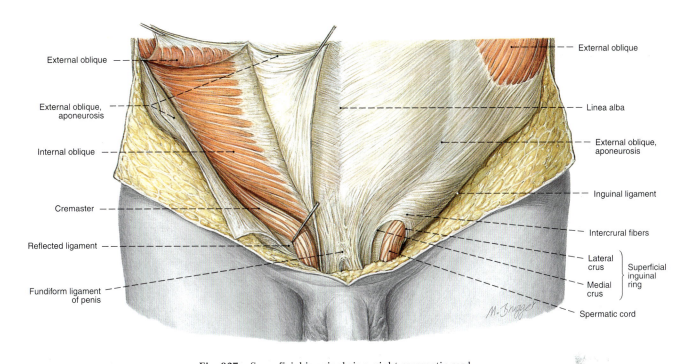

External oblique

External oblique,
aponeurosis

Internal oblique

Cremaster

Reflected ligament

Fundiform ligament
of penis

External oblique

Linea alba

External oblique,
aponeurosis

Inguinal ligament

Intercrural fibers

Lateral
crus

Medial
crus

Superficial
inguinal
ring

Spermatic cord

Fig. 827   Superficial inguinal ring; right spermatic cord
retracted by a hook; aponeurosis of external oblique
opened on the right; anterior aspect.
Compare Fig. 835.

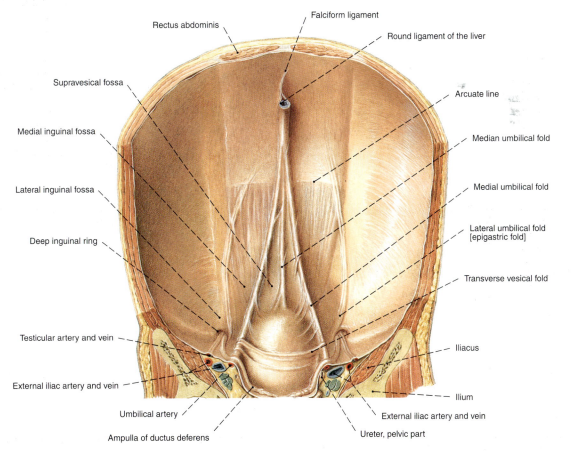

Rectus abdominis

Falciform ligament

Round ligament of the liver

Supravesical fossa

Arcuate line

Medial inguinal fossa

Median umbilical fold

Lateral inguinal fossa

Medial umbilical fold

Deep inguinal ring

Lateral umbilical fold
[epigastric fold]

Transverse vesical fold

Testicular artery and vein

External iliac artery and vein

Iliacus

Umbilical artery

Ilium

Ampulla of ductus deferens

External iliac artery and vein

Ureter, pelvic part

Fig. 828   Anterior abdominal wall of a newborn; posterior
aspect.
The umbilical vein degenerates after birth. In cases of portal
hypertension the vein may enlarge again. Compare Fig. 1029,
portocaval anastomoses.

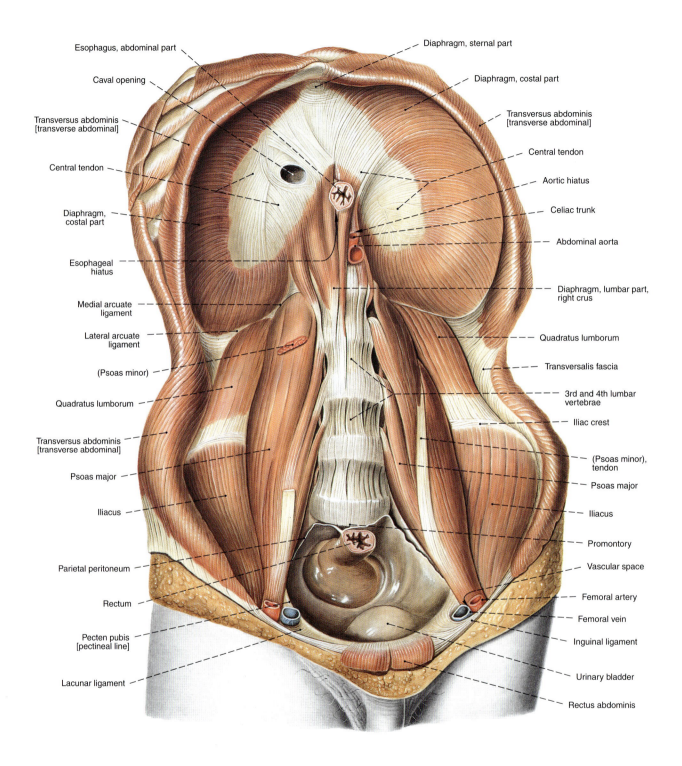

Esophagus, abdominal part

Caval opening

Transversus abdominis [transverse abdominal]

Central tendon

Diaphragm, costal part

Esophageal hiatus

Medial arcuate ligament

Lateral arcuate ligament

(Psoas minor)

Quadratus lumborum

Transversus abdominis [transverse abdominal]

Psoas major

Iliacus

Parietal peritoneum

Rectum

Pecten pubis [pectineal line]

Lacunar ligament

Diaphragm, sternal part

Diaphragm, costal part

Transversus abdominis [transverse abdominal]

Central tendon

Aortic hiatus

Celiac trunk

Abdominal aorta

Diaphragm, lumbar part, right crus

Quadratus lumborum

Transversalis fascia

3rd and 4th lumbar vertebrae

Iliac crest

(Psoas minor), tendon

Psoas major

Iliacus

Promontory

Vascular space

Femoral artery

Femoral vein

Inguinal ligament

Urinary bladder

Rectus abdominis

Fig. 829   Diaphragm; muscles of abdomen; anterior aspect.

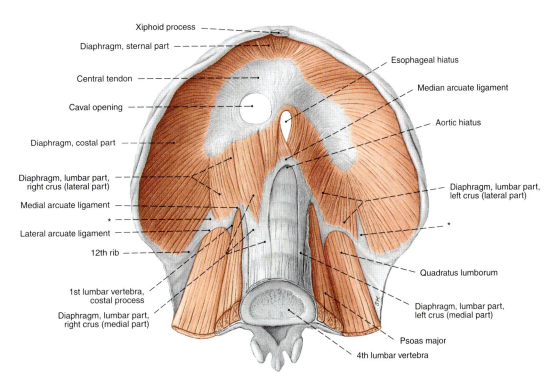

Fig. 830 Diaphragm; and posterior abdominal wall; anterior aspect.

The right crus (medial part) frequently consists of three components and extends further distally than the left crus.
* Clinically: BOCHDALEK's triangle.

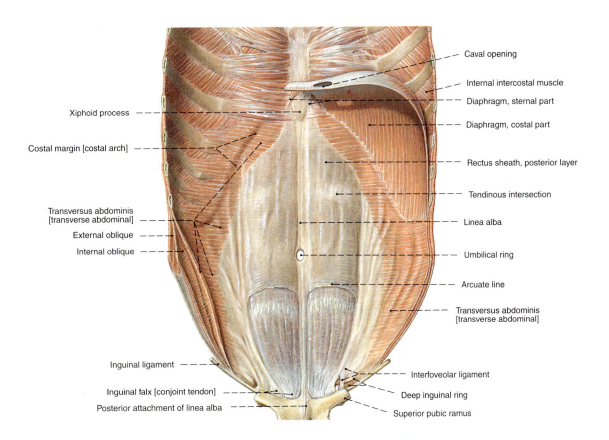

Fig. 831 Anterior abdominal wall and parts of diaphragm; posterior aspect.

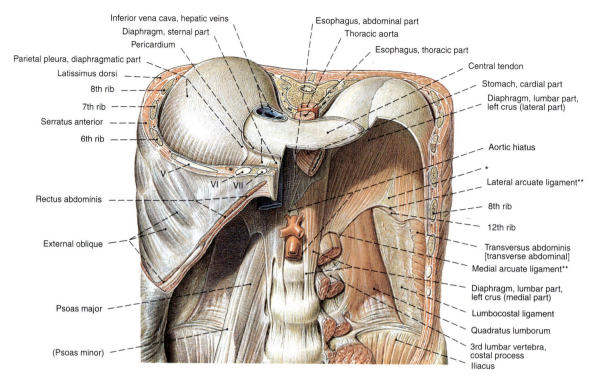

Inferior vena cava, hepatic veins
Diaphragm, sternal part
Pericardium
Parietal pleura, diaphragmatic part
Latissimus dorsi
8th rib
7th rib
Serratus anterior
6th rib

Esophagus, abdominal part
Thoracic aorta
Esophagus, thoracic part
Central tendon
Stomach, cardial part
Diaphragm, lumbar part, left crus (lateral part)
Aortic hiatus
*
Lateral arcuate ligament**
8th rib
12th rib
Transversus abdominis [transverse abdominal]
Medial arcuate ligament**
Diaphragm, lumbar part, left crus (medial part)
Lumbocostal ligament
Quadratus lumborum
3rd lumbar vertebra, costal process
Iliacus

V
VI VII
Rectus abdominis
External oblique
Psoas major
(Psoas minor)

Fig. 832 Diaphragm with openings and muscles of posterior abdominal wall; trunk sectioned at level of 10th thoracic vertebra; anterior aspect.

* Clinically: BOCHDALEK's triangle, lumbocostal triangle, area without muscles.
** Also arches of psoas and quadratus, HALLER's arches.

Diaphragm (Fig. 832)

The diaphragm separates the thoracic and the abdominal cavities. Its dome forms the floor of the right and left pleural cavities. The lumbar part borders the retroperitoneal space and—strictly speaking—is part of the posterior abdominal wall.

Muscle *Innervation*	Origin	Insertion	Function
Diaphragm *Phrenic nerve (cervical plexus)*	**Sternal part:** xiphoid process (inner surface), rectus sheath (aponeurosis of transversus abdominis [transverse abdominal]) **Costal part:** 12th-6th costal cartilage (inner surface, interdigitates with origin of transversus abdominis [transverse abdominal]) **Lumbar part, right crus:** - Medial part: bodies of 1st-3rd lumbar vertebrae, intervertebral discs - Lateral part: medial and lateral arcuate ligaments **Lumbar part, left crus:** - Medial part: bodies of 1st-4th lumbar vertebrae, intervertebral discs - Lateral part: medial and lateral arcuate ligaments	All parts unite in the central tendon. Weak spaces and openings: sternocostal triangle, lumbocostal triangle, caval opening, aortic hiatus, esophageal hiatus	Diaphragmatic respiration (inspiration), increases abdominal pressure

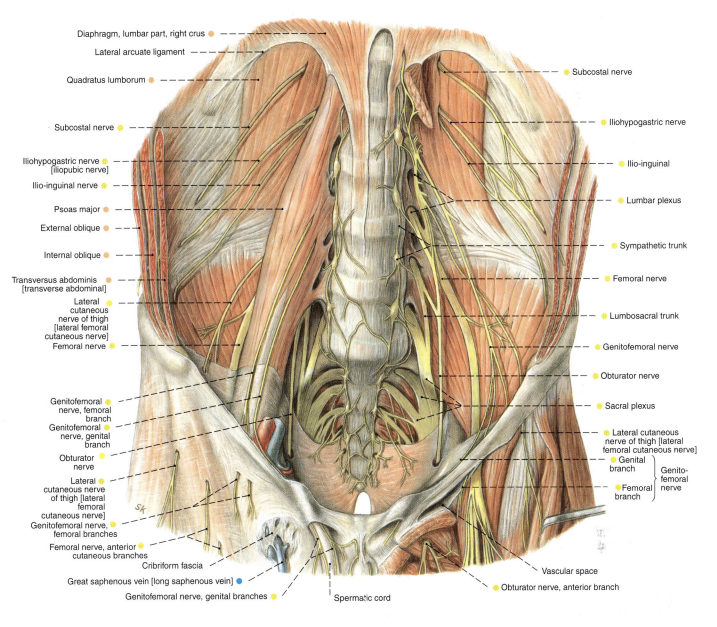

Diaphragm, lumbar part, right crus
Lateral arcuate ligament
Quadratus lumborum
Subcostal nerve
Iliohypogastric nerve [iliopubic nerve]
Ilio-inguinal nerve
Psoas major
External oblique
Internal oblique
Transversus abdominis [transverse abdominal]
Lateral cutaneous nerve of thigh [lateral femoral cutaneous nerve]
Femoral nerve
Genitofemoral nerve, femoral branch
Genitofemoral nerve, genital branch
Obturator nerve
Lateral cutaneous nerve of thigh [lateral femoral cutaneous nerve]
Genitofemoral nerve, femoral branches
Femoral nerve, anterior cutaneous branches
Cribriform fascia
Great saphenous vein [long saphenous vein]
Genitofemoral nerve, genital branches
Spermatic cord

Subcostal nerve
Iliohypogastric nerve
Ilio-inguinal
Lumbar plexus
Sympathetic trunk
Femoral nerve
Lumbosacral trunk
Genitofemoral nerve
Obturator nerve
Sacral plexus
Lateral cutaneous nerve of thigh [lateral femoral cutaneous nerve]
Genital branch
Femoral branch
Genitofemoral nerve
Vascular space
Obturator nerve, anterior branch

Fig. 833 Lumbosacral plexus;
after removal of psoas major, pectineus, and adductor
longus on the left; anterior aspect.

Diaphragmatic openings

Name	Position	Structures
Aortic hiatus	Lumbar part, between right crus and left crus	Aorta; thoracic duct
Esophageal hiatus	Lumbar part, right crus	Esophagus; vagus nerves; phrenic nerve; left phrenico-abdominal branch
Caval opening	Central tendon	Inferior vena cava; phrenic nerve; right phrenico-abdominal branch
LARREY's cleft [triangle of MORGAGNI]	Between sternal part and costal part	Superior epigastric artery and vein
Unnamed	Lumbar part, right/left crus, (medial part)	Greater and lesser splanchnic nerves; azygos vein; hemi-azygos vein [inferior hemi-azygos vein]
Unnamed	Lumbar part, between medial part and lateral part	Sympathetic trunk

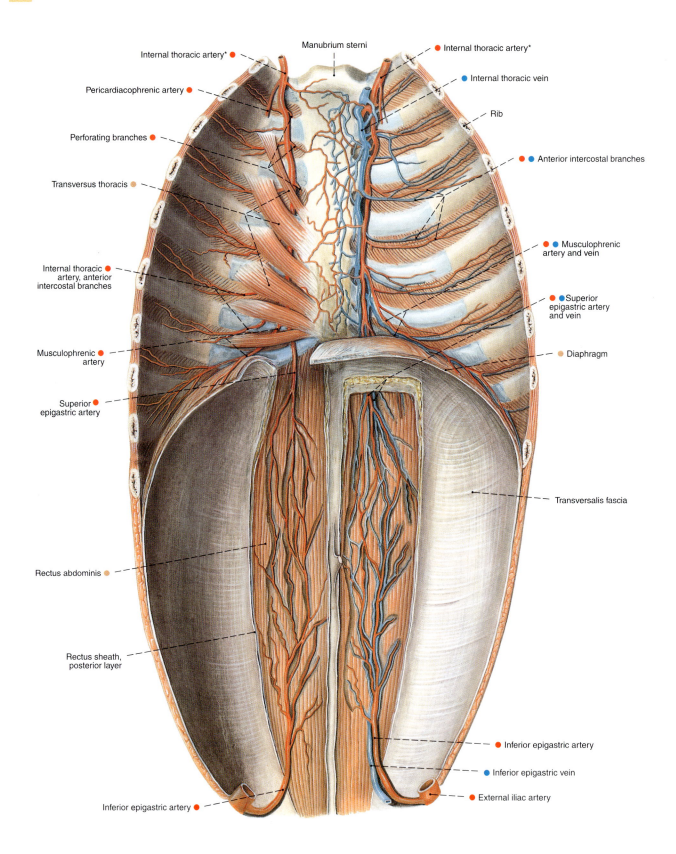

Internal thoracic artery* ●
Pericardiacophrenic artery ●
Perforating branches ●
Transversus thoracis ●
Internal thoracic artery, anterior intercostal branches ●
Musculophrenic artery ●
Superior epigastric artery ●
Rectus abdominis ●
Rectus sheath, posterior layer
Inferior epigastric artery ●

Manubrium sterni

● Internal thoracic artery*
● Internal thoracic vein
Rib
● ● Anterior intercostal branches
● ● Musculophrenic artery and vein
● ● Superior epigastric artery and vein
● Diaphragm
Transversalis fascia
● Inferior epigastric artery
● Inferior epigastric vein
● External iliac artery

Fig. 834   Blood vessels of anterior thoracic and abdominal walls;
transversus thoracis removed on the right; posterior aspect.

* Clinically: internal mammary artery.

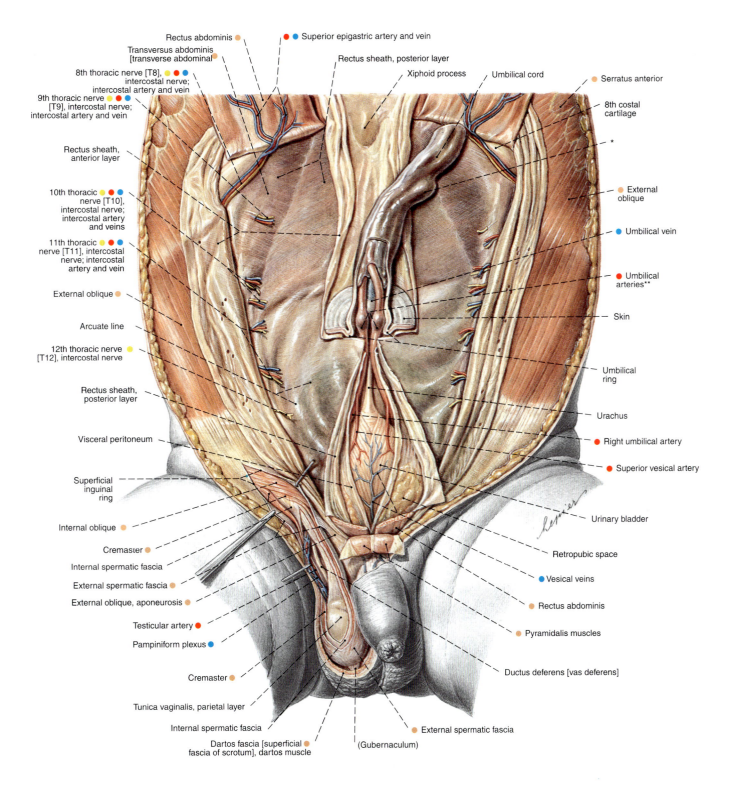

Rectus abdominis
Transversus abdominis [transverse abdominal]
8th thoracic nerve [T8], intercostal nerve; intercostal artery and vein
9th thoracic nerve [T9], intercostal nerve; intercostal artery and vein
Rectus sheath, anterior layer
10th thoracic nerve [T10], intercostal nerve; intercostal artery and veins
11th thoracic nerve [T11], intercostal nerve; intercostal artery and vein
External oblique
Arcuate line
12th thoracic nerve [T12], intercostal nerve
Rectus sheath, posterior layer
Visceral peritoneum
Superficial inguinal ring
Internal oblique
Cremaster
Internal spermatic fascia
External spermatic fascia
External oblique, aponeurosis
Testicular artery
Pampiniform plexus
Cremaster
Tunica vaginalis, parietal layer
Internal spermatic fascia
Dartos fascia [superficial fascia of scrotum], dartos muscle

Superior epigastric artery and vein
Rectus sheath, posterior layer
Xiphoid process
Umbilical cord
Serratus anterior
8th costal cartilage
*
External oblique
Umbilical vein
Umbilical arteries**
Skin
Umbilical ring
Urachus
Right umbilical artery
Superior vesical artery
Urinary bladder
Retropubic space
Vesical veins
Rectus abdominis
Pyramidalis muscles
Ductus deferens [vas deferens]
External spermatic fascia
(Gubernaculum)

Fig. 835 Anterior abdominal wall of a newborn; rectus abdominis muscles reflected upward and abdominal cavity opened in the median plane to expose urinary bladder and urachus; inguinal canal dissected on the right; anterior aspect.

* Thickening formed by loops of umbilical blood vessels (false umbilical cord knot).
** Thrombus in umbilical arteries.

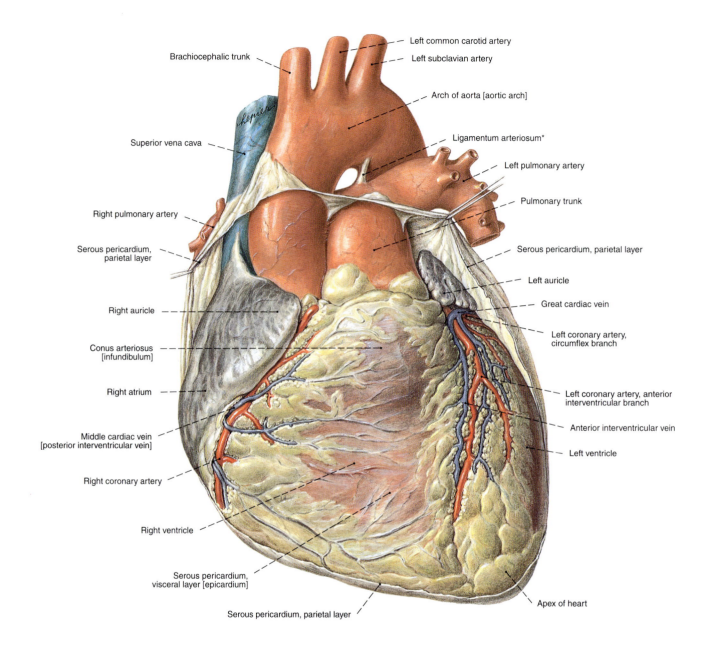

Brachiocephalic trunk

Left common carotid artery

Left subclavian artery

Arch of aorta [aortic arch]

Ligamentum arteriosum*

Superior vena cava

Left pulmonary artery

Pulmonary trunk

Right pulmonary artery

Serous pericardium, parietal layer

Serous pericardium, parietal layer

Left auricle

Right auricle

Great cardiac vein

Conus arteriosus [infundibulum]

Left coronary artery, circumflex branch

Right atrium

Left coronary artery, anterior interventricular branch

Middle cardiac vein [posterior interventricular vein]

Anterior interventricular vein

Left ventricle

Right coronary artery

Right ventricle

Serous pericardium, visceral layer [epicardium]

Apex of heart

Serous pericardium, parietal layer

Fig. 839 Heart; pericardium opened and parietal layer
mostly removed; larger branches of coronary blood vessels
dissected; visceral layer [epicardium] not shown on descending
aorta and pulmonary trunk; ventral aspect.

* BOTALLO's ligament formed from the remnants of the fetal ductus arteriosus
[BOTALLO's duct].

Fibrous pericardium	
Serous pericardium	**Pericardium**
Parietal layer	
Visceral layer = **Epicardium**	

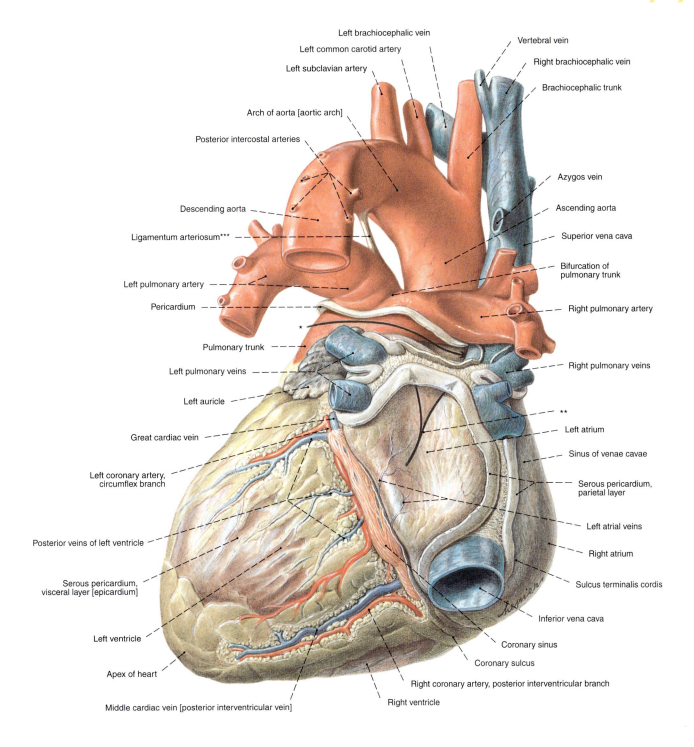

Left brachiocephalic vein
Left common carotid artery
Left subclavian artery
Vertebral vein
Right brachiocephalic vein
Brachiocephalic trunk
Arch of aorta [aortic arch]
Posterior intercostal arteries
Azygos vein
Descending aorta
Ascending aorta
Ligamentum arteriosum***
Superior vena cava
Bifurcation of pulmonary trunk
Left pulmonary artery
Pericardium
Right pulmonary artery
*
Pulmonary trunk
Left pulmonary veins
Right pulmonary veins
Left auricle
**
Great cardiac vein
Left atrium
Sinus of venae cavae
Left coronary artery, circumflex branch
Serous pericardium, parietal layer
Left atrial veins
Posterior veins of left ventricle
Right atrium
Serous pericardium, visceral layer [epicardium]
Sulcus terminalis cordis
Inferior vena cava
Left ventricle
Coronary sinus
Apex of heart
Coronary sulcus
Right coronary artery, posterior interventricular branch
Middle cardiac vein [posterior interventricular vein]
Right ventricle

Fig. 840 Heart and great blood vessels; pericardium severed next to the great blood vessels; larger branches of coronary blood vessels dissected; dorsal aspect.

*   Arrow in transverse pericardial sinus.
**   Double arrows in oblique pericardial sinus.
*** BOTALLO's ligament formed from the remnants of the fetal ductus arteriosus [BOTALLO's duct].

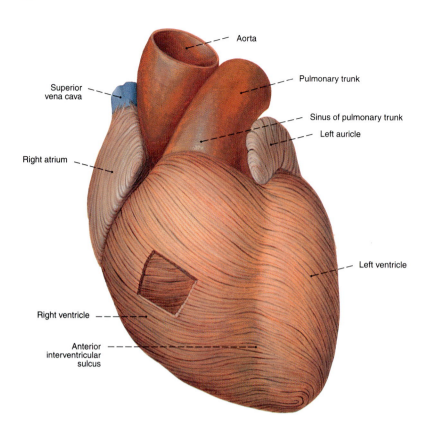

Aorta

Superior
vena cava

Pulmonary trunk

Sinus of pulmonary trunk

Left auricle

Right atrium

Left ventricle

Right ventricle

Anterior
interventricular
sulcus

Fig. 841   Myocardium; parts of the
superficial muscle layer of the right
ventricle removed to expose the deep
layer; ventral aspect.

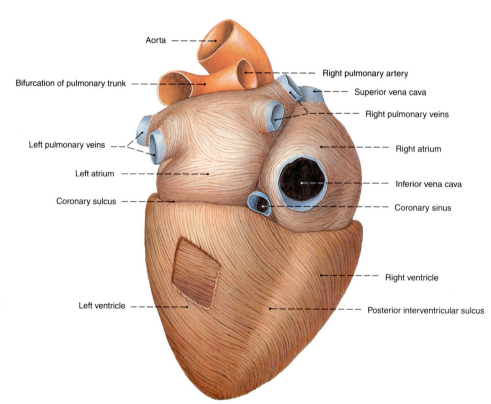

Aorta

Bifurcation of pulmonary trunk

Right pulmonary artery

Superior vena cava

Right pulmonary veins

Left pulmonary veins

Right atrium

Left atrium

Inferior vena cava

Coronary sulcus

Coronary sinus

Right ventricle

Left ventricle

Posterior interventricular sulcus

Fig. 842   Myocardium; parts of the
superficial muscle layer of the left
ventricle removed to expose the
deep layer; the intersection of
myocardium after removal of
coronary sinus is not shown;
dorsocaudal aspect.

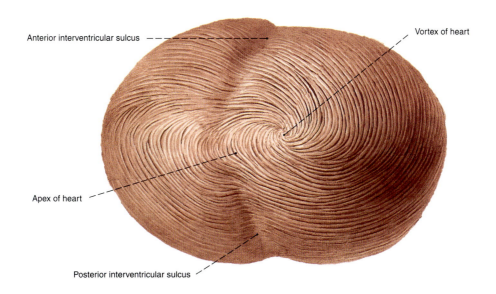

Anterior interventricular sulcus

Vortex of heart

Apex of heart

Posterior interventricular sulcus

Fig. 843   Myocardium; viewed from the apex.

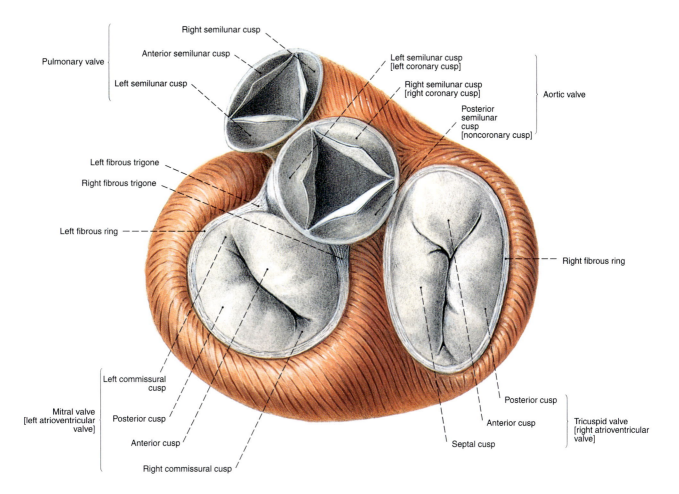

Right semilunar cusp

Anterior semilunar cusp

Pulmonary valve

Left semilunar cusp

Left semilunar cusp
[left coronary cusp]

Right semilunar cusp
[right coronary cusp]

Posterior
semilunar
cusp
[noncoronary cusp]

Aortic valve

Left fibrous trigone

Right fibrous trigone

Left fibrous ring

Right fibrous ring

Left commissural
cusp

Posterior cusp

Mitral valve
[left atrioventricular
valve]

Anterior cusp

Right commissural cusp

Posterior cusp

Anterior cusp

Tricuspid valve
[right atrioventricular
valve]

Septal cusp

Fig. 844   Myocardium; cardiac valves; surface of cut interatrial
septum and opening for bundle of HIS not shown; systolic
phase with open arterial and closed atrioventricular valves;
cranial aspect.

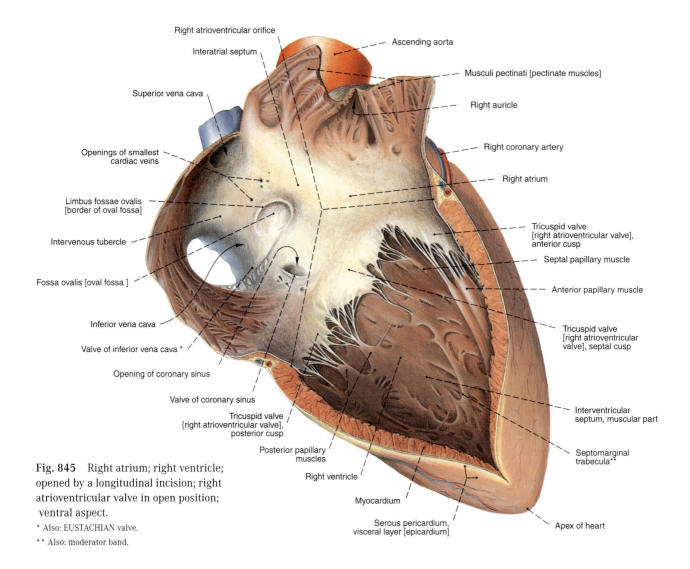

Fig. 845 Right atrium; right ventricle; opened by a longitudinal incision; right atrioventricular valve in open position; ventral aspect.

* Also: EUSTACHIAN valve.

** Also: moderator band.

Right atrioventricular orifice

Interatrial septum

Superior vena cava

Openings of smallest cardiac veins

Limbus fossae ovalis [border of oval fossa]

Intervenous tubercle

Fossa ovalis [oval fossa]

Inferior vena cava

Valve of inferior vena cava *

Opening of coronary sinus

Valve of coronary sinus

Tricuspid valve [right atrioventricular valve], posterior cusp

Posterior papillary muscles

Right ventricle

Myocardium

Serous pericardium, visceral layer [epicardium]

Ascending aorta

Musculi pectinati [pectinate muscles]

Right auricle

Right coronary artery

Right atrium

Tricuspid valve [right atrioventricular valve], anterior cusp

Septal papillary muscle

Anterior papillary muscle

Tricuspid valve [right atrioventricular valve], septal cusp

Interventricular septum, muscular part

Septomarginal trabecula**

Apex of heart

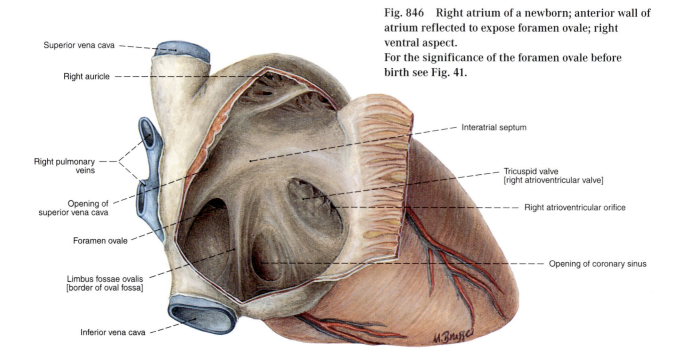

Fig. 846 Right atrium of a newborn; anterior wall of atrium reflected to expose foramen ovale; right ventral aspect.
For the significance of the foramen ovale before birth see Fig. 41.

Superior vena cava

Right auricle

Right pulmonary veins

Opening of superior vena cava

Foramen ovale

Limbus fossae ovalis [border of oval fossa]

Inferior vena cava

Interatrial septum

Tricuspid valve [right atrioventricular valve]

Right atrioventricular orifice

Opening of coronary sinus

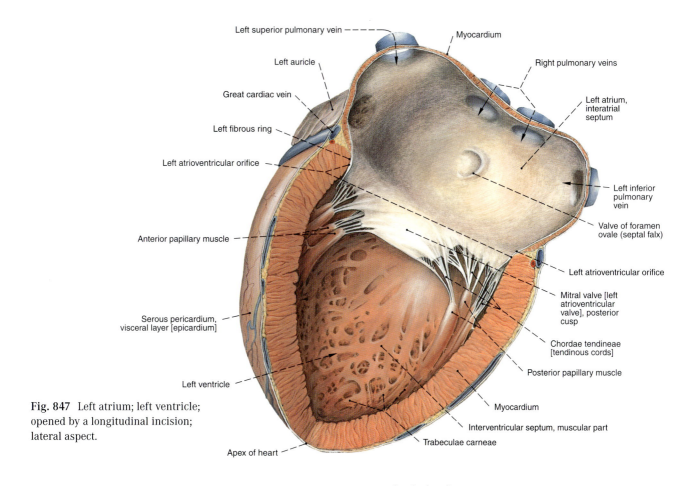

Left superior pulmonary vein
Myocardium
Left auricle
Right pulmonary veins
Great cardiac vein
Left atrium, interatrial septum
Left fibrous ring
Left atrioventricular orifice
Left inferior pulmonary vein
Valve of foramen ovale (septal falx)
Anterior papillary muscle
Left atrioventricular orifice
Mitral valve [left atrioventricular valve], posterior cusp
Serous pericardium, visceral layer [epicardium]
Chordae tendineae [tendinous cords]
Posterior papillary muscle
Left ventricle
Myocardium
Apex of heart
Interventricular septum, muscular part
Trabeculae carneae

Fig. 847 Left atrium; left ventricle; opened by a longitudinal incision; lateral aspect.

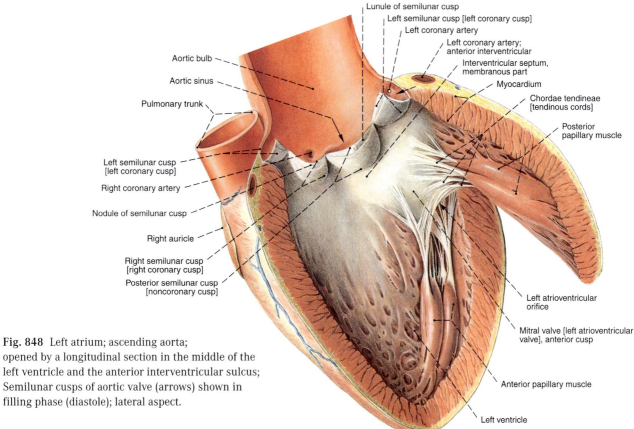

Lunule of semilunar cusp
Left semilunar cusp [left coronary cusp]
Left coronary artery
Left coronary artery; anterior interventricular
Interventricular septum, membranous part
Aortic bulb
Myocardium
Aortic sinus
Chordae tendineae [tendinous cords]
Pulmonary trunk
Posterior papillary muscle
Left semilunar cusp [left coronary cusp]
Right coronary artery
Nodule of semilunar cusp
Right auricle
Right semilunar cusp [right coronary cusp]
Posterior semilunar cusp [noncoronary cusp]
Left atrioventricular orifice
Mitral valve [left atrioventricular valve], anterior cusp
Anterior papillary muscle
Left ventricle

Fig. 848 Left atrium; ascending aorta; opened by a longitudinal section in the middle of the left ventricle and the anterior interventricular sulcus; Semilunar cusps of aortic valve (arrows) shown in filling phase (diastole); lateral aspect.

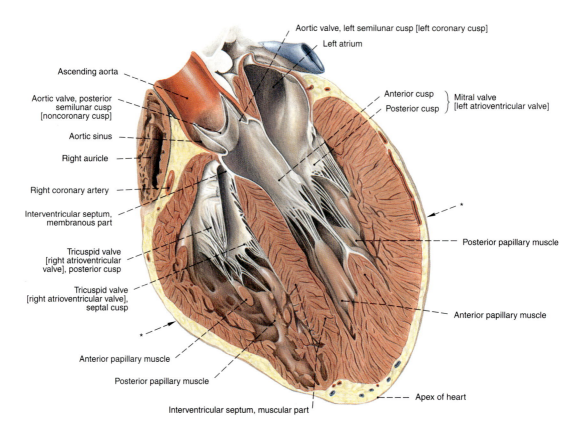

Fig. 849 Left and right ventricles; opened by a longitudinal section along the axis of the heart; left lateral ventral aspect.

Note the differences in thickness of myocardium between right and left ventricles.
* Plane of section of Fig. 850.

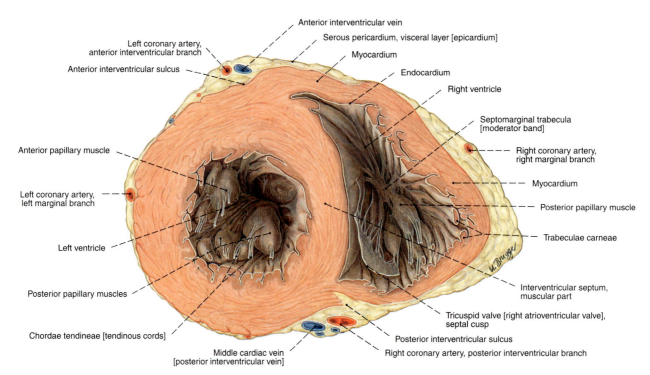

Fig. 850 Left and right ventricles; cross-section perpendicular to axis of the heart; superior aspect.

Note the differences in thickness of myocardium of right and left ventricles.

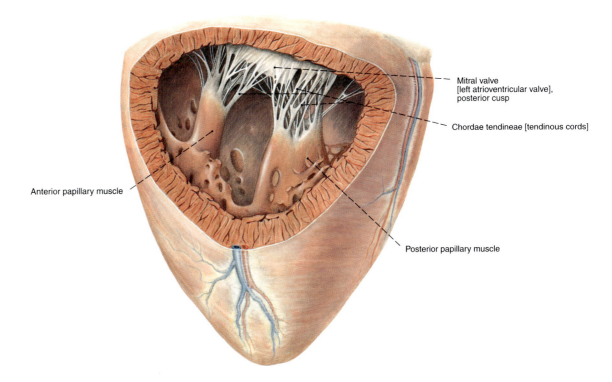

Mitral valve
[left atrioventricular valve],
posterior cusp

Chordae tendineae [tendinous cords]

Anterior papillary muscle

Posterior papillary muscle

Fig. 851 Left ventricle; window view of papillary muscles and chordae tendineae [tendinous cords]; left ventral caudal aspect.

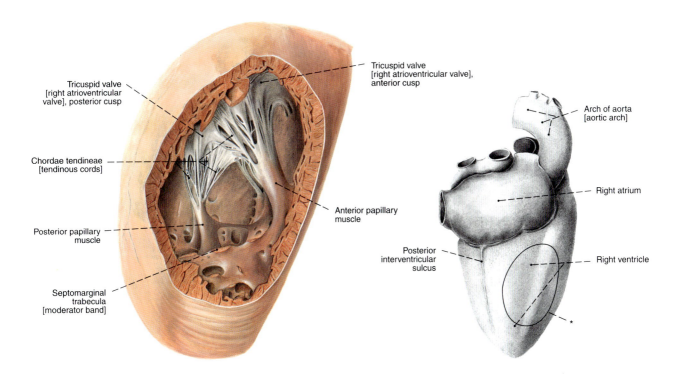

Tricuspid valve
[right atrioventricular valve],
anterior cusp

Tricuspid valve
[right atrioventricular
valve], posterior cusp

Chordae tendineae
[tendinous cords]

Posterior papillary
muscle

Septomarginal
trabecula
[moderator band]

Anterior papillary
muscle

Arch of aorta
[aortic arch]

Right atrium

Posterior
interventricular
sulcus

Right ventricle

Fig. 852 Right ventricle; window view of papillary muscles and chordae tendineae [tendinous cords]; dorsal aspect.

* Contour of window.

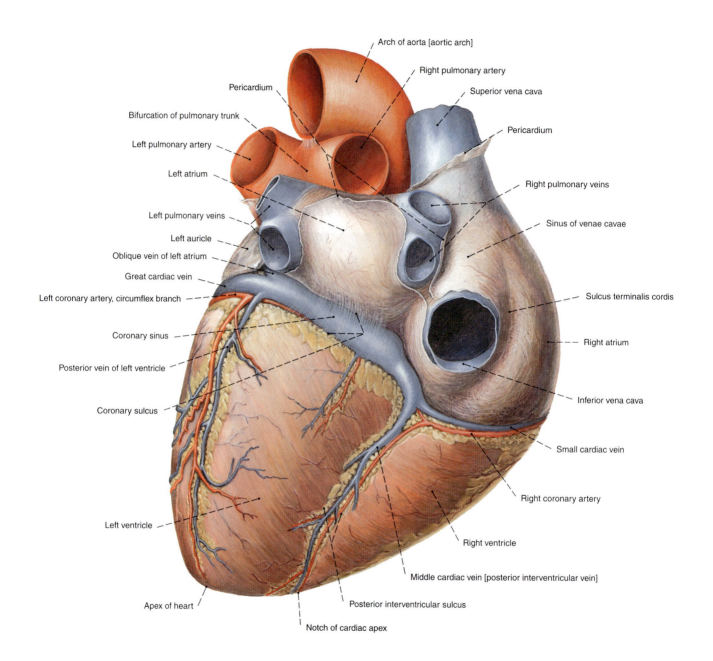

Arch of aorta [aortic arch]

Right pulmonary artery

Superior vena cava

Pericardium

Pericardium

Bifurcation of pulmonary trunk

Left pulmonary artery

Left atrium

Right pulmonary veins

Left pulmonary veins

Sinus of venae cavae

Left auricle

Oblique vein of left atrium

Great cardiac vein

Sulcus terminalis cordis

Left coronary artery, circumflex branch

Coronary sinus

Right atrium

Posterior vein of left ventricle

Coronary sulcus

Inferior vena cava

Small cardiac vein

Right coronary artery

Left ventricle

Right ventricle

Middle cardiac vein [posterior interventricular vein]

Apex of heart

Posterior interventricular sulcus

Notch of cardiac apex

Fig. 865   Cardiac veins; pericardium removed up to the great blood vessels; dorsocaudal aspect.
The coronary sinus is frequently covered with thin muscular fibers (compare Fig. 840).

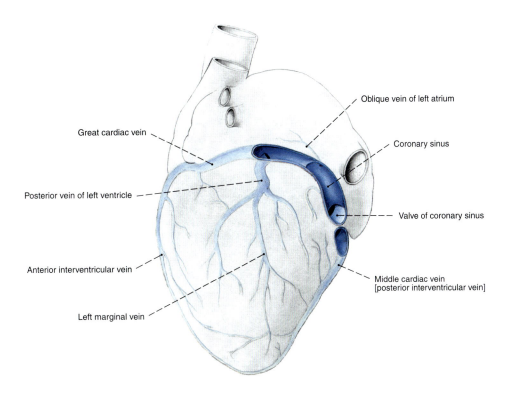

Fig. 866 Cardiac veins; branches of large cardiac veins schematically (from VON LÜDINGHAUSEN); left caudal aspect.
Size and course of cardiac veins vary considerably.

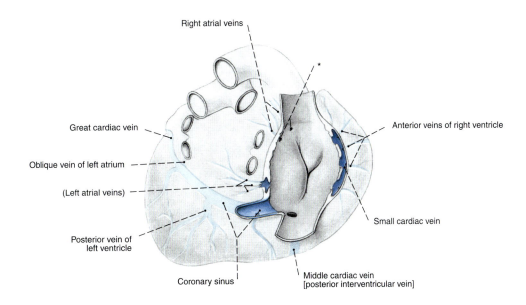

Fig. 867 Cardiac veins; right atrium removed to expose orifices of cardiac veins (from VON LÜDINGHAUSEN); cranial aspect.

* Orifices of anterior atrial veins (LANNELONGUE's crypts). Orifices of cardiac veins vary considerably.

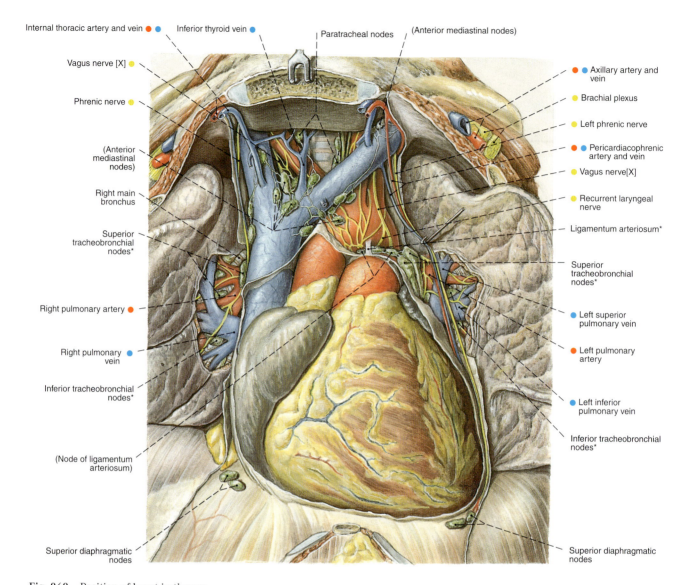

Internal thoracic artery and vein ●●
Inferior thyroid vein ●
Paratracheal nodes
(Anterior mediastinal nodes)

Vagus nerve [X] ●

Phrenic nerve ●

(Anterior mediastinal nodes)

Right main bronchus

Superior tracheobronchial nodes*

Right pulmonary artery ●

Right pulmonary vein ●

Inferior tracheobronchial nodes*

(Node of ligamentum arteriosum)

Superior diaphragmatic nodes

●● Axillary artery and vein
● Brachial plexus
● Left phrenic nerve
●● Pericardiacophrenic artery and vein
● Vagus nerve[X]
● Recurrent laryngeal nerve
Ligamentum arteriosum*
Superior tracheobronchial nodes*
● Left superior pulmonary vein
● Left pulmonary artery
● Left inferior pulmonary vein
Inferior tracheobronchial nodes*
Superior diaphragmatic nodes

Fig. 868 Position of heart in thorax; thymus removed; manubrium of sternum retracted cranially; pericardium partially removed and hilum of lung dissected to expose mediastinal lymph nodes; ventral aspect.
* Clinically: hilar lymph nodes.
** Clinically: BOTALLO's ligament formed from the remnants of the fetal ductus arteriosus [BOTALLO's duct].

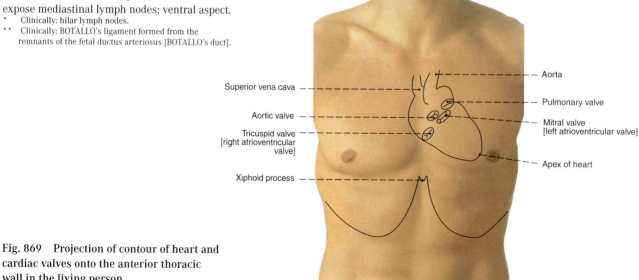

Superior vena cava
Aortic valve
Tricuspid valve [right atrioventricular valve]
Xiphoid process

Aorta
Pulmonary valve
Mitral valve [left atrioventricular valve]
Apex of heart

Fig. 869 Projection of contour of heart and cardiac valves onto the anterior thoracic wall in the living person.

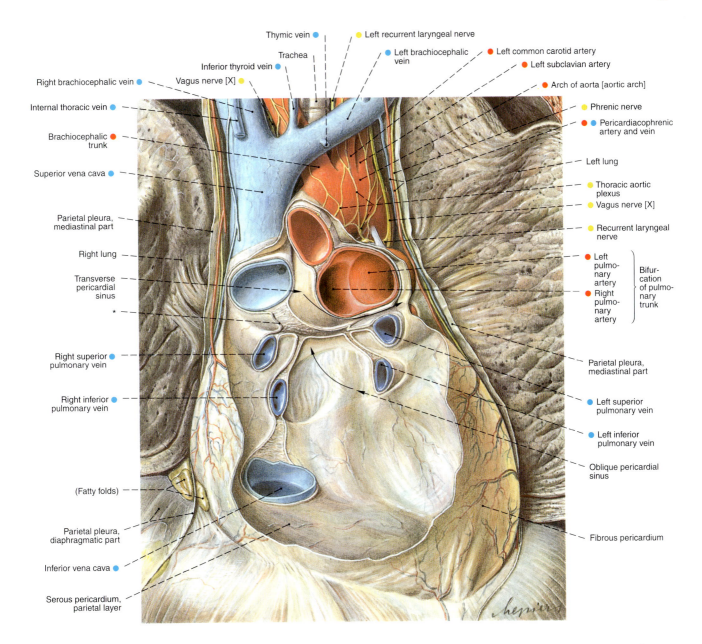

Thymic vein ●
Left recurrent laryngeal nerve ●
Trachea
Left brachiocephalic vein ●
Left common carotid artery ●
Inferior thyroid vein ●
Left subclavian artery ●
Vagus nerve [X] ●
Arch of aorta [aortic arch] ●
Right brachiocephalic vein ●
Internal thoracic vein ●
Phrenic nerve ●
Pericardiacophrenic artery and vein ● ●
Brachiocephalic trunk ●
Superior vena cava ●
Left lung
Thoracic aortic plexus ●
Vagus nerve [X] ●
Parietal pleura, mediastinal part
Recurrent laryngeal nerve ●
Right lung
Left pulmonary artery ●
Transverse pericardial sinus
Right pulmonary artery ●
Bifurcation of pulmonary trunk
*
Parietal pleura, mediastinal part
Right superior pulmonary vein ●
Left superior pulmonary vein ●
Right inferior pulmonary vein ●
Left inferior pulmonary vein ●
Oblique pericardial sinus
(Fatty folds)
Parietal pleura, diaphragmatic part
Fibrous pericardium
Inferior vena cava ●
Serous pericardium, parietal layer

Fig. 870 Pericardium; anterior parts of pericardium as well as heart and great blood vessels removed; ventral aspect.

* Reflection of visceral layer [epicardium] into parietal layer of serous pericardium.

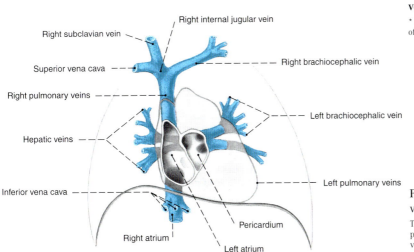

Right internal jugular vein
Right subclavian vein
Right brachiocephalic vein
Superior vena cava
Right pulmonary veins
Left brachiocephalic vein
Hepatic veins
Left pulmonary veins
Inferior vena cava
Right atrium
Pericardium
Left atrium

Fig. 871 Great veins draining into the heart; ventral aspect.

The so-called "venous cross" is formed by the horizontal pulmonary veins and the vertical superior and inferior venae cavae.

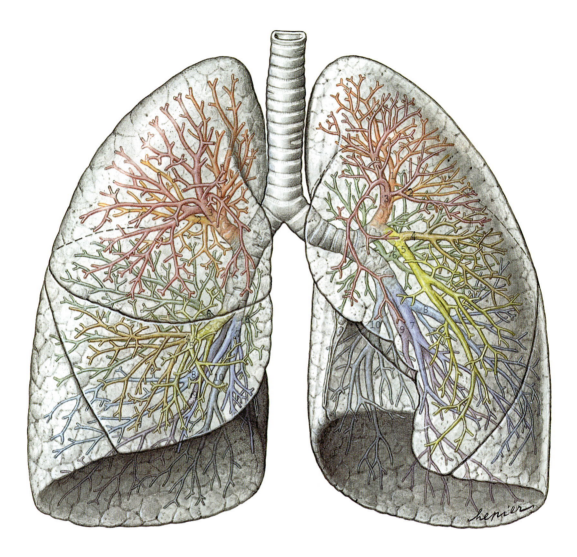

Fig. 874   Lungs, bronchi; lobar and segmental bronchi
projected onto the lung in different colors; ventral aspect.
Numbers refer to segmental bronchi (compare page 92).
In the left lung the segments S I and S II frequently arise
from a common bronchus; the medial basal segment
S VII is frequently missing.

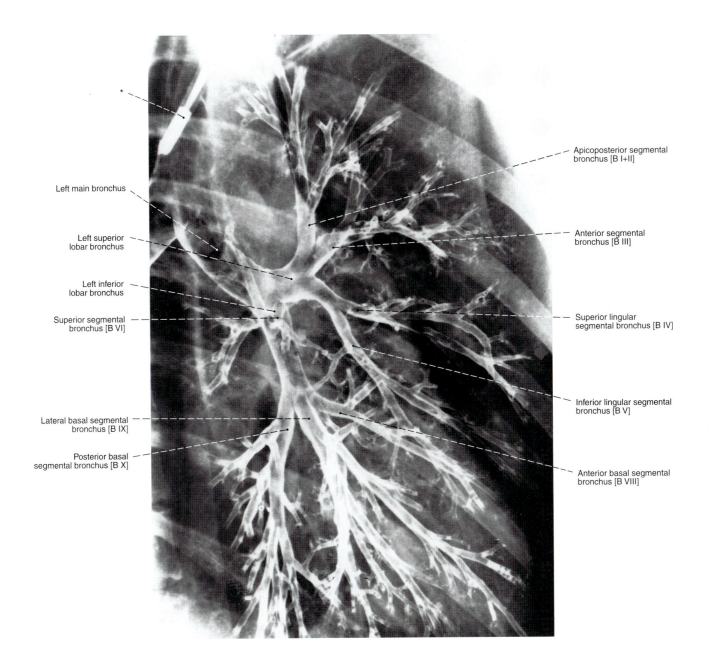

Apicoposterior segmental
bronchus [B I+II]

Anterior segmental
bronchus [B III]

Superior lingular
segmental bronchus [B IV]

Inferior lingular segmental
bronchus [B V]

Anterior basal segmental
bronchus [B VIII]

Left main bronchus

Left superior
lobar bronchus

Left inferior
lobar bronchus

Superior segmental
bronchus [B VI]

Lateral basal segmental
bronchus [B IX]

Posterior basal
segmental bronchus [B X]

Fig. 875 Left bronchi; AP bronchogram (bronchial
tree is visualized by administration of contrast
medium powder); ventral aspect.

* Bronchography catheter in trachea.

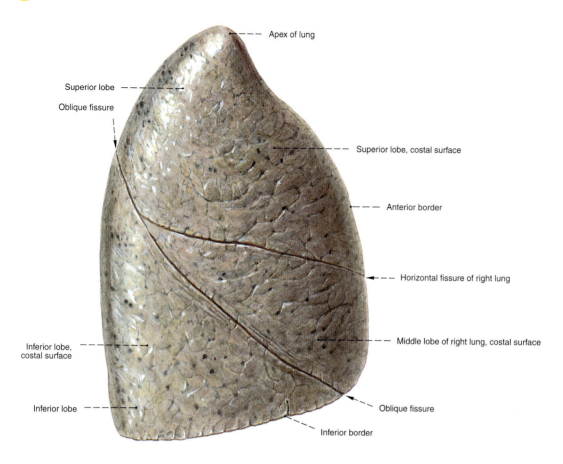

Apex of lung

Superior lobe

Oblique fissure

Superior lobe, costal surface

Anterior border

Horizontal fissure of right lung

Inferior lobe, costal surface

Middle lobe of right lung, costal surface

Inferior lobe

Oblique fissure

Inferior border

Fig. 876   Right lung; lateral aspect.
Note the grey-black spots of the lung, that are caused
by deposits of inhaled dust particles ("anthracotic
pigment" under the visceral pleura.

Apex of lung

Superior lobe, costal surface

Oblique fissure

Anterior border

Superior lobe

Inferior lobe, costal surface

Cardiac notch of left lung

Lingula of left lung

Oblique fissure

Inferior border

Fig. 877   Left lung; lateral aspect.

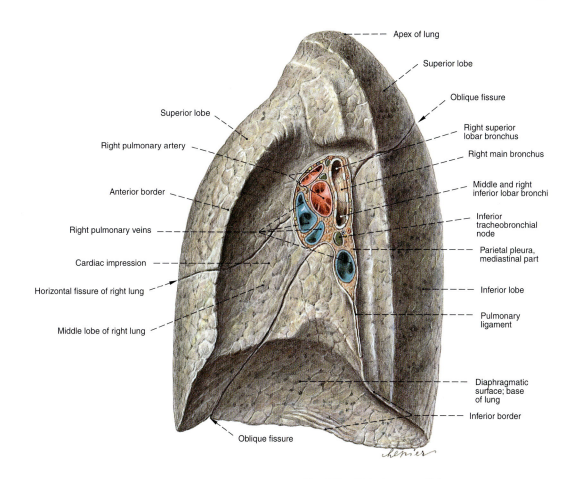

Apex of lung

Superior lobe

Oblique fissure

Right superior lobar bronchus

Right main bronchus

Middle and right inferior lobar bronchi

Inferior tracheobronchial node

Parietal pleura, mediastinal part

Inferior lobe

Pulmonary ligament

Diaphragmatic surface; base of lung

Inferior border

Superior lobe

Right pulmonary artery

Anterior border

Right pulmonary veins

Cardiac impression

Horizontal fissure of right lung

Middle lobe of right lung

Oblique fissure

Fig. 878 Right lung; medial aspect.
In older people or in persons heavily exposed to dust in the workplace the hilar lymph nodes are blackened by deposits of inhaled soot or other particles ("anthracotic nodes").

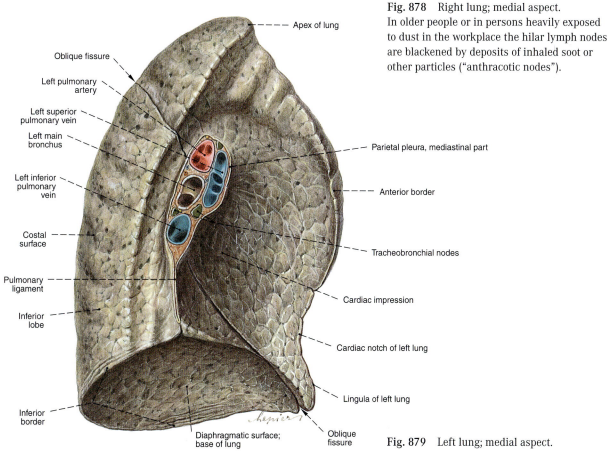

Apex of lung

Oblique fissure

Left pulmonary artery

Left superior pulmonary vein

Left main bronchus

Left inferior pulmonary vein

Costal surface

Pulmonary ligament

Inferior lobe

Inferior border

Diaphragmatic surface; base of lung

Parietal pleura, mediastinal part

Anterior border

Tracheobronchial nodes

Cardiac impression

Cardiac notch of left lung

Lingula of left lung

Oblique fissure

Fig. 879 Left lung; medial aspect.

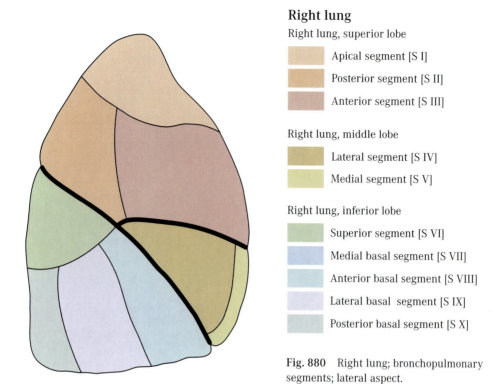

Right lung

Right lung, superior lobe

Apical segment [S I]

Posterior segment [S II]

Anterior segment [S III]

Right lung, middle lobe

Lateral segment [S IV]

Medial segment [S V]

Right lung, inferior lobe

Superior segment [S VI]

Medial basal segment [S VII]

Anterior basal segment [S VIII]

Lateral basal segment [S IX]

Posterior basal segment [S X]

Fig. 880   Right lung; bronchopulmonary segments; lateral aspect.

Left lung

Left lung, superior lobe

Apicoposterior segment [S I+II]

Anterior segment [S III]

Superior lingular segment [S IV]

Inferior lingular segment [S V]

Left lung, inferior lobe

Superior segment [S VI]

Medial basal segment [S VII] *

Anterior basal segment [S VIII]

Lateral basal segment [S IX]

Posterior basal segment [S X]

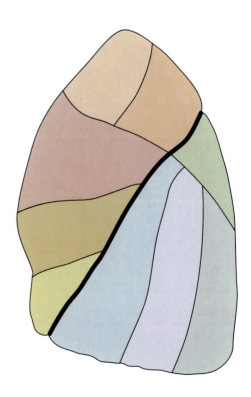

Fig. 881   Left lung; bronchopulmonary segments; lateral aspect.

*Generally this segment is not a separate unit, but fused with the anterior basal segment.

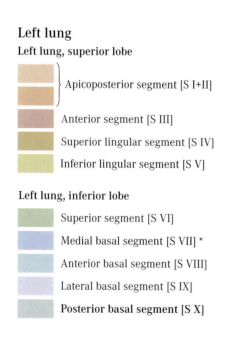

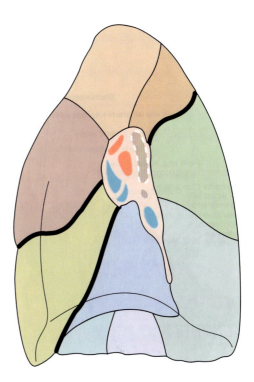

Fig. 882 Right lung; bronchopulmonary segments; medial aspect.
For color code and names of segments see page 98.

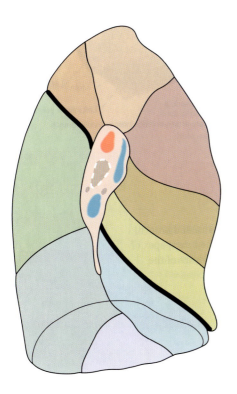

Fig. 883 Left lung; bronchopulmonary segments; medial aspect.
For color code and names of segments see page 98.

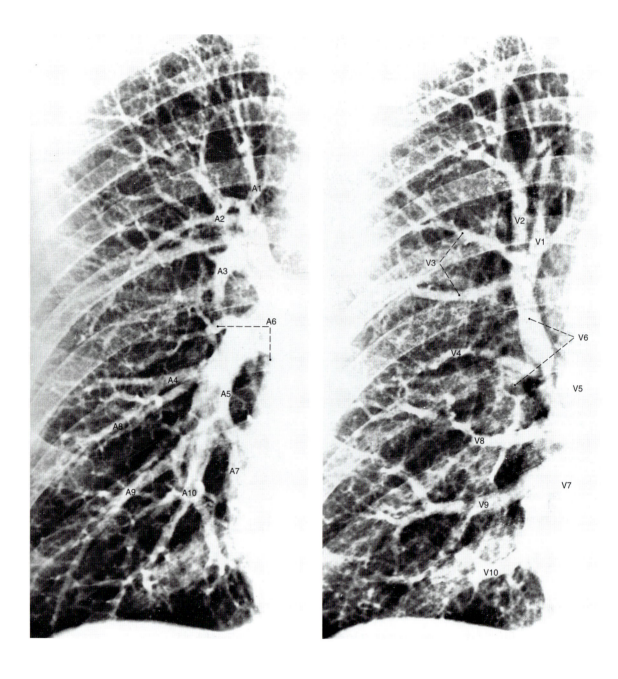

Fig. 886　Arteries of right lung; right pulmonary arteries; AP radiograph (pulmonary angiogram); injection of contrast medium into the right ventricle; ventral aspect.
Note the similar course of arteries and bronchi (Figs. 874, 875). Numbers refer to respective segmental arteries.

Fig. 887　Veins of right lung; right pulmonary veins; AP radiograph (reflux of contrast medium from the lung after injection into the right ventricle); ventral aspect.
Note the different course of the veins compared to the pulmonary arteries (Fig. 886).

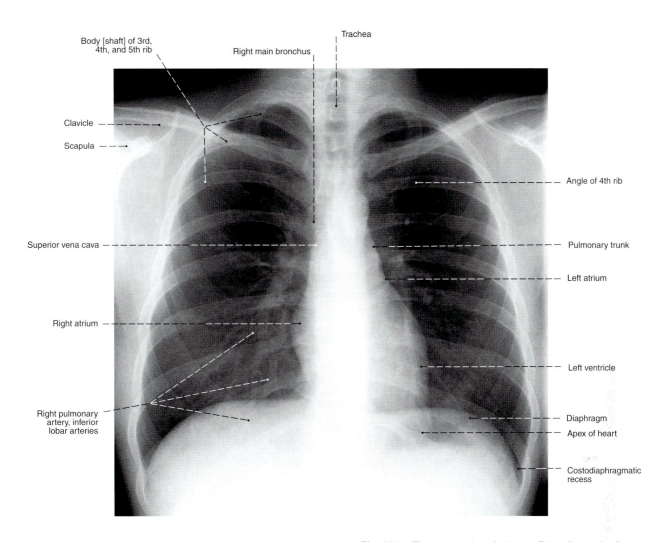

Body [shaft] of 3rd, 4th, and 5th rib

Right main bronchus

Trachea

Clavicle

Scapula

Angle of 4th rib

Superior vena cava

Pulmonary trunk

Left atrium

Right atrium

Left ventricle

Right pulmonary artery, inferior lobar arteries

Diaphragm

Apex of heart

Costodiaphragmatic recess

Fig. 888 Thoracic cage and viscera; PA radiograph of a 27-years-old male; beam directed sagittally onto the center of the sternum.

Position and size of the heart, the lung, and the bony structures of the thoracic cage as well as the vertebral column can be viewed.

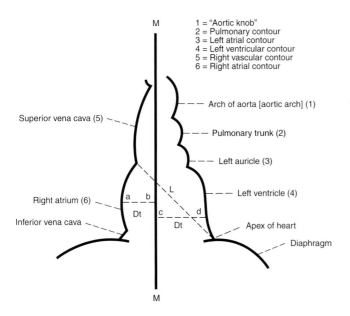

M

1 = "Aortic knob"
2 = Pulmonary contour
3 = Left atrial contour
4 = Left ventricular contour
5 = Right vascular contour
6 = Right atrial contour

Arch of aorta [aortic arch] (1)

Superior vena cava (5)

Pulmonary trunk (2)

Left auricle (3)

L

Left ventricle (4)

Right atrium (6)

a   b

Dt

Inferior vena cava

c   d

Dt

Apex of heart

Diaphragm

M

Fig. 889 Diagram of silhouette of heart in the radiograph,

Dt = Transverse diameter, ab + cd = 13-14 cm

L = Longitudinal axis of heart (from superior end of right atrial contour to apex of heart) = 15-16 cm

M = Median plane of body

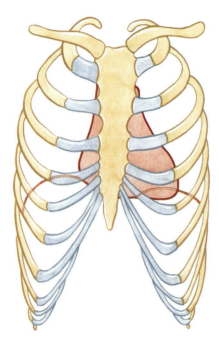

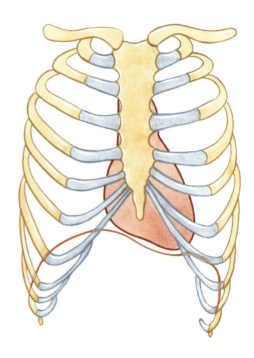

Fig. 890 Position of heart in the thorax during expiration; ventral aspect.

Fig. 891 Position of heart in the thorax during inspiration; ventral aspect.
The heart is positioned more vertical; the apex of heart is directed medially and caudally.

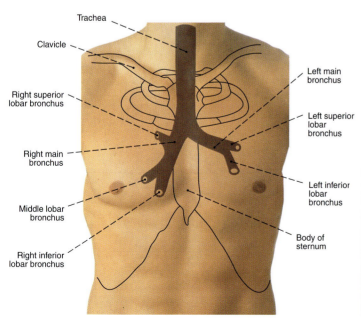

Trachea

Clavicle

Right superior lobar bronchus

Right main bronchus

Middle lobar bronchus

Right inferior lobar bronchus

Left main bronchus

Left superior lobar bronchus

Left inferior lobar bronchus

Body of sternum

Fig. 892 Trachea and bronchi in a living person; projection onto the anterior thoracic wall.

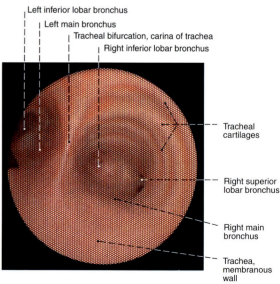

Left inferior lobar bronchus

Left main bronchus

Tracheal bifurcation, carina of trachea

Right inferior lobar bronchus

Tracheal cartilages

Right superior lobar bronchus

Right main bronchus

Trachea, membranous wall

Fig. 893 Tracheal bifurcation; endoscopic view (bronchoscopy).

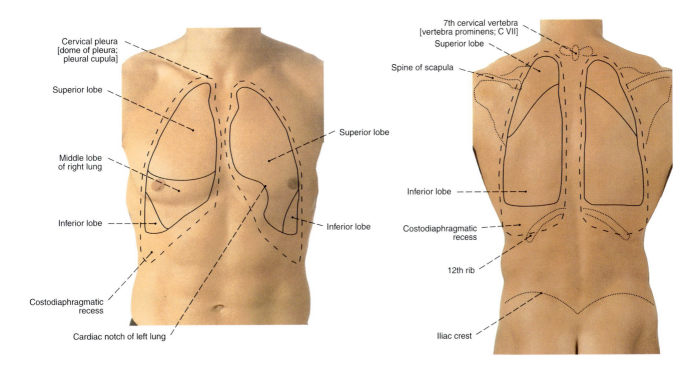

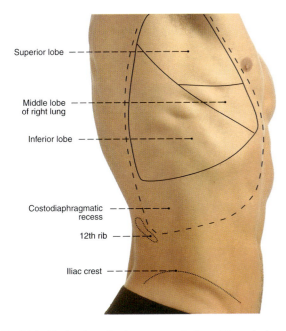

Fig. 894 Projection of pulmonary and pleural boundaries onto the anterior thoracic wall; ventral aspect.
Pulmonary boundaries are solid lines; pleural boundaries are broken lines.

Fig. 895 Projection of pulmonary and pleural boundaries onto the anterior thoracic wall; dorsal aspect.
Pulmonary boundaries are solid lines; pleural boundaries are broken lines.

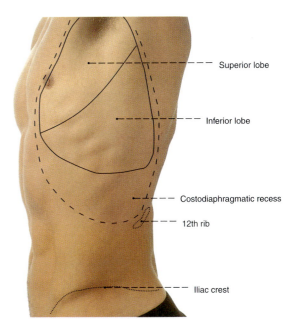

Fig. 896 Projection of pulmonary and pleural boundaries onto the anterior thoracic wall; right lateral aspect.
Pulmonary boundaries are solid lines; pleural boundaries are broken lines.

Fig. 897 Projection of pulmonary and pleural boundaries onto the anterior thoracic wall; left lateral aspect.
Pulmonary boundaries are solid lines; pleural boundaries are broken lines.

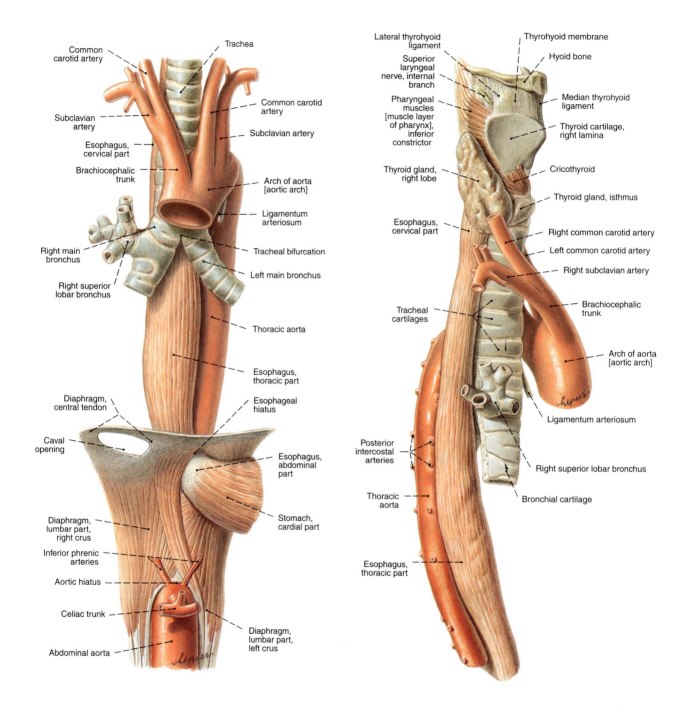

Fig. 898 Esophagus, trachea; thoracic aorta; parts of diaphragm retained to show openings for aorta, inferior vena cava, and esophagus; ventral aspect.

Fig. 899 Esophagus, trachea; thoracic aorta; right lateral aspect.

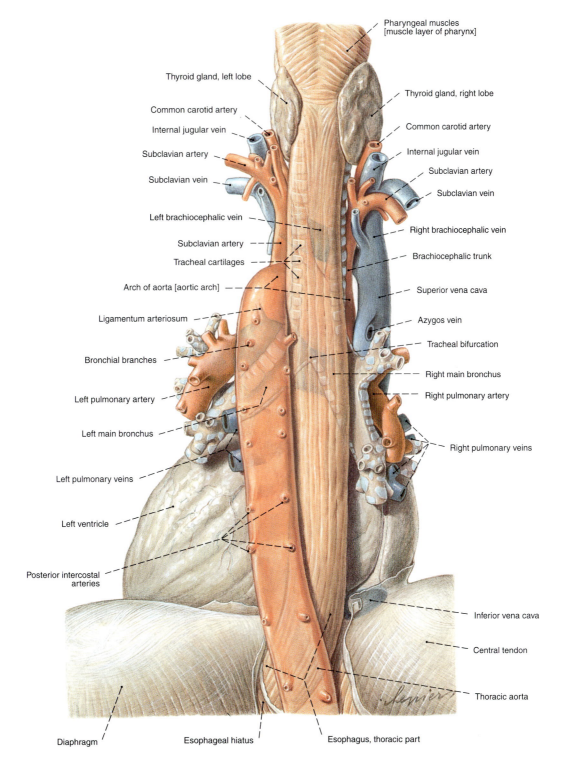

Pharyngeal muscles
[muscle layer of pharynx]

Thyroid gland, left lobe

Thyroid gland, right lobe

Common carotid artery

Internal jugular vein

Common carotid artery

Subclavian artery

Internal jugular vein

Subclavian vein

Subclavian artery

Subclavian vein

Left brachiocephalic vein

Right brachiocephalic vein

Subclavian artery

Brachiocephalic trunk

Tracheal cartilages

Arch of aorta [aortic arch]

Superior vena cava

Ligamentum arteriosum

Azygos vein

Bronchial branches

Tracheal bifurcation

Right main bronchus

Left pulmonary artery

Right pulmonary artery

Left main bronchus

Left pulmonary veins

Right pulmonary veins

Left ventricle

Posterior intercostal
arteries

Inferior vena cava

Central tendon

Thoracic aorta

Diaphragm

Esophageal hiatus

Esophagus, thoracic part

Fig. 900   Esophagus, thoracic aorta; pericardium;
dorsal aspect.

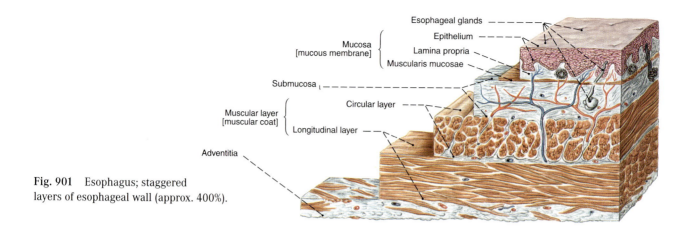

Fig. 901   Esophagus; staggered layers of esophageal wall (approx. 400%).

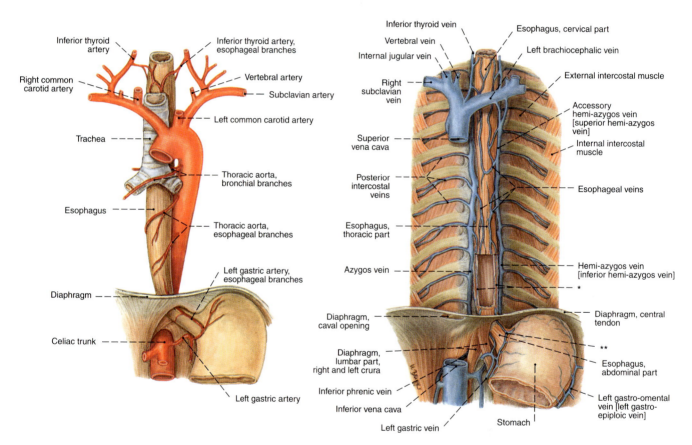

Fig. 902   Esophagus and its arterial supply; ventral aspect.

Fig. 903   Esophageal veins; parts of diaphragm and stomach removed; in the lower thoracic part anterior wall of esophagus removed.

* Veins of esophageal mucosa.

** Connecting branch between veins of stomach and esophagus.

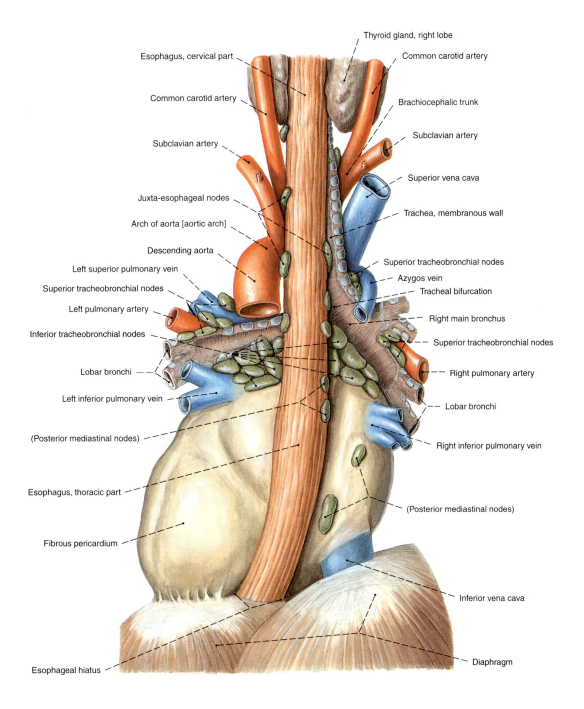

Thyroid gland, right lobe

Esophagus, cervical part

Common carotid artery

Common carotid artery

Brachiocephalic trunk

Subclavian artery

Subclavian artery

Superior vena cava

Juxta-esophageal nodes

Trachea, membranous wall

Arch of aorta [aortic arch]

Descending aorta

Superior tracheobronchial nodes

Left superior pulmonary vein

Azygos vein

Superior tracheobronchial nodes

Tracheal bifurcation

Left pulmonary artery

Right main bronchus

Inferior tracheobronchial nodes

Superior tracheobronchial nodes

Lobar bronchi

Right pulmonary artery

Left inferior pulmonary vein

Lobar bronchi

(Posterior mediastinal nodes)

Right inferior pulmonary vein

Esophagus, thoracic part

(Posterior mediastinal nodes)

Fibrous pericardium

Inferior vena cava

Esophageal hiatus

Diaphragm

Fig. 904   Thoracic lymph nodes; bronchi sectioned after division into
lobar bronchi; great blood vessels retained in mediastinum; dorsal aspect.
Lymph nodes in the healthy adult are usually smaller than shown here.

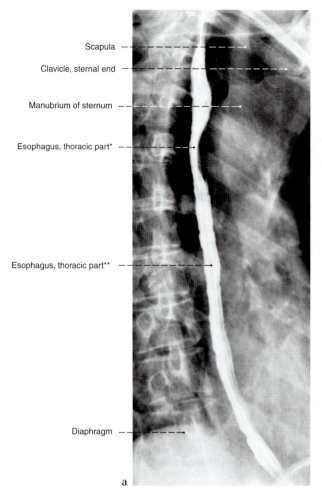

Scapula

Clavicle, sternal end

Manubrium of sternum

Esophagus, thoracic part*

Esophagus, thoracic part**

Diaphragm

a

Piriform fossa [piriform recess]

Esophagus, cervical part***

Clavicles

Arch of aorta [aortic arch]

Esophagus, thoracic part

b

Fig. 905   a, b Esophagus; radiograph (after swallowing contrast medium);
a Right anterior oblique (RAO) position (beam from left anterior to right posterior)
b Left anterior oblique (LAO) position (beam from right anterior to left posterior)

*   Thoracic constriction [broncho-aortic constriction].
**   Retrocardial part.
*** Constriction at beginning of esophagus.

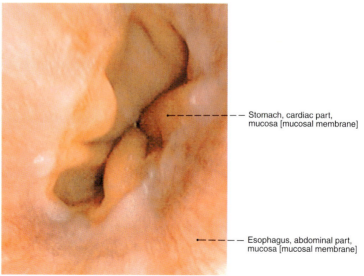

Stomach, cardiac part, mucosa [mucosal membrane]

Esophagus, abdominal part, mucosa [mucosal membrane]

Fig. 906   Esophagus; mucosa viewed by endoscope (esophagoscopy); superior aspect.

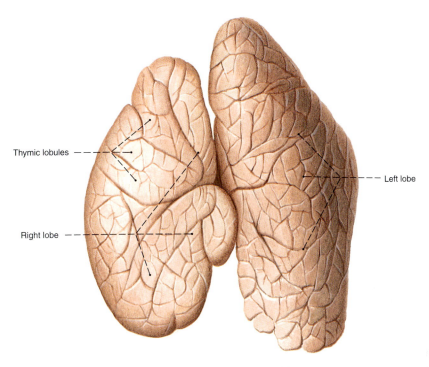

Thymic lobules

Left lobe

Right lobe

Fig. 907 Thymus of a 2-year-old child;
ventral aspect.

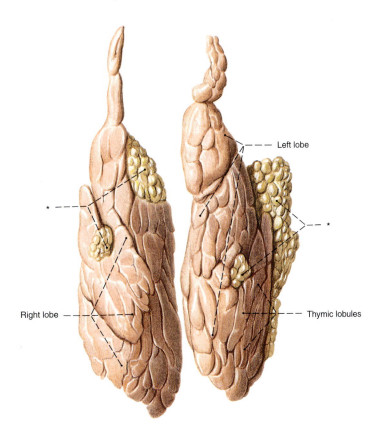

Left lobe

*

*

Right lobe

Thymic lobules

Fig. 908 Thymus of a 42-year-old; fatty tissue
extensively removed; ventral aspect.

* Parathymic fat.

In this specimen shape and size of the thymus were
unusually preserved.

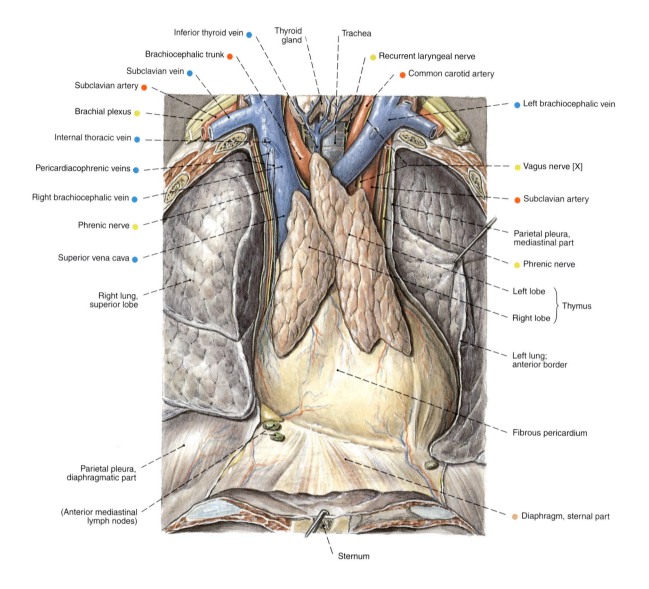

Inferior thyroid vein ●
Thyroid gland
Trachea

Brachiocephalic trunk ●
Recurrent laryngeal nerve ●

Subclavian vein ●
Common carotid artery ●

Subclavian artery ●

Brachial plexus ●
Left brachiocephalic vein ●

Internal thoracic vein ●
Vagus nerve [X] ●

Pericardiacophrenic veins ●
Subclavian artery ●

Right brachiocephalic vein ●
Parietal pleura, mediastinal part

Phrenic nerve ●
Phrenic nerve ●

Superior vena cava ●
Left lobe ⎫
Right lobe ⎭ Thymus

Right lung, superior lobe
Left lung; anterior border

Fibrous pericardium

Parietal pleura, diaphragmatic part

(Anterior mediastinal lymph nodes)
Diaphragm, sternal part ●

Sternum

Fig. 909   Thymus in the adolescent; anterior thoracic wall removed, pleural cavity opened and left lung retracted laterally; ventral aspect. Compare size of thymus of newborn (Fig. 999) and 2-year-old child (Fig. 907).

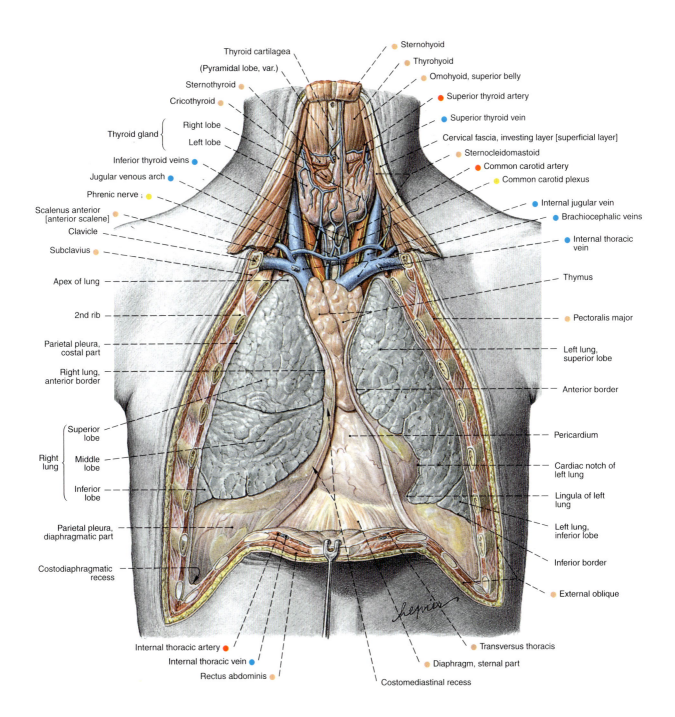

Thyroid cartilagea

(Pyramidal lobe, var.)

Sternothyroid

Cricothyroid

Thyroid gland { Right lobe / Left lobe }

Inferior thyroid veins

Jugular venous arch

Phrenic nerve ;

Scalenus anterior [anterior scalene]

Clavicle

Subclavius

Apex of lung

2nd rib

Parietal pleura, costal part

Right lung, anterior border

Right lung { Superior lobe / Middle lobe / Inferior lobe }

Parietal pleura, diaphragmatic part

Costodiaphragmatic recess

Internal thoracic artery

Internal thoracic vein

Rectus abdominis

Sternohyoid

Thyrohyoid

Omohyoid, superior belly

Superior thyroid artery

Superior thyroid vein

Cervical fascia, investing layer [superficial layer]

Sternocleidomastoid

Common carotid artery

Common carotid plexus

Internal jugular vein

Brachiocephalic veins

Internal thoracic vein

Thymus

Pectoralis major

Left lung, superior lobe

Anterior border

Pericardium

Cardiac notch of left lung

Lingula of left lung

Left lung, inferior lobe

Inferior border

External oblique

Transversus thoracis

Diaphragm, sternal part

Costomediastinal recess

Fig. 910 Thymus; pericardium; lungs; anterior thoracic wall removed, pleural cavity opened; ventral aspect. Note the size of thymus in the young adult. In the older individuals thymic tissue is almost entirely replaced by fat.

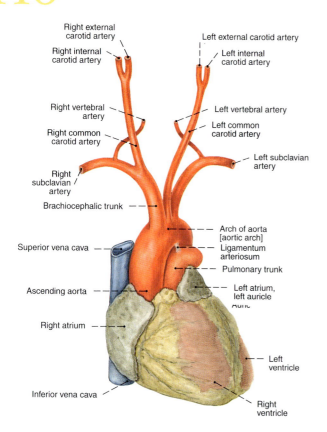

Fig. 913   Heart; arch of aorta [aortic arch] with origins of large arteries; ventral aspect.

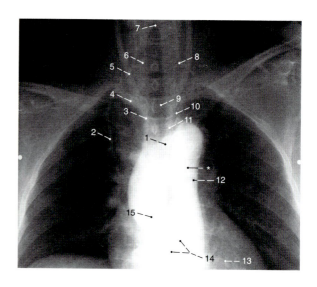

Fig. 914   Arch of aorta [aortic arch] and branches; AP radiograph (after injection of contrast medium into the aortic bulb [infundibulum]; ventral aspect.
* Catheter.

1	Arch of aorta [aortic arch]	9	Trachea
2	Internal thoracic artery	10	Left subclavian artery
3	Brachiocephalic trunk	11	Left common carotid artery
4	Right subclavian artery	12	Descending aorta
5	Right common carotid artery	13	Heart
6	Right vertebral artery	14	Aortic valve
7	Rima glottidis	15	Ascending aorta
8	Left vertebral artery		

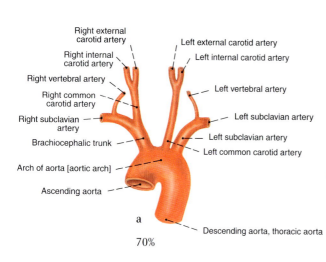

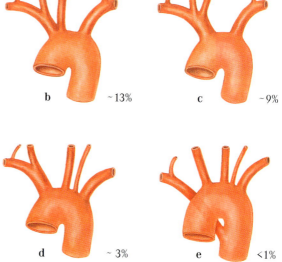

Fig. 915 a-e   Variations of origins of large arteries from arch of aorta [aortic arch].

a   "Normal case"
b   Common origin of brachiocephalic trunk and left common carotid artery
c   Common stem of brachiocephalic trunk and left common carotid artery

d   Independent origin of left vertebral artery from arch of aorta [aortic arch]
e   Right subclavian artery as the last branch of arch of aorta [aortic arch]

This abnormal artery usually crosses to the right behind the esophoagus, causing difficulties in swallowing (dysphagia lusoria).

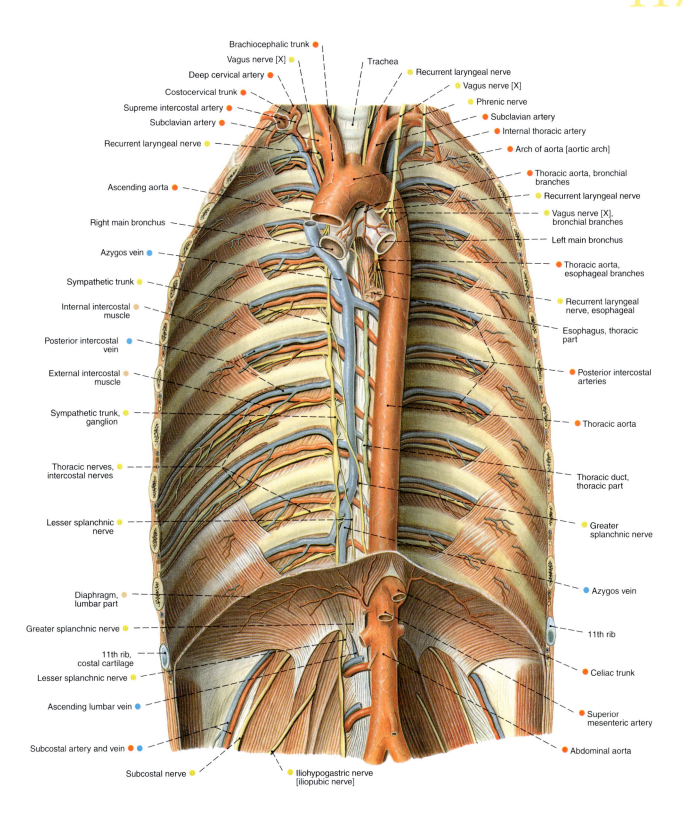

Fig. 916 Thoracic and abdominal aorta; posterior mediastinum; pleura removed to expose intercostal nerves and sympathetic trunk; ventral aspect.

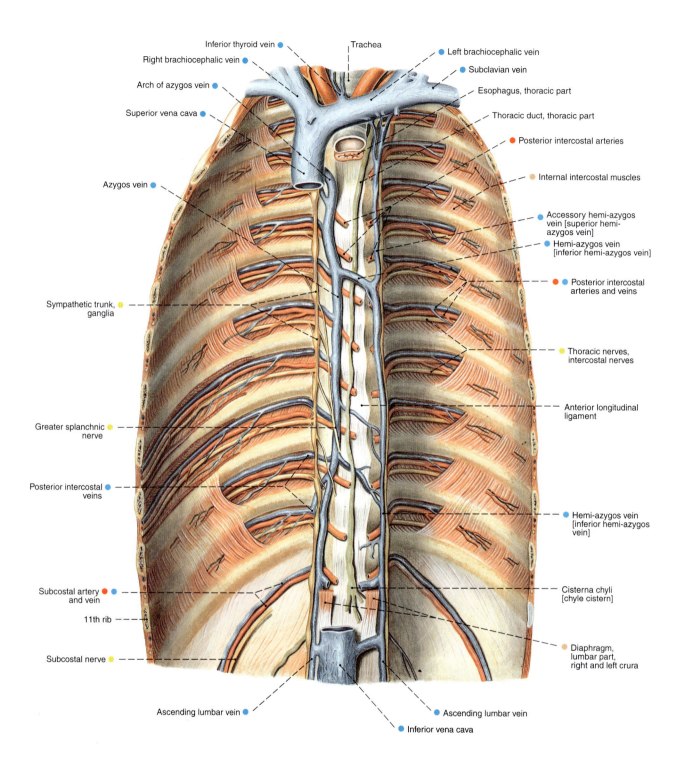

Inferior thyroid vein ●

Right brachiocephalic vein ●

Arch of azygos vein ●

Superior vena cava ●

Trachea

● Left brachiocephalic vein

● Subclavian vein

Esophagus, thoracic part

Thoracic duct, thoracic part

● Posterior intercostal arteries

● Internal intercostal muscles

Azygos vein ●

● Accessory hemi-azygos vein [superior hemi-azygos vein]

● Hemi-azygos vein [inferior hemi-azygos vein]

● ● Posterior intercostal arteries and veins

Sympathetic trunk, ganglia ●

● Thoracic nerves, intercostal nerves

Anterior longitudinal ligament

Greater splanchnic nerve ●

Posterior intercostal veins ●

● Hemi-azygos vein [inferior hemi-azygos vein]

Subcostal artery ● ● and vein

Cisterna chyli [chyle cistern]

11th rib

Subcostal nerve ●

● Diaphragm, lumbar part, right and left crura

Ascending lumbar vein ●

● Ascending lumbar vein

● Inferior vena cava

Fig. 917 Blood vessels and nerves of posterior mediastinum; pleura, aorta, and esophagus removed to expose thoracic duct, azygos vein, and intercostal blood vessels and nerves; ventral aspect.

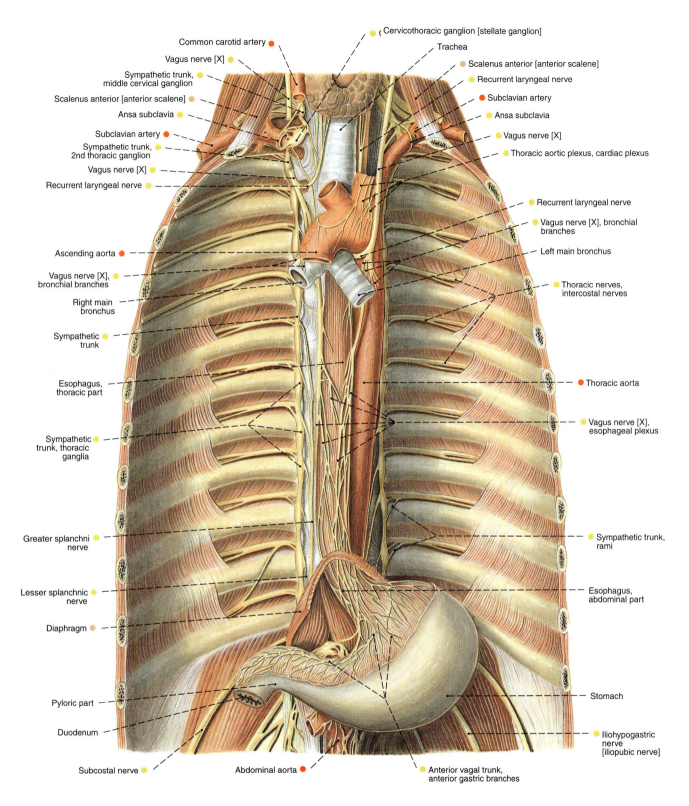

Common carotid artery

Vagus nerve [X]

Sympathetic trunk, middle cervical ganglion

Scalenus anterior [anterior scalene]

Ansa subclavia

Subclavian artery

Sympathetic trunk, 2nd thoracic ganglion

Vagus nerve [X]

Recurrent laryngeal nerve

Ascending aorta

Vagus nerve [X], bronchial branches

Right main bronchus

Sympathetic trunk

Esophagus, thoracic part

Sympathetic trunk, thoracic ganglia

Greater splanchni nerve

Lesser splanchnic nerve

Diaphragm

Pyloric part

Duodenum

Subcostal nerve

Cervicothoracic ganglion [stellate ganglion]

Trachea

Scalenus anterior [anterior scalene]

Recurrent laryngeal nerve

Subclavian artery

Ansa subclavia

Vagus nerve [X]

Thoracic aortic plexus, cardiac plexus

Recurrent laryngeal nerve

Vagus nerve [X], bronchial branches

Left main bronchus

Thoracic nerves, intercostal nerves

Thoracic aorta

Vagus nerve [X], esophageal plexus

Sympathetic trunk, rami

Esophagus, abdominal part

Stomach

Iliohypogastric nerve [iliopubic nerve]

Abdominal aorta

Anterior vagal trunk, anterior gastric branches

Fig. 918   Esophagus; aorta; autonomic division [part] of peripheral nervous system; stomach.
Only dorsal parts of diaphragm retained; pleura removed to expose sympathetic trunk and its connections to intercostal nerves; ventral aspect.

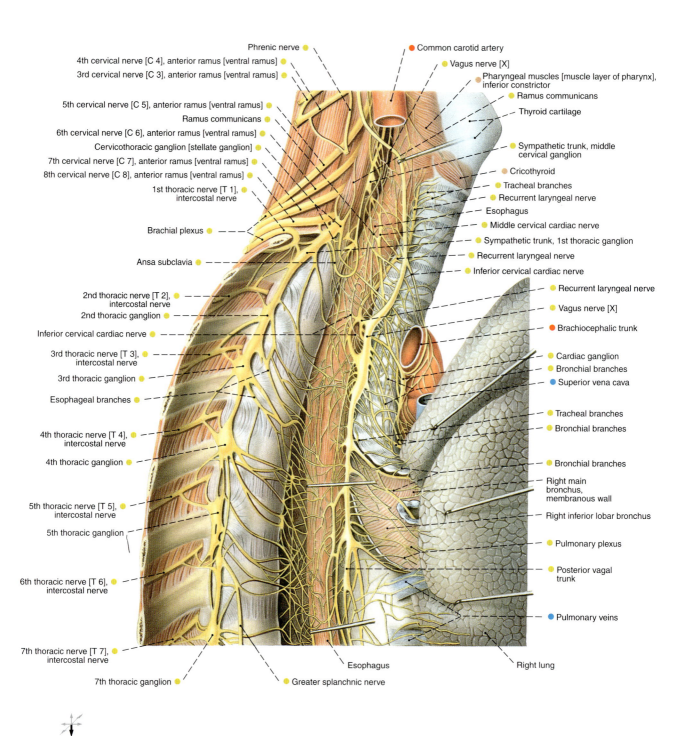

Phrenic nerve
Common carotid artery
4th cervical nerve [C 4], anterior ramus [ventral ramus]
3rd cervical nerve [C 3], anterior ramus [ventral ramus]
Vagus nerve [X]
Pharyngeal muscles [muscle layer of pharynx], inferior constrictor
Ramus communicans
5th cervical nerve [C 5], anterior ramus [ventral ramus]
Thyroid cartilage
Ramus communicans
6th cervical nerve [C 6], anterior ramus [ventral ramus]
Sympathetic trunk, middle cervical ganglion
Cervicothoracic ganglion [stellate ganglion]
Cricothyroid
7th cervical nerve [C 7], anterior ramus [ventral ramus]
Tracheal branches
8th cervical nerve [C 8], anterior ramus [ventral ramus]
Recurrent laryngeal nerve
1st thoracic nerve [T 1], intercostal nerve
Esophagus
Middle cervical cardiac nerve
Brachial plexus
Sympathetic trunk, 1st thoracic ganglion
Recurrent laryngeal nerve
Ansa subclavia
Inferior cervical cardiac nerve
Recurrent laryngeal nerve
2nd thoracic nerve [T 2], intercostal nerve
Vagus nerve [X]
2nd thoracic ganglion
Brachiocephalic trunk
Inferior cervical cardiac nerve
3rd thoracic nerve [T 3], intercostal nerve
Cardiac ganglion
Bronchial branches
3rd thoracic ganglion
Superior vena cava
Esophageal branches
Tracheal branches
Bronchial branches
4th thoracic nerve [T 4], intercostal nerve
4th thoracic ganglion
Bronchial branches
Right main bronchus, membranous wall
5th thoracic nerve [T 5], intercostal nerve
Right inferior lobar bronchus
5th thoracic ganglion
Pulmonary plexus
6th thoracic nerve [T 6], intercostal nerve
Posterior vagal trunk
Pulmonary veins
7th thoracic nerve [T 7], intercostal nerve
7th thoracic ganglion
Esophagus
Right lung
Greater splanchnic nerve

920

Fig. 919   Lower cervical and upper thoracic part of autonomic division of peripheral nervous system; vagus nerve and right lung retracted anteriorly to expose esophagus; right lateral aspect.

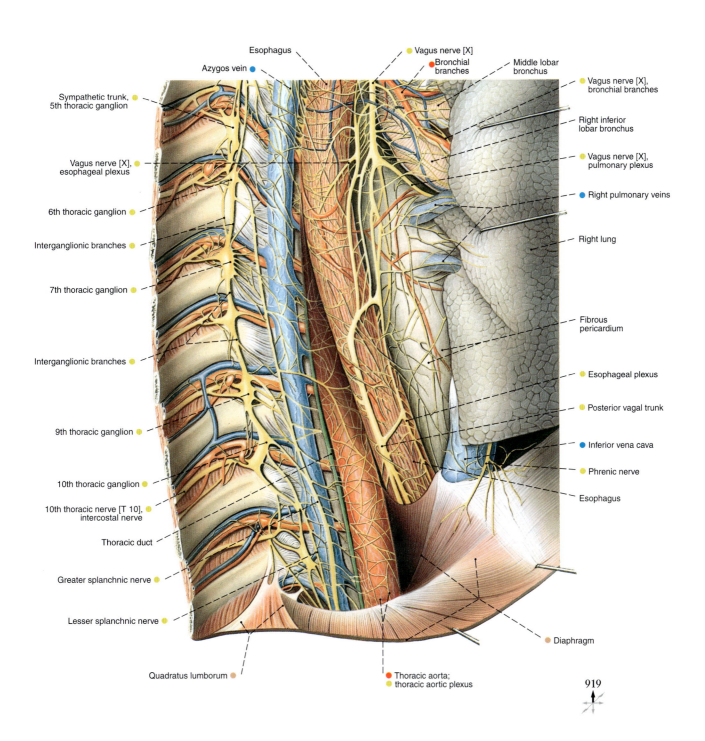

Esophagus

Vagus nerve [X]

Azygos vein ●

● Bronchial branches

Middle lobar bronchus

Sympathetic trunk, ● 5th thoracic ganglion

● Vagus nerve [X], bronchial branches

Right inferior lobar bronchus

Vagus nerve [X], ● esophageal plexus

● Vagus nerve [X], pulmonary plexus

● Right pulmonary veins

6th thoracic ganglion ●

Interganglionic branches ●

Right lung

7th thoracic ganglion ●

Fibrous pericardium

Interganglionic branches ●

● Esophageal plexus

● Posterior vagal trunk

9th thoracic ganglion ●

● Inferior vena cava

● Phrenic nerve

10th thoracic ganglion ●

Esophagus

10th thoracic nerve [T 10], ● intercostal nerve

Thoracic duct

Greater splanchnic nerve ●

Lesser splanchnic nerve ●

● Diaphragm

Quadratus lumborum ●

● Thoracic aorta; ● thoracic aortic plexus

919

Fig. 920 Lower thoracic part of autonomic division of peripheral nervous system; dissection similar to Fig.919; aorta, thoracic duct, and azygos vein, however, retained; right lateral aspect.

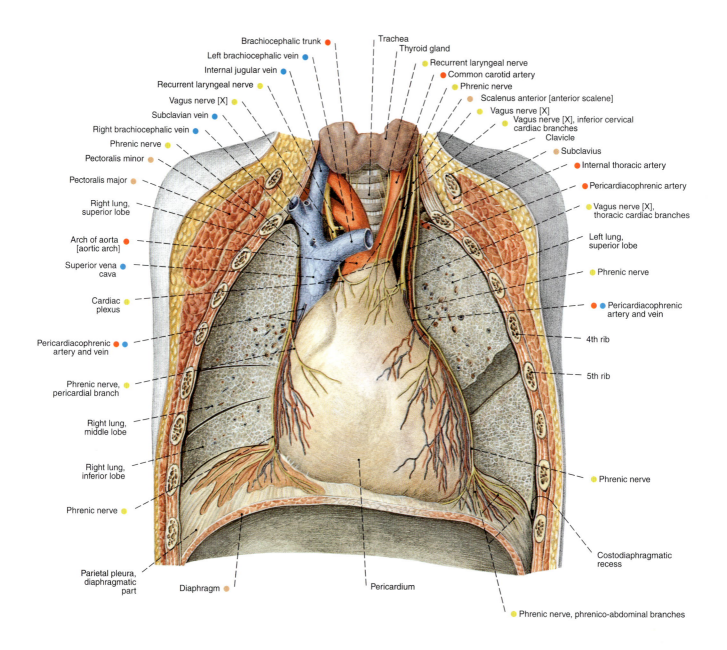

Brachiocephalic trunk ●
Left brachiocephalic vein ●
Internal jugular vein ●
Recurrent laryngeal nerve ●
Vagus nerve [X] ●
Subclavian vein ●
Right brachiocephalic vein ●
Phrenic nerve ●
Pectoralis minor ●
Pectoralis major ●
Right lung, superior lobe
Arch of aorta [aortic arch] ●
Superior vena cava ●
Cardiac plexus ●
Pericardiacophrenic artery and vein ● ●
Phrenic nerve, pericardial branch ●
Right lung, middle lobe
Right lung, inferior lobe
Phrenic nerve ●
Parietal pleura, diaphragmatic part
Diaphragm ●

Trachea
Thyroid gland
Recurrent laryngeal nerve ●
Common carotid artery ●
Phrenic nerve ●
Scalenus anterior [anterior scalene] ●
Vagus nerve [X] ●
Vagus nerve [X], inferior cervical cardiac branches ●
Clavicle
Subclavius ●
Internal thoracic artery ●
Pericardiacophrenic artery ●
Vagus nerve [X], thoracic cardiac branches ●
Left lung, superior lobe
Phrenic nerve ●
Pericardiacophrenic artery and vein ● ●
4th rib
5th rib
Phrenic nerve ●
Costodiaphragmatic recess
Phrenic nerve ●
Pericardium
Phrenic nerve, phrenico-abdominal branches ●

Fig. 921   Thoracic cavity in an adult; anterior thoracic wall removed; right and left lung sectioned in the frontal plane; mediastinal and diaphragmatic pleura removed to expose pericardiacophrenic artery and branches of phrenic nerve; ventral aspect.

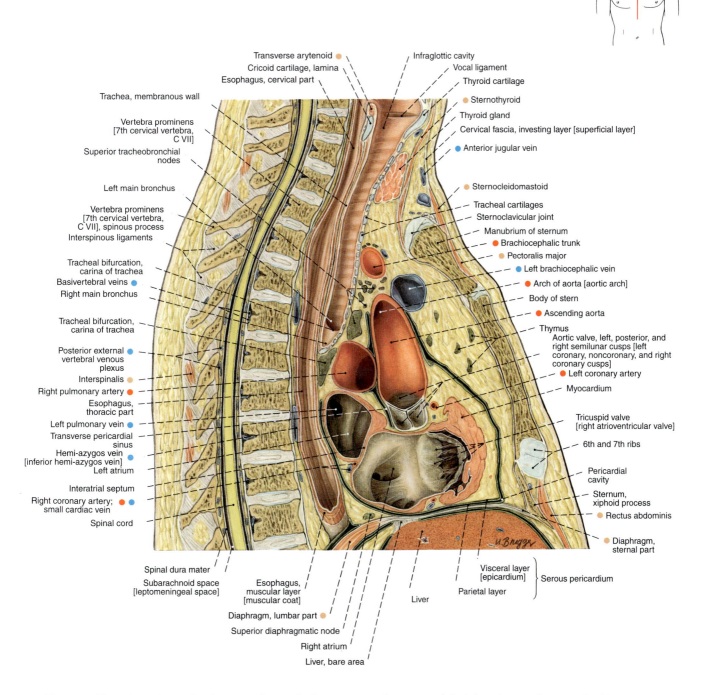

Transverse arytenoid
Cricoid cartilage, lamina
Esophagus, cervical part
Infraglottic cavity
Vocal ligament
Thyroid cartilage
Trachea, membranous wall
Sternothyroid
Thyroid gland
Vertebra prominens [7th cervical vertebra, C VII]
Cervical fascia, investing layer [superficial layer]
Superior tracheobronchial nodes
Anterior jugular vein
Left main bronchus
Sternocleidomastoid
Tracheal cartilages
Vertebra prominens [7th cervical vertebra, C VII], spinous process
Sternoclavicular joint
Interspinous ligaments
Manubrium of sternum
Tracheal bifurcation, carina of trachea
Brachiocephalic trunk
Basivertebral veins
Pectoralis major
Right main bronchus
Left brachiocephalic vein
Arch of aorta [aortic arch]
Tracheal bifurcation, carina of trachea
Body of stern
Ascending aorta
Posterior external vertebral venous plexus
Thymus
Aortic valve, left, posterior, and right semilunar cusps [left coronary, noncoronary, and right coronary cusps]
Interspinalis
Right pulmonary artery
Left coronary artery
Esophagus, thoracic part
Myocardium
Left pulmonary vein
Transverse pericardial sinus
Tricuspid valve [right atrioventricular valve]
Hemi-azygos vein [inferior hemi-azygos vein]
6th and 7th ribs
Left atrium
Interatrial septum
Pericardial cavity
Right coronary artery; small cardiac vein
Sternum, xiphoid process
Rectus abdominis
Spinal cord
Diaphragm, sternal part

Spinal dura mater
Subarachnoid space [leptomeningeal space]
Visceral layer [epicardium]
Serous pericardium
Esophagus, muscular layer [muscular coat]
Parietal layer
Diaphragm, lumbar part
Liver
Superior diaphragmatic node
Right atrium
Liver, bare area

Fig. 922 Thoracic cavity; mediastinum; median sagittal section through neck and thorax. Due to a slight asymmetry of the thorax the sternoclavicular joint is sectioned above the manubrium of sternum; right lateral aspect.
Due to the proximity of the left atrium to the esophagus, an enlargement of the left atrium can be recognized by displacement of the esophagus in the radiograph. The heart may be examined with ultrasound through the esophagus (transesophageal ultrasonography).

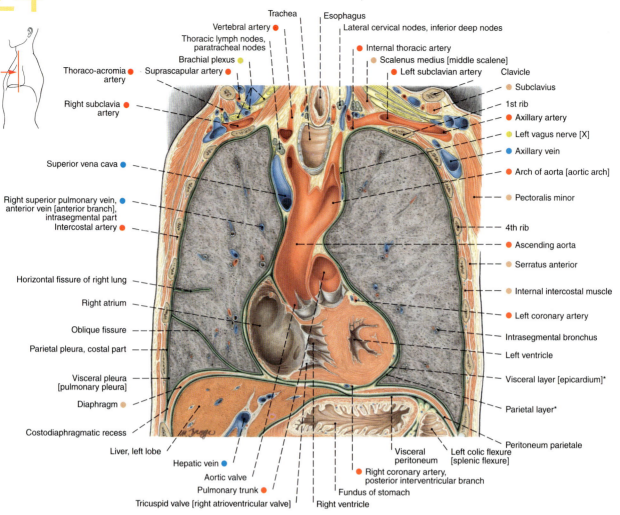

Trachea
Esophagus
Vertebral artery ●
Lateral cervical nodes, inferior deep nodes
Thoracic lymph nodes, paratracheal nodes
Internal thoracic artery ●
Brachial plexus ●
Scalenus medius [middle scalene]
Thoraco-acromia artery ●
Suprascapular artery ●
● Left subclavian artery
Clavicle
Right subclavia artery ●
Subclavius ●
1st rib
Axillary artery ●
Superior vena cava ●
● Left vagus nerve [X]
Axillary vein ●
Right superior pulmonary vein, anterior vein [anterior branch], intrasegmental part
Arch of aorta [aortic arch] ●
Intercostal artery ●
Pectoralis minor ●
4th rib
Horizontal fissure of right lung
Ascending aorta ●
Serratus anterior ●
Right atrium
Internal intercostal muscle ●
Oblique fissure
Left coronary artery ●
Parietal pleura, costal part
Intrasegmental bronchus
Visceral pleura [pulmonary pleura]
Left ventricle
Diaphragm ●
Visceral layer [epicardium]*
Costodiaphragmatic recess
Parietal layer*
Liver, left lobe
Peritoneum parietale
Hepatic vein ●
Left colic flexure [splenic flexure]
Aortic valve
Visceral peritoneum
Pulmonary trunk ●
Right coronary artery, posterior interventricular branch
Tricuspid valve [right atrioventricular valve]
Fundus of stomach
Right ventricle

Fig. 923 Thoracic cavity; frontal section; ventral aspect.

* Serous pericardium.

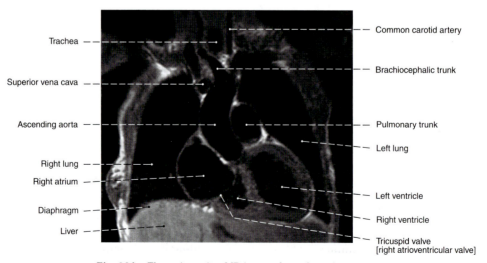

Trachea
Common carotid artery
Superior vena cava
Brachiocephalic trunk
Ascending aorta
Pulmonary trunk
Left lung
Right lung
Right atrium
Left ventricle
Diaphragm
Right ventricle
Liver
Tricuspid valve [right atrioventricular valve]

Fig. 924 Thoracic cavity; MR image; frontal section at level of superior vena cava; ventral aspect. Compare Fig. 913.

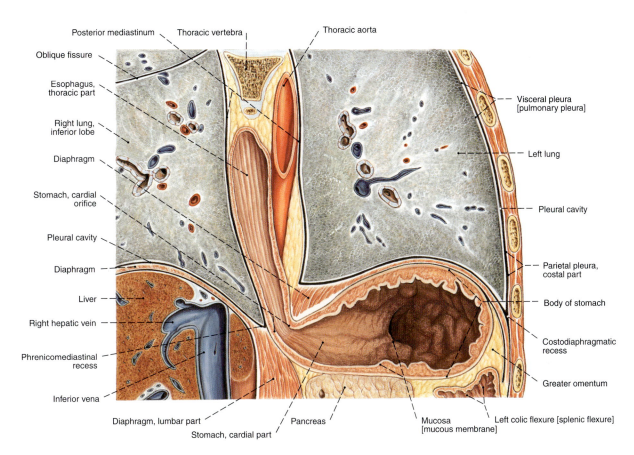

Posterior mediastinum — Thoracic vertebra — Thoracic aorta

Oblique fissure

Esophagus, thoracic part

Right lung, inferior lobe

Diaphragm

Stomach, cardial orifice

Pleural cavity

Diaphragm

Liver

Right hepatic vein

Phrenicomediastinal recess

Inferior vena

Visceral pleura [pulmonary pleura]

Left lung

Pleural cavity

Parietal pleura, costal part

Body of stomach

Costodiaphragmatic recess

Greater omentum

Diaphragm, lumbar part — Pancreas — Mucosa [mucous membrane] — Left colic flexure [splenic flexure]

Stomach, cardial part

Fig. 925 Diaphragm; esophagus and junction to stomach; frontal section through lower part of thoracic and upper part of abdominal cavities; ventral aspect.

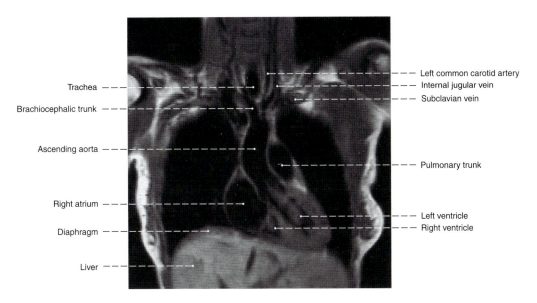

Trachea

Brachiocephalic trunk

Ascending aorta

Right atrium

Diaphragm

Liver

Left common carotid artery
Internal jugular vein
Subclavian vein

Pulmonary trunk

Left ventricle
Right ventricle

Fig. 926 Thoracic cavity; MR image; frontal section at level of aortic valve; ventral aspect. Compare Figs. 913 and 923.

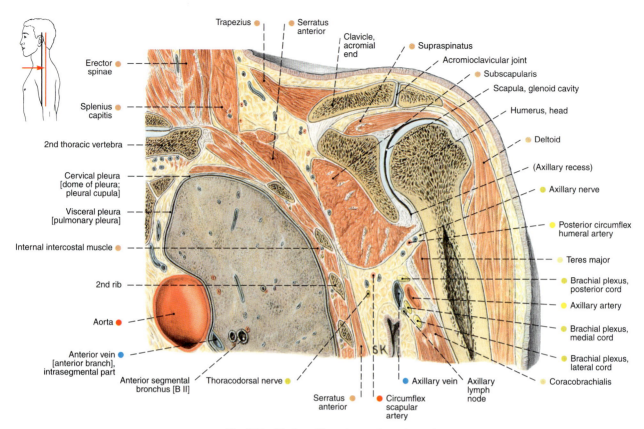

Trapezius
Serratus anterior
Clavicle, acromial end
Supraspinatus
Acromioclavicular joint
Subscapularis
Scapula, glenoid cavity
Humerus, head
Deltoid
(Axillary recess)
Axillary nerve
Posterior circumflex humeral artery
Teres major
Brachial plexus, posterior cord
Axillary artery
Brachial plexus, medial cord
Brachial plexus, lateral cord
Coracobrachialis

Erector spinae
Splenius capitis
2nd thoracic vertebra
Cervical pleura [dome of pleura; pleural cupula]
Visceral pleura [pulmonary pleura]
Internal intercostal muscle
2nd rib
Aorta
Anterior vein [anterior branch], intrasegmental part
Anterior segmental bronchus [B II]
Thoracodorsal nerve
Serratus anterior
Circumflex scapular artery
Axillary vein
Axillary lymph node

Fig. 927   Neck; axillary fossa; thoracic cavity; frontal section of left side; ventral aspect.

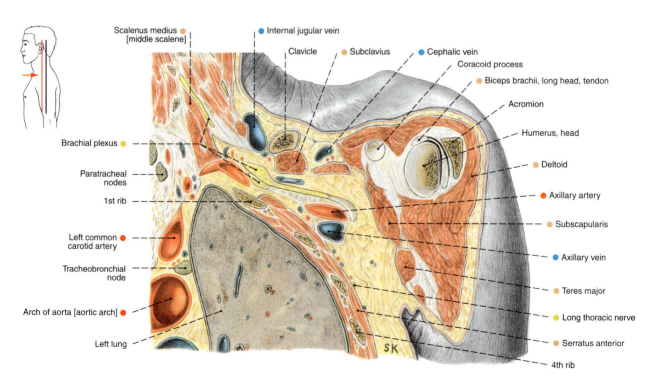

Scalenus medius [middle scalene]
Internal jugular vein
Clavicle
Subclavius
Cephalic vein
Coracoid process
Biceps brachii, long head, tendon
Acromion
Humerus, head
Deltoid
Axillary artery
Subscapularis
Axillary vein
Teres major
Long thoracic nerve
Serratus anterior
4th rib

Brachial plexus
Paratracheal nodes
1st rib
Left common carotid artery
Tracheobronchial node
Arch of aorta [aortic arch]
Left lung

Fig. 928   Neck; axillary fossa; thoracic cavity; frontal section of left side; ventral aspect.

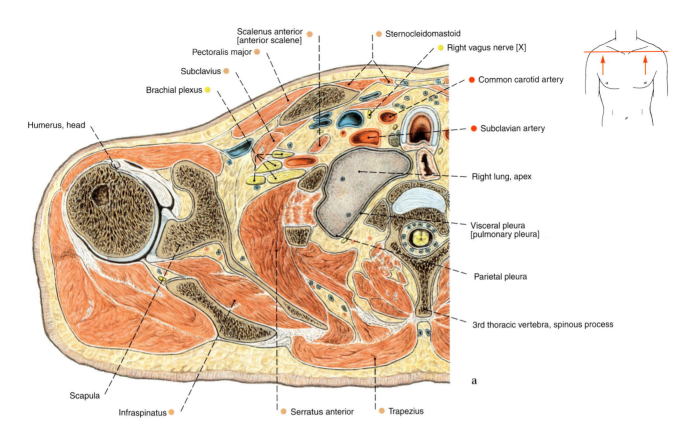

Scalenus anterior [anterior scalene]

Pectoralis major

Subclavius

Brachial plexus

Sternocleidomastoid

Right vagus nerve [X]

Common carotid artery

Subclavian artery

Humerus, head

Right lung, apex

Visceral pleura [pulmonary pleura]

Parietal pleura

3rd thoracic vertebra, spinous process

Scapula

Infraspinatus

Serratus anterior

Trapezius

a

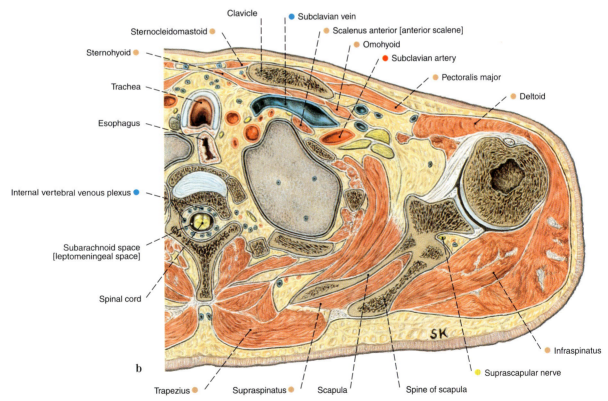

Clavicle

Subclavian vein

Sternocleidomastoid

Scalenus anterior [anterior scalene]

Sternohyoid

Omohyoid

Subclavian artery

Trachea

Pectoralis major

Esophagus

Deltoid

Internal vertebral venous plexus

Subarachnoid space [leptomeningeal space]

Spinal cord

Infraspinatus

Suprascapular nerve

Trapezius

Supraspinatus

Scapula

Spine of scapula

b

SK

Fig. 929 a, b   Thoracic cavity; horizontal section to expose cervical pleura [dome of pleura; pleural cupula] and apices of lungs; caudal aspect.

a   Right side of body
b   Left side of body

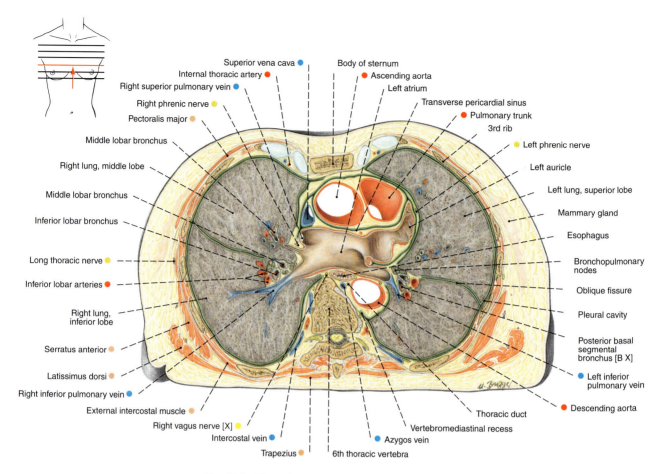

Superior vena cava

Internal thoracic artery

Right superior pulmonary vein

Right phrenic nerve

Pectoralis major

Middle lobar bronchus

Right lung, middle lobe

Middle lobar bronchus

Inferior lobar bronchus

Long thoracic nerve

Inferior lobar arteries

Right lung, inferior lobe

Serratus anterior

Latissimus dorsi

Right inferior pulmonary vein

External intercostal muscle

Right vagus nerve [X]

Intercostal vein

Trapezius

Body of sternum

Ascending aorta

Left atrium

Transverse pericardial sinus

Pulmonary trunk

3rd rib

Left phrenic nerve

Left auricle

Left lung, superior lobe

Mammary gland

Esophagus

Bronchopulmonary nodes

Oblique fissure

Pleural cavity

Posterior basal segmental bronchus [B X]

Left inferior pulmonary vein

Descending aorta

Thoracic duct

Vertebromediastinal recess

Azygos vein

6th thoracic vertebra

Fig. 934   Thoracic cavity; horizontal section at level of left atrium; caudal aspect.

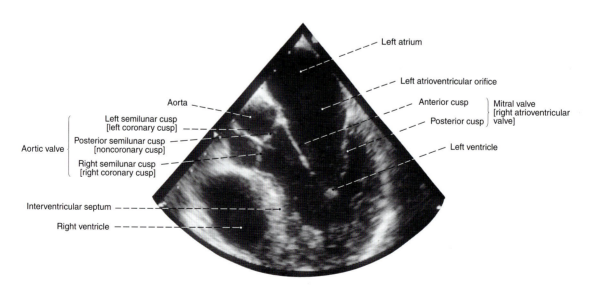

Left atrium

Left atrioventricular orifice

Aorta

Anterior cusp

Mitral valve [right atrioventricular valve]

Left semilunar cusp [left coronary cusp]

Posterior cusp

Posterior semilunar cusp [noncoronary cusp]

Aortic valve

Left ventricle

Right semilunar cusp [right coronary cusp]

Interventricular septum

Right ventricle

Fig. 935   Thoracic cavity; ultrasound image; transducer in the esophagus via endoscope to visualize the left heart and its valves; transducer at top of triangle; superior left aspect.

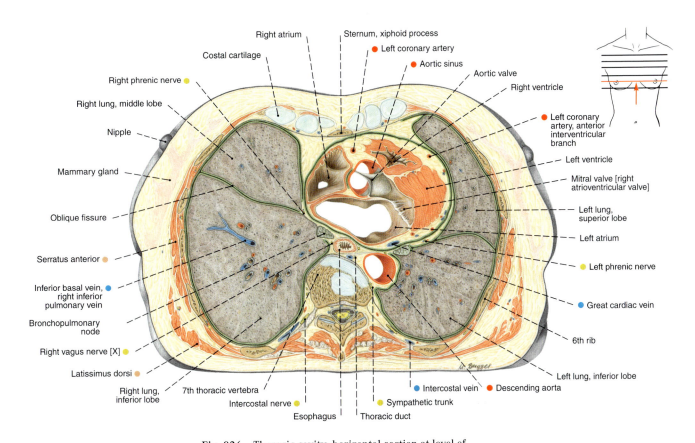

Right atrium — Sternum, xiphoid process — Left coronary artery — Aortic sinus — Aortic valve — Right ventricle
Costal cartilage
Right phrenic nerve
Right lung, middle lobe
Nipple — Left coronary artery, anterior interventricular branch
Mammary gland — Left ventricle — Mitral valve [right atrioventricular valve]
Oblique fissure — Left lung, superior lobe
— Left atrium
Serratus anterior — Left phrenic nerve
Inferior basal vein, right inferior pulmonary vein — Great cardiac vein
Bronchopulmonary node — 6th rib
Right vagus nerve [X]
Latissimus dorsi — Left lung, inferior lobe
Right lung, inferior lobe — 7th thoracic vertebra — Intercostal vein — Descending aorta
Intercostal nerve — Sympathetic trunk
Esophagus — Thoracic duct

Fig. 936   Thoracic cavity; horizontal section at level of 7th thoracic vertebra; caudal aspect.

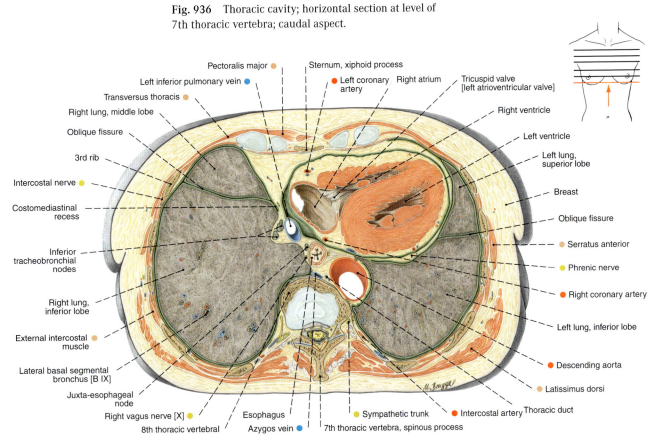

Pectoralis major — Sternum, xiphoid process — Left coronary artery — Right atrium — Tricuspid valve [left atrioventricular valve]
Left inferior pulmonary vein
Transversus thoracis — Right ventricle
Right lung, middle lobe
Oblique fissure — Left ventricle
3rd rib — Left lung, superior lobe
Intercostal nerve — Breast
Costomediastinal recess — Oblique fissure
— Serratus anterior
Inferior tracheobronchial nodes — Phrenic nerve
— Right coronary artery
Right lung, inferior lobe — Left lung, inferior lobe
External intercostal muscle — Descending aorta
Lateral basal segmental bronchus [B IX] — Latissimus dorsi
Juxta-esophageal node — Intercostal artery — Thoracic duct
Right vagus nerve [X] — Esophagus — Sympathetic trunk
8th thoracic vertebral — Azygos vein — 7th thoracic vertebra, spinous process

Fig. 937   Thoracic cavity; horizontal section at level of 8th thoracic vertebra; caudal aspect.

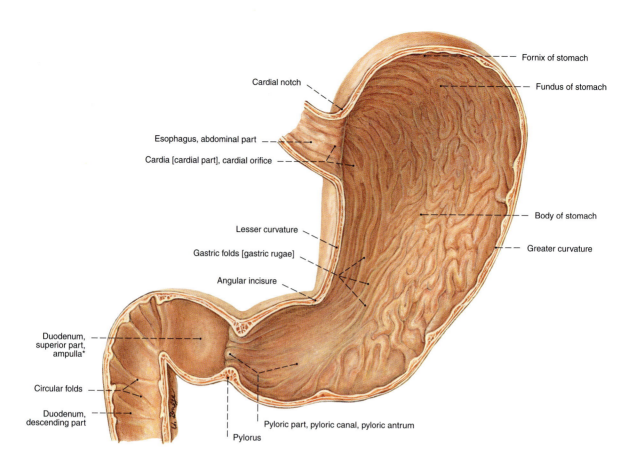

Fornix of stomach

Fundus of stomach

Cardial notch

Esophagus, abdominal part

Cardia [cardial part], cardial orifice

Body of stomach

Lesser curvature

Greater curvature

Gastric folds [gastric rugae]

Angular incisure

Duodenum, superior part, ampulla*

Circular folds

Duodenum, descending part

Pyloric part, pyloric canal, pyloric antrum

Pylorus

Fig. 938 Stomach; duodenum; anterior wall removed to expose folds of gastric and intestinal mucosa [mucous membrane]; ventral aspect.
The circular muscular layer is especially pronounced at the pylorus.

*Clinically: duodenal cap [duodenal bulb].

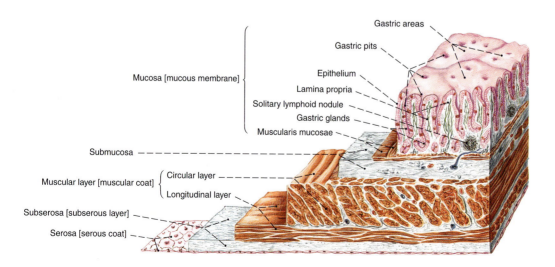

Gastric areas

Gastric pits

Epithelium

Lamina propria

Solitary lymphoid nodule

Gastric glands

Muscularis mucosae

Mucosa [mucous membrane]

Submucosa

Muscular layer [muscular coat]

Circular layer

Longitudinal layer

Subserosa [subserous layer]

Serosa [serous coat]

Fig. 939 Diagram of staggered wall of stomach; low power magnification.

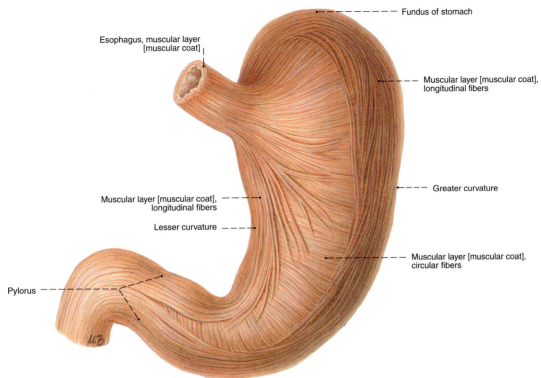

Fundus of stomach

Esophagus, muscular layer [muscular coat]

Muscular layer [muscular coat], longitudinal fibers

Muscular layer [muscular coat], longitudinal fibers

Lesser curvature

Greater curvature

Pylorus

Muscular layer [muscular coat], circular fibers

Fig. 940 Stomach; peritoneum removed to expose external muscular layers of anterior wall of stomach; ventral aspect.

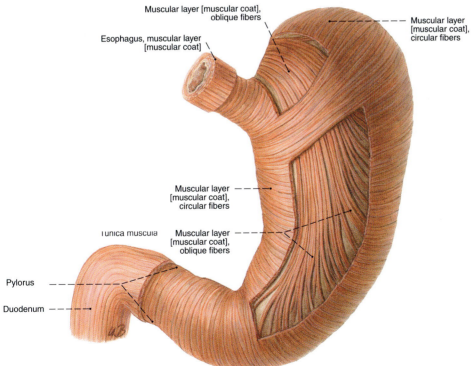

Muscular layer [muscular coat], oblique fibers

Esophagus, muscular layer [muscular coat]

Muscular layer [muscular coat], circular fibers

Muscular layer [muscular coat], circular fibers

Tunica muscula

Muscular layer [muscular coat], oblique fibers

Pylorus

Duodenum

Fig. 941 Stomach; peritoneum removed; external muscular layer partially resected to expose oblique fibers internally; ventral aspect.

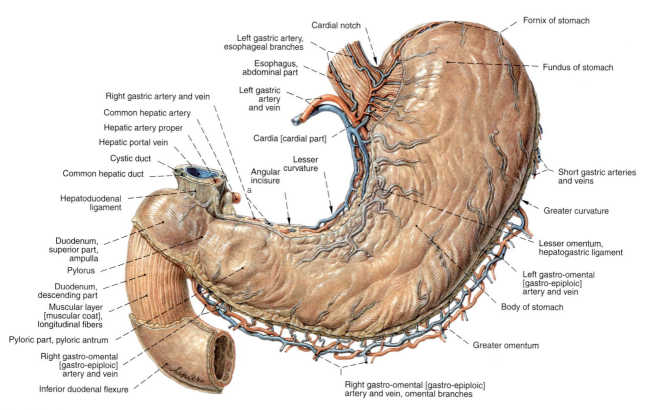

Cardial notch

Fornix of stomach

Left gastric artery, esophageal branches

Fundus of stomach

Esophagus, abdominal part

Right gastric artery and vein

Left gastric artery and vein

Common hepatic artery

Hepatic artery proper

Cardia [cardial part]

Hepatic portal vein

Cystic duct

Lesser curvature

Common hepatic duct

Angular incisure
a

Short gastric arteries and veins

Hepatoduodenal ligament

Greater curvature

Duodenum, superior part, ampulla

Lesser omentum, hepatogastric ligament

Pylorus

Left gastro-omental [gastro-epiploic] artery and vein

Duodenum, descending part

Muscular layer [muscular coat], longitudinal fibers

Body of stomach

Pyloric part, pyloric antrum

Greater omentum

Right gastro-omental [gastro-epiploic] artery and vein

Inferior duodenal flexure

Right gastro-omental [gastro-epiploic] artery and vein, omental branches

Fig. 942   Stomach; duodenum; peritoneum partially removed; ventral aspect.

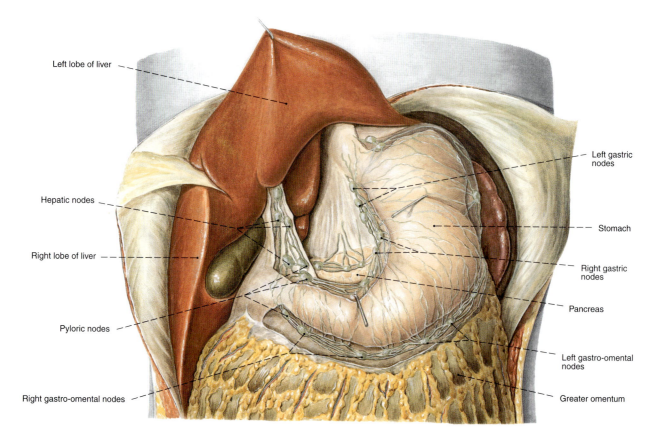

Left lobe of liver

Left gastric nodes

Hepatic nodes

Stomach

Right lobe of liver

Right gastric nodes

Pancreas

Pyloric nodes

Left gastro-omental nodes

Right gastro-omental nodes

Greater omentum

Fig. 943   Stomach and liver, with lymph nodes; left lobe of liver retracted superiorly; peritoneum removed from the lesser and the greater curvatures to expose the lymph nodes; ventral aspect.
Number and size of gastric lymph nodes vary considerable.

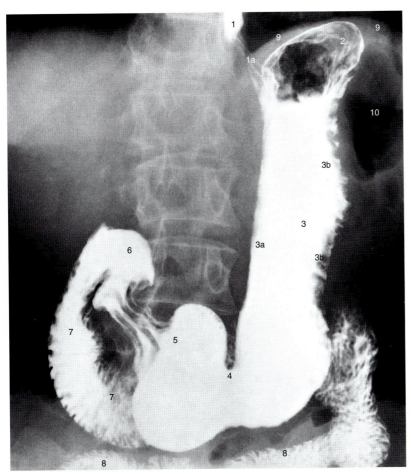

1 = Esophagus with contrast medium. In the passage (1a) to the fundus of the stomach the grooves between the folds are visible as dark stripes.
2 = Fundus of stomach with air bubble
3 = Body of stomach
3a = Lesser curvature
3b = Greater curvature.
  At the boundary between 3a and 3b notches according to the relief of the mucosa are visible.
4 = Peristaltic contraction at angular incisure
5 = Pyloric part just before progression of a portion of the contents of the stomach.
6 = Duodenum, superior part, ampulla
7 = Duodenum, descending part with circular folds
8 = Jejunum
9 = Left dome of diaphragm
10 = Left colic flexure [splenic flexure] (with air)

Fig. 944 Stomach; duodenum; AP radiograph after oral intake of contrast medium in upright position; ventral aspect.
In the radiograph of an upright patient an air bubble can be seen in the fundus of stomach, which is bordered by a fluid balance inferiorly.

The stripes in the junction between the esophagus and the stomach and in the pylorus are caused by longitudinal folds of the mucosa.

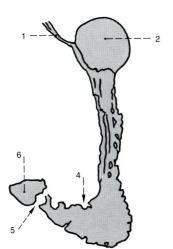

Fig. 945 Stomach; line drawing of relief of mucosa from an AP radiograph in an upright patient; ventral aspect.
The pyloric part is constricted; the wall of the pyloric antrum is relaxed.

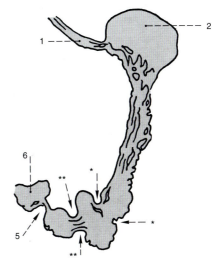

Fig. 946 Stomach; line drawing of relief of mucosa from an AP radiograph in an upright patient; ventral aspect.
The two constrictions at the angular incisure (*) and in the area of the pyloric antrum (**) indicate a peristaltic wave.

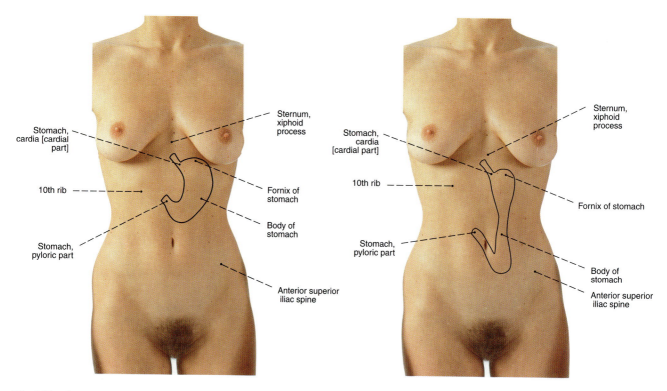

Stomach, cardia [cardial part]

Sternum, xiphoid process

10th rib

Fornix of stomach

Stomach, pyloric part

Body of stomach

Anterior superior iliac spine

Stomach, cardia [cardial part]

Sternum, xiphoid process

10th rib

Fornix of stomach

Stomach, pyloric part

Body of stomach

Anterior superior iliac spine

Fig. 947 Stomach; projection of "normal" stomach onto the anterior abdominal wall in the upright position.

Fig. 948 Stomach; projection of "long" stomach onto the anterior abdominal wall in the upright position. The stomach is fixed at its inlet and its outlet. Size and position of the other parts of the stomach largely depend on filling status and body position. Moreover, there are many variations among individuals.

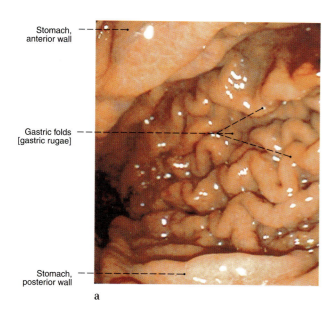

Stomach, anterior wall

Gastric folds [gastric rugae]

Stomach, posterior wall

a

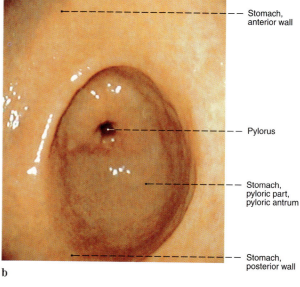

Stomach, anterior wall

Pylorus

Stomach, pyloric part, pyloric antrum

Stomach, posterior wall

b

Fig. 949a, b Stomach; endoscopic view of stomach (gastroscopy); superior aspect.

a Body of stomach with well-developed longitudinal folds of mucosa (gastric folds [gastric rugae]).
b Pyloric antrum with mainly smooth mucosa.

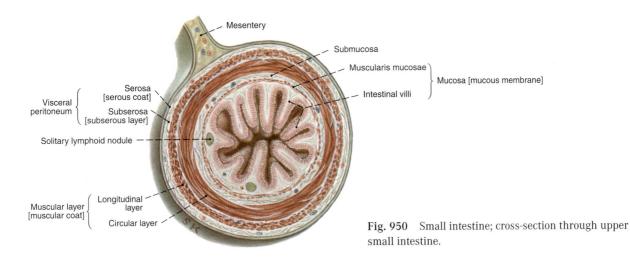

Mesentery

Submucosa

Muscularis mucosae

Mucosa [mucous membrane]

Intestinal villi

Visceral peritoneum

Serosa [serous coat]

Subserosa [subserous layer]

Solitary lymphoid nodule

Muscular layer [muscular coat]

Longitudinal layer

Circular layer

Fig. 950   Small intestine; cross-section through upper small intestine.

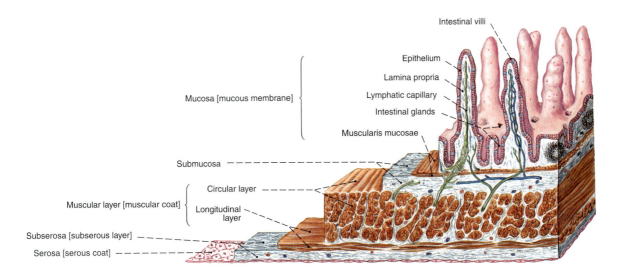

Intestinal villi

Epithelium

Lamina propria

Lymphatic capillary

Intestinal glands

Muscularis mucosae

Mucosa [mucous membrane]

Submucosa

Circular layer

Muscular layer [muscular coat]

Longitudinal layer

Subserosa [subserous layer]

Serosa [serous coat]

Fig. 951   Small intestine; staggered layers of wall; low-power magnification.

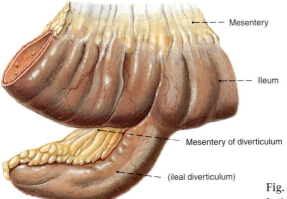

Mesentery

Ileum

Mesentery of diverticulum

(ileal diverticulum)

Fig. 952   MECKEL's diverticulum (ileal diverticulum). In 1-3% of people, such a diverticulum is present as a residuum of the vitelline duct (yolk stalk).

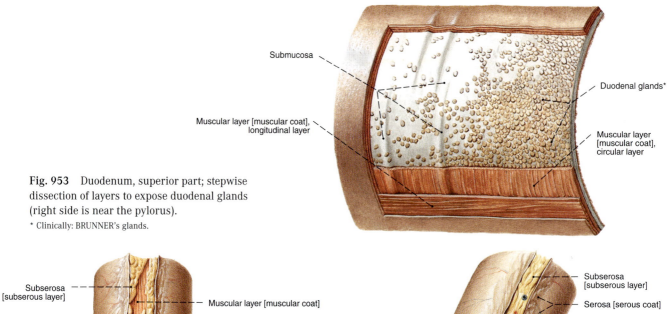

Submucosa

Muscular layer [muscular coat], longitudinal layer

Duodenal glands*

Muscular layer [muscular coat], circular layer

Fig. 953 Duodenum, superior part; stepwise dissection of layers to expose duodenal glands (right side is near the pylorus).

* Clinically: BRUNNER's glands.

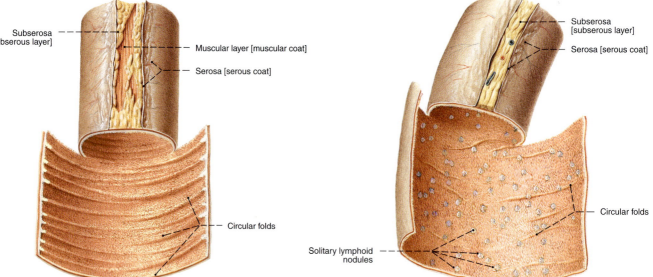

Subserosa [subserous layer]

Muscular layer [muscular coat]

Serosa [serous coat]

Circular folds

Subserosa [subserous layer]

Serosa [serous coat]

Circular folds

Solitary lymphoid nodules

Fig. 954 Upper small intestine: jejunum; wall partially opened along the attachment of the mesentery to expose the mucosa [mucous membrane]. Compare number of folds in Fig. 955.

Fig. 955 Lower small intestine: ileum; wall partially opened along the attachment of the mesentery to expose the mucosa [mucous membrane]. Compare with Fig. 954.

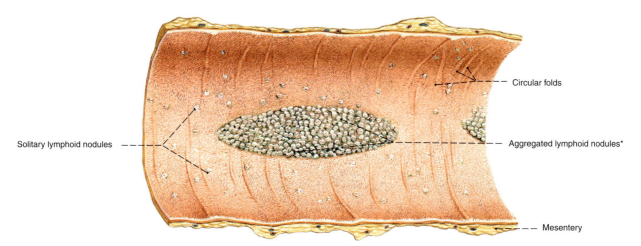

Solitary lymphoid nodules

Circular folds

Aggregated lymphoid nodules*

Mesentery

Fig. 956 Lowest small intestine: terminal ileum; wall opened along the attachment of the mesentery. PEYER'S patches are also found in the duodenum and the jejunum and are not characteristic of the ileum.

* Clinically: PEYER'S patches.

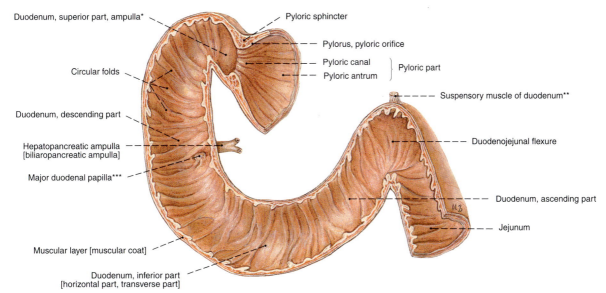

Duodenum, superior part, ampulla*

Pyloric sphincter

Pylorus, pyloric orifice

Pyloric canal

Pyloric antrum

Pyloric part

Circular folds

Suspensory muscle of duodenum**

Duodenum, descending part

Duodenojejunal flexure

Hepatopancreatic ampulla [biliaropancreatic ampulla]

Major duodenal papilla***

Duodenum, ascending part

Jejunum

Muscular layer [muscular coat]

Duodenum, inferior part [horizontal part, transverse part]

Fig. 957 Duodenum; anterior wall removed to expose the mucosa [mucous membrane]; ventral aspect.

The superior part courses from the stomach dorsocranially to the right; ND at the duodenojejunal flexure the duodenum swings ventrocaudally.

*   Clinically: Duodenal cap [bulb].

**   Clinically: muscle of TREITZ.

***   Clinically: tubercle of VATER.

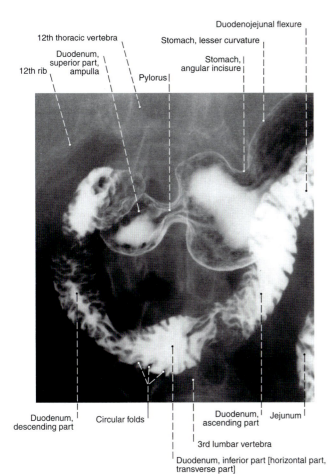

12th thoracic vertebra

Duodenojejunal flexure

Stomach, lesser curvature

Duodenum, superior part, ampulla

Stomach, angular incisure

12th rib

Pylorus

Duodenum, descending part

Circular folds

Duodenum, ascending part

Jejunum

3rd lumbar vertebra

Duodenum, inferior part [horizontal part, transverse part]

Fig. 958 Duodenum; AP radiograph after oral application of contrast medium; upright position; ventral aspect.

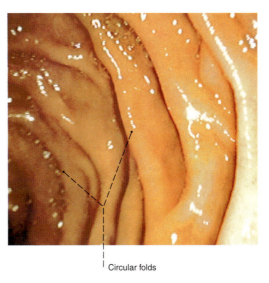

Circular folds

Fig. 959 Duodenum; endoscopic view of the mucosa [mucous membrane] with circular folds; superior aspect.

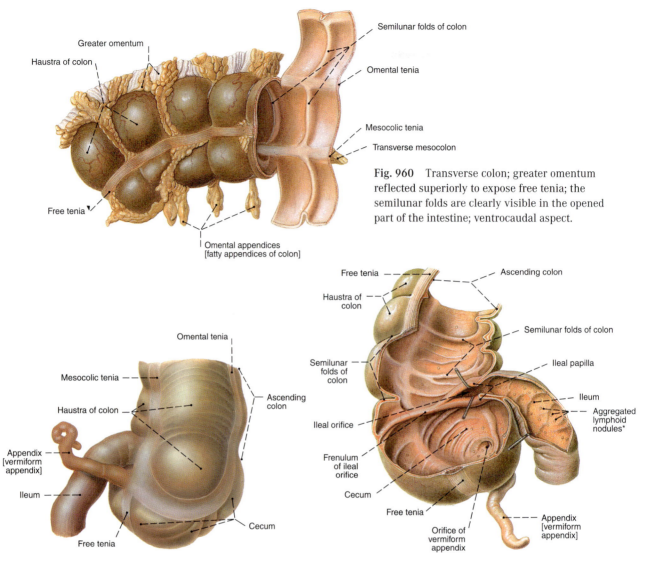

Greater omentum

Haustra of colon

Semilunar folds of colon

Omental tenia

Mesocolic tenia

Transverse mesocolon

Free tenia

Omental appendices [fatty appendices of colon]

Fig. 960   Transverse colon; greater omentum reflected superiorly to expose free tenia; the semilunar folds are clearly visible in the opened part of the intestine; ventrocaudal aspect.

Omental tenia

Mesocolic tenia

Haustra of colon

Appendix [vermiform appendix]

Ileum

Free tenia

Ascending colon

Cecum

Fig. 961   Cecum; appendix [vermiform appendix]; terminal ileum; dorsal aspect.

Free tenia

Haustra of colon

Semilunar folds of colon

Ileal orifice

Frenulum of ileal orifice

Cecum

Free tenia

Orifice of vermiform appendix

Ascending colon

Semilunar folds of colon

Ileal papilla

Ileum

Aggregated lymphoid nodules*

Appendix [vermiform appendix]

Fig. 962   Ascending colon; cecum; appendix [vermiform appendix]; intestine opened by a frontal section to expose ileal orifice [orifice of ileal papilla; BAUHIN's valve]; orifice is held open with hooks; ventral aspect.
*PEYER's patches.

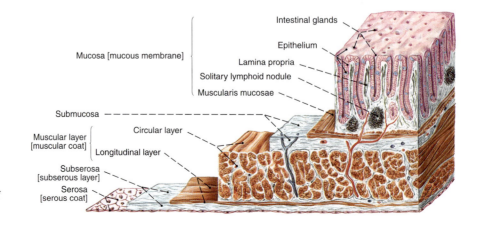

Mucosa [mucous membrane]

Submucosa

Muscular layer [muscular coat]

Subserosa [subserous layer]

Serosa [serous coat]

Circular layer

Longitudinal layer

Intestinal glands

Epithelium

Lamina propria

Solitary lymphoid nodule

Muscularis mucosae

Fig. 963   Colon; staggered layers of wall; low-power magnification.

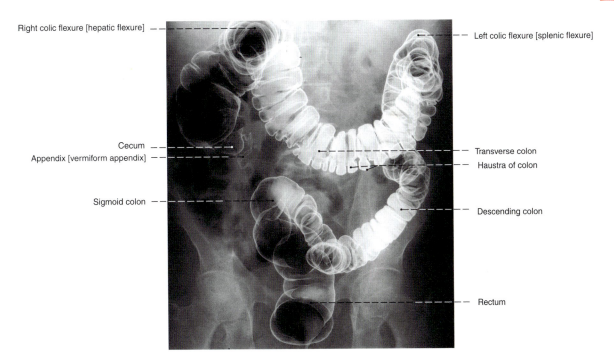

Right colic flexure [hepatic flexure]

Cecum

Appendix [vermiform appendix]

Sigmoid colon

Left colic flexure [splenic flexure]

Transverse colon

Haustra of colon

Descending colon

Rectum

Fig. 964 Colon; rectum; AP radiograph after filling with contrast agent and air (double-contrast method). Compare the topography of colon in Figs. 1005 and 1008.

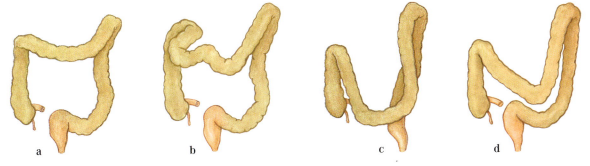

a   b   c   d

Fig. 965 a-d Transverse colon; frequent variations.
a normal position; **b** twisted, **c** U-shaped; **d** V-shaped.

The position of the transverse colon also depends on filling status and on body position; ventral aspect.

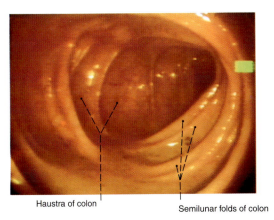

Haustra of colon

Semilunar folds of colon

Fig. 966 Ascending colon; endoscopic (colonoscopic) view; endoscope inserted via rectum, sigmoid, and descending colon.

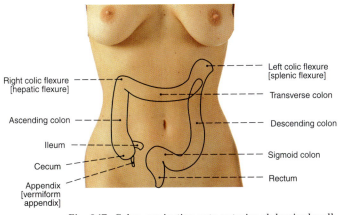

Right colic flexure [hepatic flexure]

Ascending colon

Ileum

Cecum

Appendix [vermiform appendix]

Left colic flexure [splenic flexure]

Transverse colon

Descending colon

Sigmoid colon

Rectum

Fig. 967 Colon; projection onto anterior abdominal wall. Position of transverse and sigmoid colon vary considerably (compare Fig. 965).

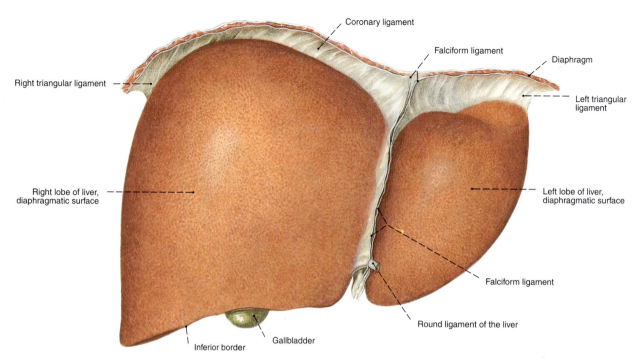

Fig. 968   Liver; parts of diaphragm retained to expose its attachment to the liver; the falciform ligament and the round ligament of the liver severed; ventral aspect.

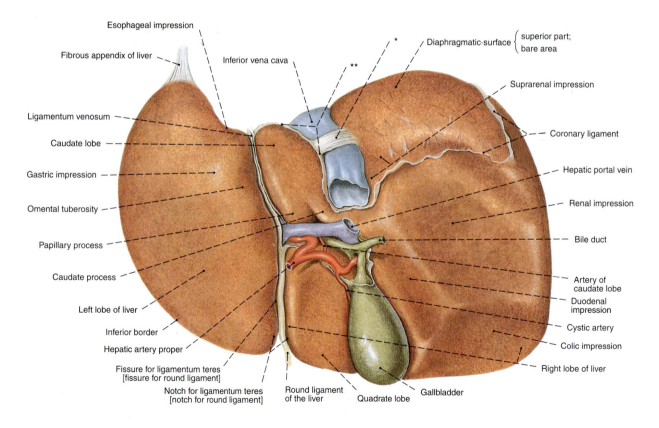

Fig. 969   Liver; porta hepatis; ligaments of the liver and blood vessels severed; dorsal aspect.

* Also: ligament of vena cava.

** Boundary of superior recess of omental bursa [lesser sac].

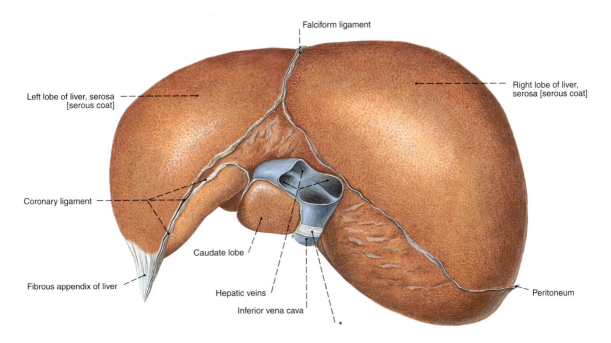

Falciform ligament

Left lobe of liver, serosa
[serous coat]

Right lobe of liver,
serosa [serous coat]

Coronary ligament

Caudate lobe

Hepatic veins

Inferior vena cava

Peritoneum

*

Fig. 970 Liver; reflections of peritoneum sectioned; cranial aspect.

The bare area without peritoneum can be recognized by its roughened surface.

* Also: ligament of vena cava.

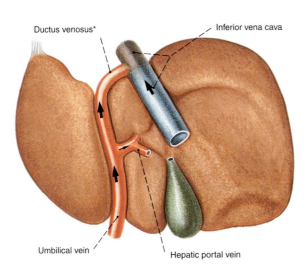

Ductus venosus*

Inferior vena cava

Umbilical vein

Hepatic portal vein

Fig. 971 Liver of a fetus; colors indicate oxygen content of blood , arrows indicate direction of blood flow; dorsal aspect. The liver parenchyma is bypassed by the ductus venosus, that carries oxygen-rich blood from the placenta to the inferior vena cava.

* Also: ARTANTIUS' duct.

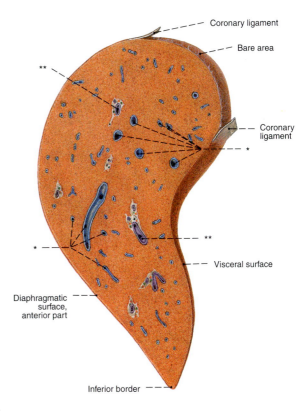

Coronary ligament

Bare area

**

Coronary
ligament

*

**

Visceral surface

Diaphragmatic
surface,
anterior part

*

Inferior border

Fig. 972 Liver of a fetus; sagittal section through right lobe of liver to expose branches of both hepatic and portal veins.

*   Intrahepatic branches of hepatic veins.

** Intrahepatic branches of hepatic portal vein and hepatic artery.

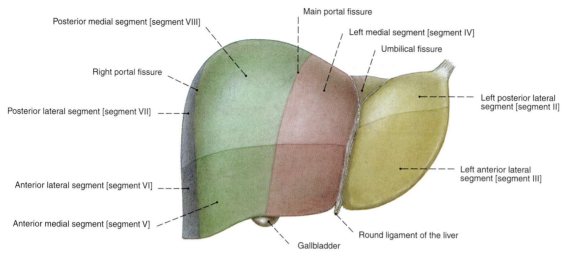

Fig. 973   Liver; colors indicate different liver segments; ventral aspect.

Surgically, the 4th segment is divided into an upper (IV a) and lower (IV b) subsegment.

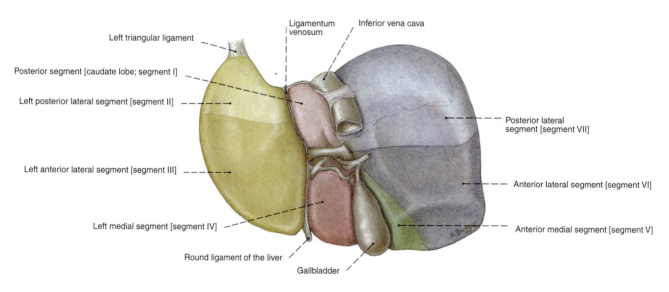

Fig. 974   Liver; colors indicate same liver segments as in Fig. 973; dorsal aspect.

Hepatic segmentation

Left liver [left part of liver]	Posterior liver [posterior part of liver, caudate lobe]	Posterior segment [caudate lobe; segment I]
	Left lateral division	Left posterior lateral segment [segment II]
		Left anterior lateral segment [segment III]
	Left medial division	Left medial segment [segment IV]
Right liver [right part of liver]	Right medial division	Anterior medial segment [segment V]
		Posterior medial segment [segment VIII]
	Right lateral division	Anterior lateral segment [segment VI]
		Posterior lateral segment [segment VII]

Traditionally, the liver is divided into a right and a left lobe with regard to the falciform ligament. The classification in parts and divisions, however, based on the branching pattern of hepatic artery, hepatic portal vein, and hepatic duct, are based on practical aspects, e.g. the requirements for surgical resection of parts of the liver. Moreover, in this classification also developmental aspects are taken into account.

The separate parts are divided by fissures, which do not correspond to superficially visible clefts.

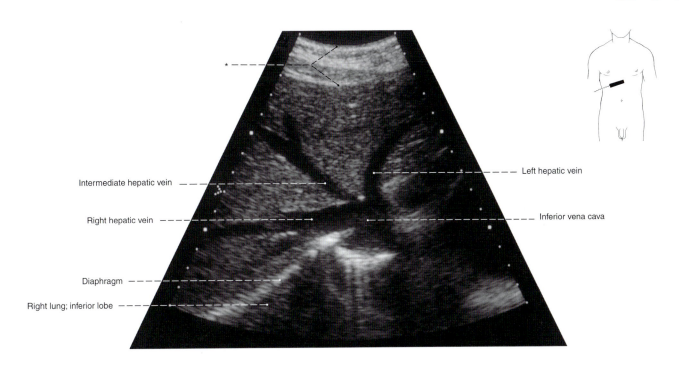

Fig. 975 Hepatic veins; ultrasound scan of openings
of hepatic veins into inferior vena cava; inferior aspect.
* Abdominal wall.

Intermediate hepatic vein

Right hepatic vein

Diaphragm

Right lung; inferior lobe

Left hepatic vein

Inferior vena cava

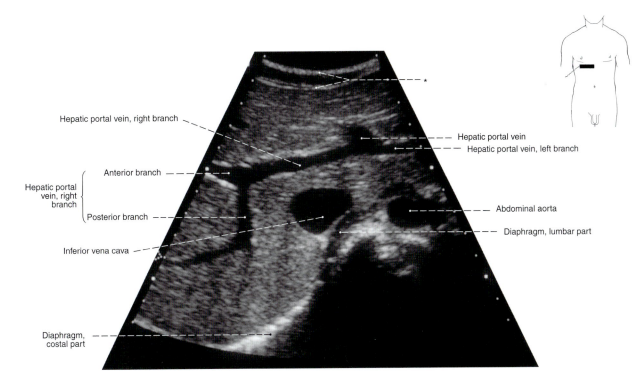

Hepatic portal vein, right branch

Hepatic portal
vein, right
branch {
  Anterior branch
  Posterior branch
}

Inferior vena cava

Diaphragm,
costal part

Hepatic portal vein

Hepatic portal vein, left branch

Abdominal aorta

Diaphragm, lumbar part

Fig. 976 Hepatic portal vein; ultrasound scan
of division of hepatic portal vein into main
branches; inferior aspect.
Compare Fig. 982.
* Abdominal wall.

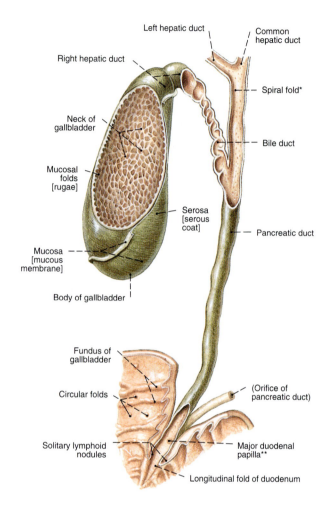

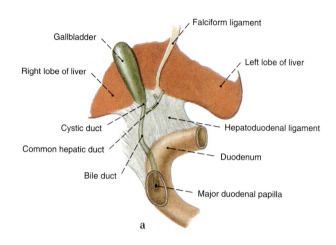

Fig. 977 Gallbladder; biliary duct system; parts of anterior wall of gallbladder, biliary duct system, and duodenum removed to expose mucosa [mucous membrane]; ventral aspect.

* Clinically: HEISTER's valve.

** Clinically: Tubercle of VATER.

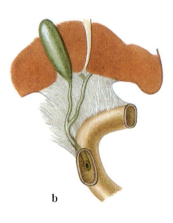

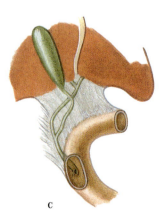

Fig. 978 a-c Variability of biliary duct system, common hepatic duct, bile duct.

a High union of common hepatic duct and cystic duct

b Low union of common hepatic duct and cystic duct

c Low union after cystic duct crossing over common hepatic duct

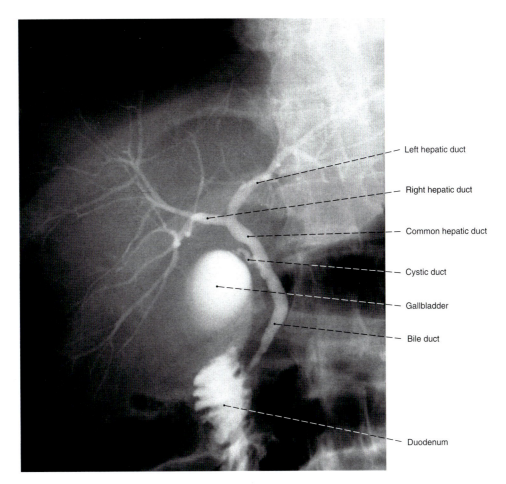

Left hepatic duct

Right hepatic duct

Common hepatic duct

Cystic duct

Gallbladder

Bile duct

Duodenum

Fig. 979   Biliary duct system; AP radiograph after administration of contrast medium; upright position; ventral aspect.

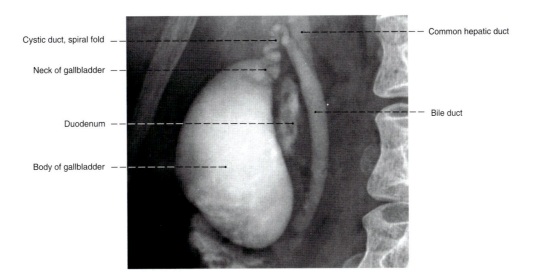

Cystic duct, spiral fold

Neck of gallbladder

Duodenum

Body of gallbladder

Common hepatic duct

Bile duct

Fig. 980   Gallbladder and biliary duct system; AP radiograph after administration of contrast medium; upright position; ventral aspect.

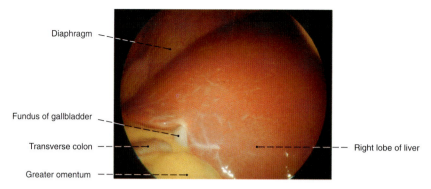

Diaphragm

Fundus of gallbladder

Transverse colon

Greater omentum

Right lobe of liver

Fig. 981   Liver; gallbladder; endoscopy (laparoscopy) allows visualization of color, surface, and shape of the liver; ventral, left inferior aspect.

Insufflation of gas into the peritoneal cavity causes a space between the diaphragm and the liver, thus, allowing a comprehensive exploration of liver and gallbladder.

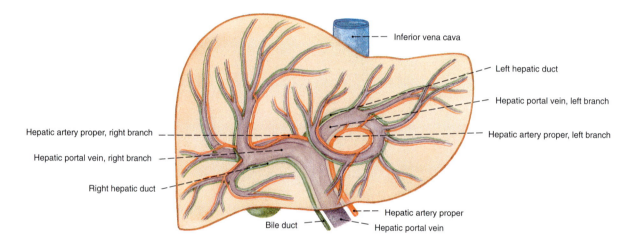

Inferior vena cava

Left hepatic duct

Hepatic portal vein, left branch

Hepatic artery proper, right branch

Hepatic artery proper, left branch

Hepatic portal vein, right branch

Right hepatic duct

Hepatic artery proper

Bile duct

Hepatic portal vein

Fig. 982   Liver; hepatic portal vein; diagram of branching pattern of hepatic portal vein projected onto the surface of the liver; ventral aspect.

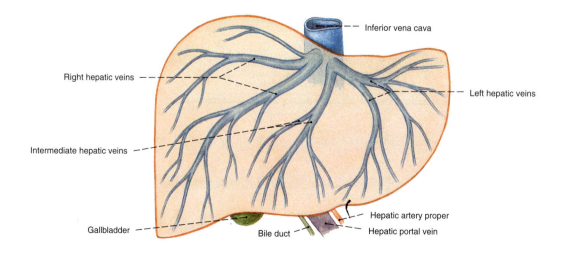

Inferior vena cava

Right hepatic veins

Left hepatic veins

Intermediate hepatic veins

Gallbladder

Hepatic artery proper

Bile duct

Hepatic portal vein

Fig. 983   Liver; hepatic veins; diagram of branching pattern of hepatic veins projected onto the surface of the liver; ventral aspect.

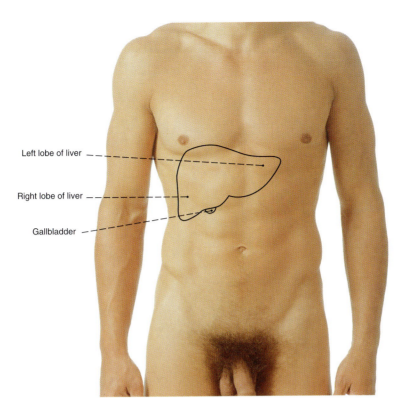

Left lobe of liver

Right lobe of liver

Gallbladder

Fig. 984 Liver; projection onto the anterior abdominal wall; in midrespiratory position. Position of the liver highly depends on the respiratory cycle. In inspiration the diaphragm flattens and the diaphragmatic dome descends caudally. This pushes the healthy liver caudally to the costal margin [costal arch], and the inferior border becomes palpable.

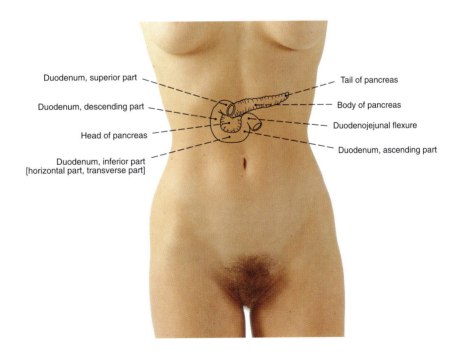

Duodenum, superior part

Duodenum, descending part

Head of pancreas

Duodenum, inferior part [horizontal part, transverse part]

Tail of pancreas

Body of pancreas

Duodenojejunal flexure

Duodenum, ascending part

Fig. 985 Duodenum; pancreas; projection onto the anterior abdominal wall.

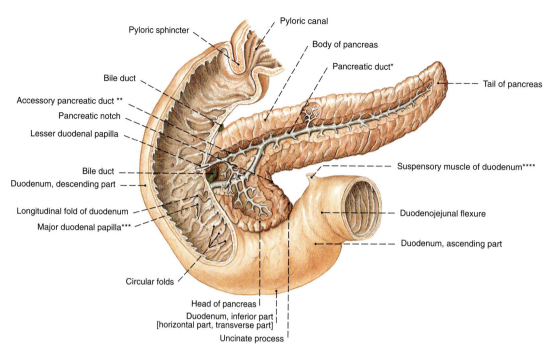

Pyloric sphincter
Pyloric canal
Body of pancreas
Pancreatic duct*
Bile duct
Tail of pancreas
Accessory pancreatic duct **
Pancreatic notch
Lesser duodenal papilla
Bile duct
Duodenum, descending part
Suspensory muscle of duodenum****
Longitudinal fold of duodenum
Duodenojejunal flexure
Major duodenal papilla***
Duodenum, ascending part
Circular folds
Head of pancreas
Duodenum, inferior part
[horizontal part, transverse part]
Uncinate process

Fig. 986 Duodenum; pancreas; parts of anterior wall of duodenum removed to expose the opening of the pancreatic duct; pancreatic duct dissected; ventral aspect.

Shape and size of the accessory pancreatic duct vary considerably (in ~30% adjacent branch, in less than 10% main excretory duct).
* Clinically: duct of WIRSUNG.
** Clinically: SANTORINI's duct.
*** Clinically: muscle of TREITZ.
**** Clinically: tubercle of VATER.

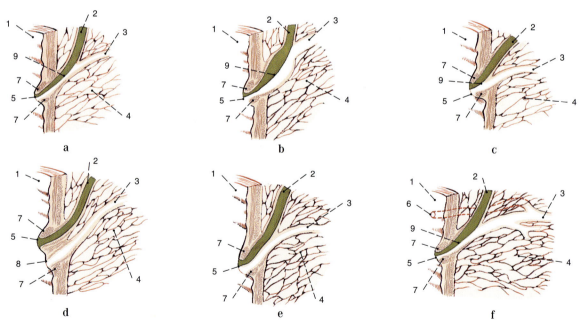

a

b

c

d

e

f

Fig. 987 a-f   Variability of opening of bile duct and pancreatic duct.

a   Long common section
b   Ampullar enlargement of terminal part
c   Short common section
d   Separate openings
e   Common opening with septum in the common section
f   Additional duct, accessory pancreatic duct

1 = Duodenum
2 = Bile duct
3 = Pancreatic duct
4 = Pancreas
5 = Major duodenal papilla
6 = Minor duodenal papilla, accessory pancreatic duct
7 = Sphincter of ampulla
8 = Pancreatic duct (in bipartite papilla)
9 = Hepatopancreatic ampulla [biliaropancreatic ampulla]

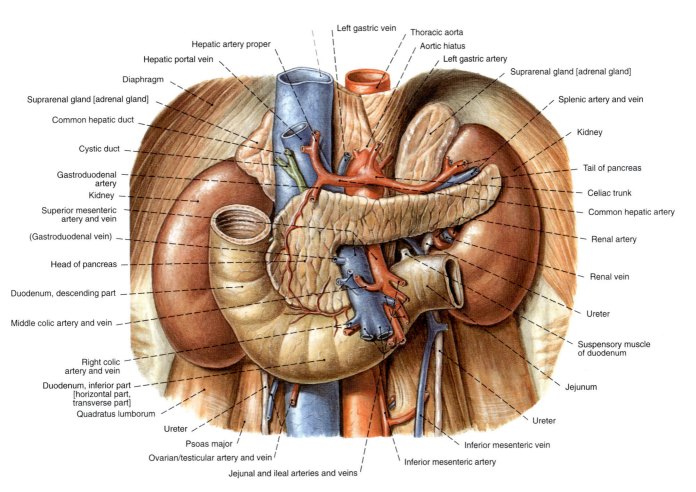

Left gastric vein
Thoracic aorta
Aortic hiatus
Hepatic artery proper
Left gastric artery
Hepatic portal vein
Suprarenal gland [adrenal gland]
Diaphragm
Splenic artery and vein
Suprarenal gland [adrenal gland]
Kidney
Common hepatic duct
Tail of pancreas
Cystic duct
Celiac trunk
Gastroduodenal artery
Common hepatic artery
Kidney
Renal artery
Superior mesenteric artery and vein
(Gastroduodenal vein)
Renal vein
Head of pancreas
Duodenum, descending part
Ureter
Middle colic artery and vein
Suspensory muscle of duodenum
Right colic artery and vein
Jejunum
Duodenum, inferior part [horizontal part, transverse part]
Quadratus lumborum
Ureter
Psoas major
Inferior mesenteric vein
Ovarian/testicular artery and vein
Inferior mesenteric artery
Jejunal and ileal arteries and veins

Fig. 988 Retroperitoneal organs and blood vessels of upper abdomen; ventral aspect. Lymph nodes are not shown.

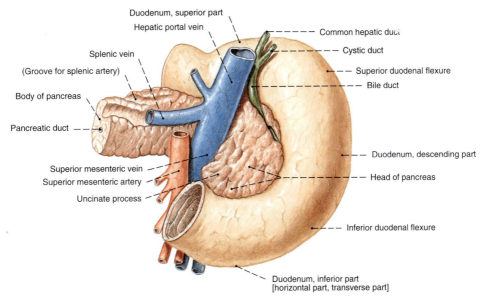

Duodenum, superior part
Hepatic portal vein
Common hepatic duct
Cystic duct
Splenic vein
Superior duodenal flexure
(Groove for splenic artery)
Bile duct
Body of pancreas
Pancreatic duct
Duodenum, descending part
Superior mesenteric vein
Head of pancreas
Superior mesenteric artery
Uncinate process
Inferior duodenal flexure
Duodenum, inferior part [horizontal part, transverse part]

Fig. 989 Duodenum; pancreas; body of pancreas severed to expose pancreatic duct; dorsal aspect.

The bile duct courses through the pancreas; the head of pancreas embraces the superior mesenteric vein.

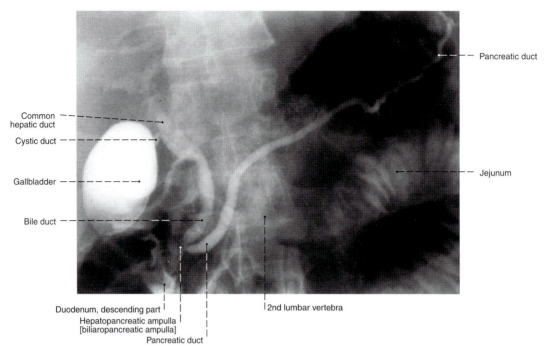

Common hepatic duct

Cystic duct

Gallbladder

Bile duct

Pancreatic duct

Jejunum

Duodenum, descending part

Hepatopancreatic ampulla [biliaropancreatic ampulla]

Pancreatic duct

2nd lumbar vertebra

Fig. 990 Pancreatic duct; bile duct; gallbladder; AP radiograph; supine position; after endoscopic cannulation of the common excretory duct of pancreas and liver and injection of contrast medium; ventral aspect.

Clinically: ERCP (endoscopic retrograde cholangio-pancreatography). The pancreatic duct is visible throughout its entire length up to the splenic hilum and shows a typical oblique course superiorly toward the left. Some contrast medium has flowed into the small intestine; thus, parts of duodenum and jejunum are also visible. When the contrast medium is injected with higher pressure also, the side branches of the pancreatic duct are visible (compare Fig. 986). This, however, may lead to damage of the pancreas.

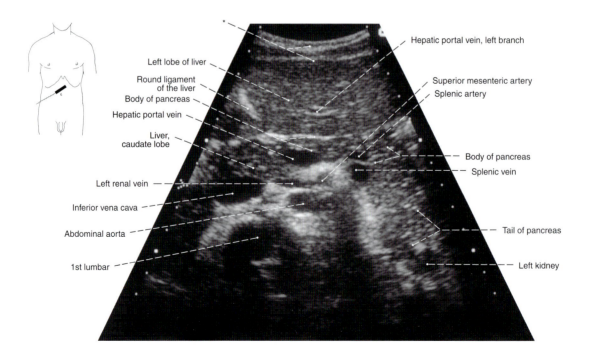

Left lobe of liver

Round ligament of the liver

Body of pancreas

Hepatic portal vein

Liver, caudate lobe

Left renal vein

Inferior vena cava

Abdominal aorta

1st lumbar

Hepatic portal vein, left branch

Superior mesenteric artery

Splenic artery

Body of pancreas

Splenic vein

Tail of pancreas

Left kidney

Fig. 991 Pancreas; ultrasound scan visualizing pancreas and neighboring blood vessels in deep inspiration; the tail of pancreas extends far dorsally; inferior aspect.
* Abdominal wall.

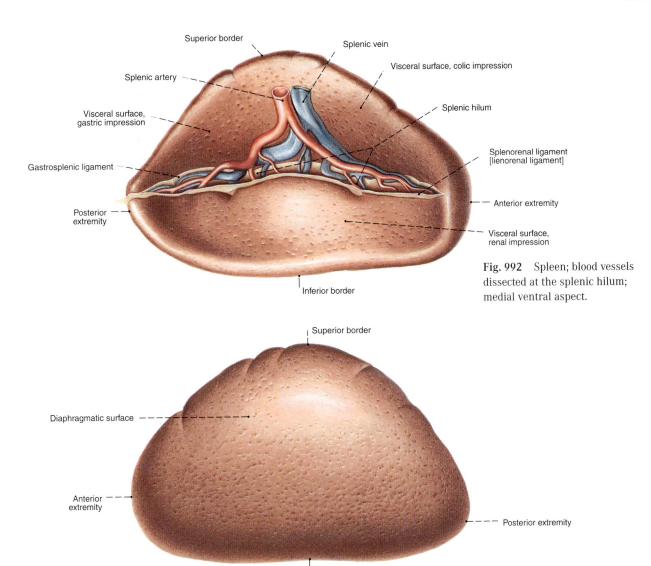

Superior border

Splenic vein

Visceral surface, colic impression

Splenic artery

Splenic hilum

Visceral surface, gastric impression

Splenorenal ligament [lienorenal ligament]

Gastrosplenic ligament

Anterior extremity

Posterior extremity

Visceral surface, renal impression

Inferior border

Fig. 992   Spleen; blood vessels dissected at the splenic hilum; medial ventral aspect.

Superior border

Diaphragmatic surface

Anterior extremity

Posterior extremity

Inferior border

Fig. 993   Spleen; lateral cranial aspect.

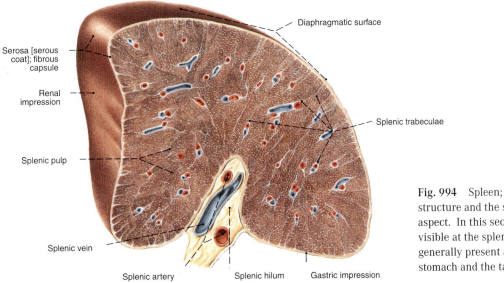

Diaphragmatic surface

Serosa [serous coat]; fibrous capsule

Renal impression

Splenic trabeculae

Splenic pulp

Splenic vein

Splenic artery

Splenic hilum

Gastric impression

Fig. 994   Spleen; cross-section exposing the structure and the splenic hilum; medial cranial aspect. In this section no lymph nodes are visible at the splenic hilum, although they are generally present at the hilum, draining the stomach and the tail of pancreas.

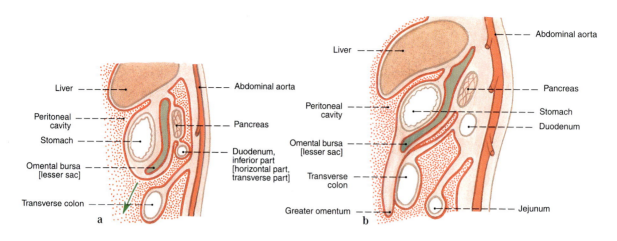

Fig. 995 a, b   Development of peritoneal cavity and relationship of peritoneum; schematic median section; lateral aspect.
a   Early development
b   During formation of greater omentum

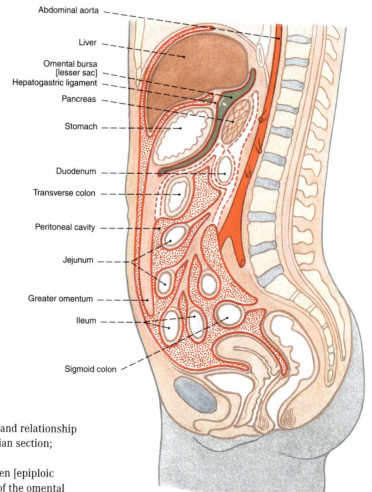

Fig. 996   Development of peritoneal cavity and relationship of peritoneum in the female; schematic median section; lateral aspect.

The arrow indicates the omental foramen [epiploic foramen]; the arrowhead is in the vestibule of the omental bursa [lesser sac].

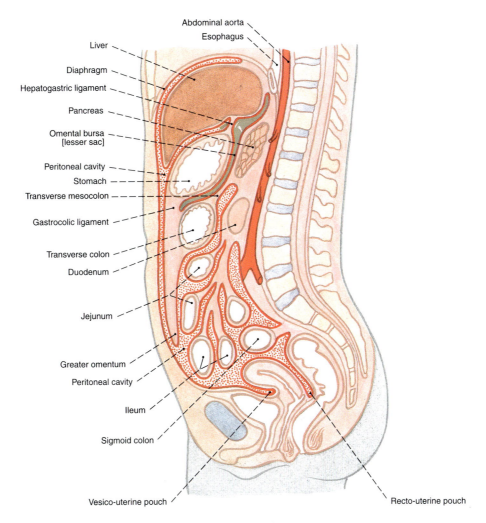

Abdominal aorta

Esophagus

Liver

Diaphragm

Hepatogastric ligament

Pancreas

Omental bursa
[lesser sac]

Peritoneal cavity

Stomach

Transverse mesocolon

Gastrocolic ligament

Transverse colon

Duodenum

Jejunum

Greater omentum

Peritoneal cavity

Ileum

Sigmoid colon

Vesico-uterine pouch

Recto-uterine pouch

Fig. 997 Development of peritoneal cavity and relationship
of peritoneum in the female; final state of peritoneal cavity
with fixation of the transverse colon to the greater omentum;
schematic median section; lateral aspect.

* Clinically: pouch of DOUGLAS.

Figs. 995-997   The development of the intestines is presented
highly schematically; in fact, several developmental steps take
place at the same time. The peritoneal cavity is enlarged for
didactic reasons. In reality, the organs lie tightly adjacent to
each other, separated only by a small capillary space. The
volume of the peritoneal fluid is only a few milliliters.

Peritoneal cavity: dotted red; omental bursa [lesser
sac]: olive; red dotted line: original arrangement of
peritoneum. Arrow in omental foramen [epiploic foramen].

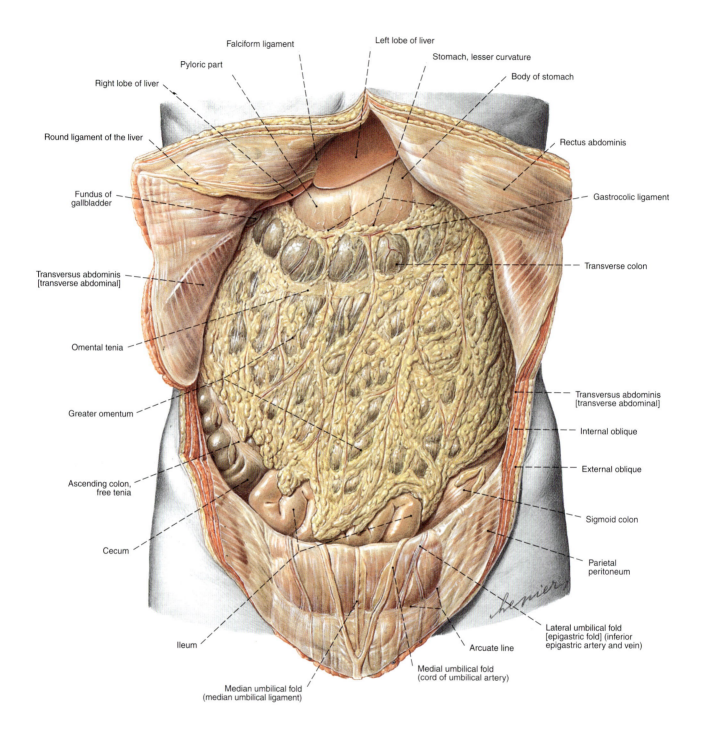

Falciform ligament

Left lobe of liver

Pyloric part

Stomach, lesser curvature

Right lobe of liver

Body of stomach

Round ligament of the liver

Rectus abdominis

Fundus of gallbladder

Gastrocolic ligament

Transversus abdominis [transverse abdominal]

Transverse colon

Omental tenia

Transversus abdominis [transverse abdominal]

Internal oblique

Greater omentum

External oblique

Ascending colon, free tenia

Sigmoid colon

Cecum

Parietal peritoneum

Ileum

Lateral umbilical fold [epigastric fold] (inferior epigastric artery and vein)

Arcuate line

Medial umbilical fold (cord of umbilical artery)

Median umbilical fold (median umbilical ligament)

Fig. 998 Position of abdominal viscera; greater omentum; ventral aspect.
The lower part of the peritoneal cavity is also called "intestinal abdomen."

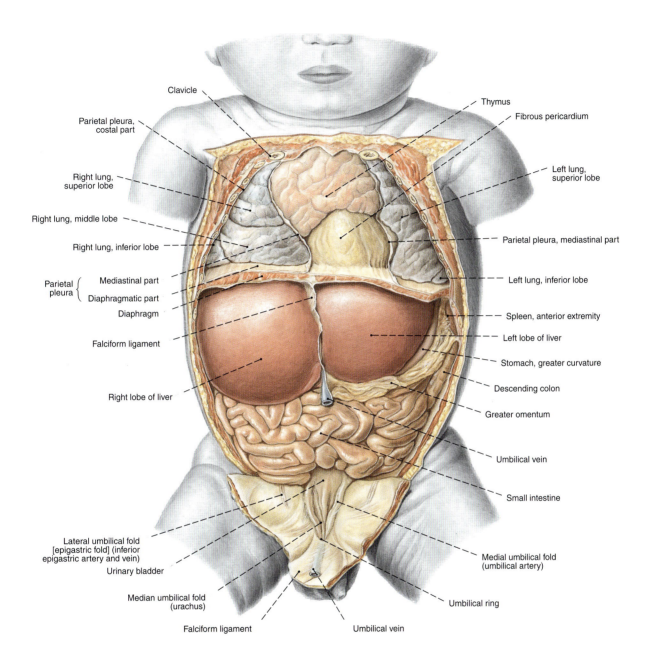

Clavicle

Parietal pleura,
costal part

Right lung,
superior lobe

Right lung, middle lobe

Right lung, inferior lobe

Parietal { Mediastinal part
pleura { Diaphragmatic part

Diaphragm

Falciform ligament

Right lobe of liver

Lateral umbilical fold
[epigastric fold] (inferior
epigastric artery and vein)

Urinary bladder

Median umbilical fold
(urachus)

Falciform ligament

Thymus

Fibrous pericardium

Left lung,
superior lobe

Parietal pleura, mediastinal part

Left lung, inferior lobe

Spleen, anterior extremity

Left lobe of liver

Stomach, greater curvature

Descending colon

Greater omentum

Umbilical vein

Small intestine

Medial umbilical fold
(umbilical artery)

Umbilical ring

Umbilical vein

Fig. 999 Position of viscera in the newborn; anterior
thoracic and abdominal walls, as well as parts of
diaphragm, removed; ventral aspect.
Note the relative size of the liver, the limited extension of
the greater omentum, and the size of the medial
umbilical folds and the umbilical vein compared to that of
the adult (Fig. 998).

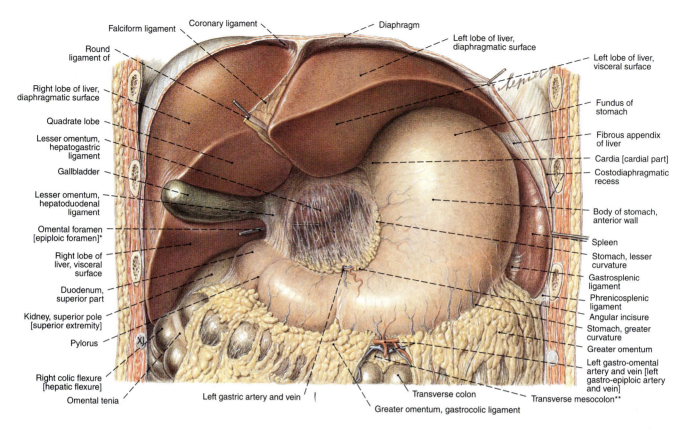

Falciform ligament
Coronary ligament
Diaphragm
Left lobe of liver, diaphragmatic surface
Left lobe of liver, visceral surface
Round ligament of
Right lobe of liver, diaphragmatic surface
Quadrate lobe
Lesser omentum, hepatogastric ligament
Gallbladder
Lesser omentum, hepatoduodenal ligament
Omental foramen [epiploic foramen]*
Right lobe of liver, visceral surface
Duodenum, superior part
Kidney, superior pole [superior extremity]
Pylorus
Right colic flexure [hepatic flexure]
Omental tenia
Left gastric artery and vein
Greater omentum, gastrocolic ligament
Transverse colon
Transverse mesocolon**
Fundus of stomach
Fibrous appendix of liver
Cardia [cardial part]
Costodiaphragmatic recess
Body of stomach, anterior wall
Spleen
Stomach, lesser curvature
Gastrosplenic ligament
Phrenicosplenic ligament
Angular incisure
Stomach, greater curvature
Greater omentum
Left gastro-omental artery and vein [left gastro-epiploic artery and vein]

Fig. 1000   Position of viscera in the upper abdomen; anterior thoracic and abdominal walls, as well as parts of diaphragm, removed; ventral aspect.

This part of the peritoneal cavity is also called "glandular abdomen."

* Also: foramen of WINSLOW.

** Omental bursa [lesser sac] partially opened.

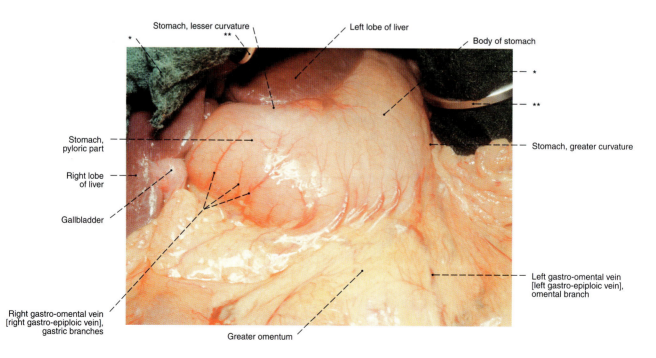

Stomach, lesser curvature
Left lobe of liver
Body of stomach
Stomach, pyloric part
Right lobe of liver
Gallbladder
Right gastro-omental vein [right gastro-epiploic vein], gastric branches
Greater omentum
Stomach, greater curvature
Left gastro-omental vein [left gastro-epiploic vein], omental branch

Fig. 1001   Stomach; greater omentum; intra-operative photograph; organs in natural positions; ventral aspect.

* Surgical drape.

** Surgical hook.

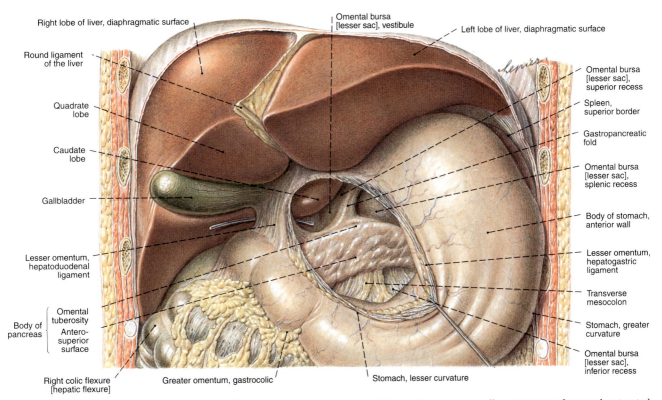

Right lobe of liver, diaphragmatic surface
Round ligament of the liver
Quadrate lobe
Caudate lobe
Gallbladder
Lesser omentum, hepatoduodenal ligament
Body of pancreas
{ Omental tuberosity
Antero-superior surface }
Right colic flexure [hepatic flexure]
Greater omentum, gastrocolic

Omental bursa [lesser sac], vestibule
Left lobe of liver, diaphragmatic surface
Omental bursa [lesser sac], superior recess
Spleen, superior border
Gastropancreatic fold
Omental bursa [lesser sac], splenic recess
Body of stomach, anterior wall
Lesser omentum, hepatogastric ligament
Transverse mesocolon
Stomach, greater curvature
Omental bursa [lesser sac], inferior recess
Stomach, lesser curvature

Fig. 1002 Upper abdominal viscera; parts of lesser omentum (hepatogastric ligament) removed to expose omental bursa [lesser sac] and body of pancreas; smaller curvature of stomach retracted inferiorly to the right; ventral aspect.

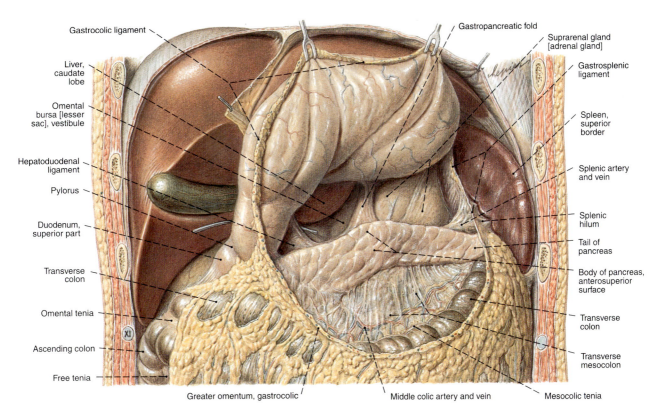

Gastrocolic ligament
Liver, caudate lobe
Omental bursa [lesser sac], vestibule
Hepatoduodenal ligament
Pylorus
Duodenum, superior part
Transverse colon
Omental tenia
Ascending colon
Free tenia
Greater omentum, gastrocolic

Gastropancreatic fold
Suprarenal gland [adrenal gland]
Gastrosplenic ligament
Spleen, superior border
Splenic artery and vein
Splenic hilum
Tail of pancreas
Body of pancreas, anterosuperior surface
Transverse colon
Transverse mesocolon
Middle colic artery and vein
Mesocolic tenia

Fig. 1003 Liver; stomach; pancreas; spleen; greater omentum severed in the gastrocolic ligament; greater curvature of stomach retracted superiorly by a hook to expose omental bursa [lesser sac]; ventral aspect.

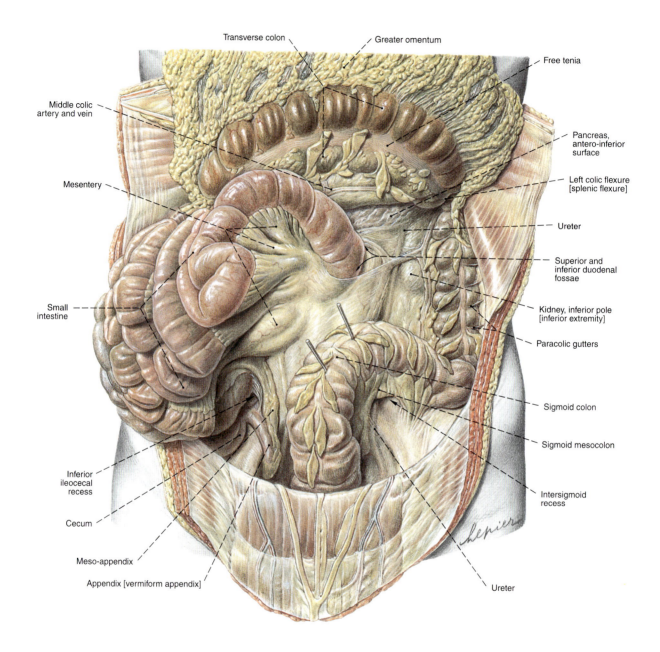

Transverse colon

Greater omentum

Free tenia

Middle colic artery and vein

Pancreas, antero-inferior surface

Mesentery

Left colic flexure [splenic flexure]

Ureter

Superior and inferior duodenal fossae

Small intestine

Kidney, inferior pole [inferior extremity]

Paracolic gutters

Sigmoid colon

Sigmoid mesocolon

Inferior ileocecal recess

Intersigmoid recess

Cecum

Meso-appendix

Appendix [vermiform appendix]

Ureter

Fig. 1006   Small and large intestines; greater omentum and transverse colon reflected cranially, small intestine retracted laterally to the right; sigmoid colon retracted to the right by a hook; ventral aspect.

The recesses/ fossae/ spaces at the changes between retroperitoneal and intraperitoneal parts of the intestine vary considerably.

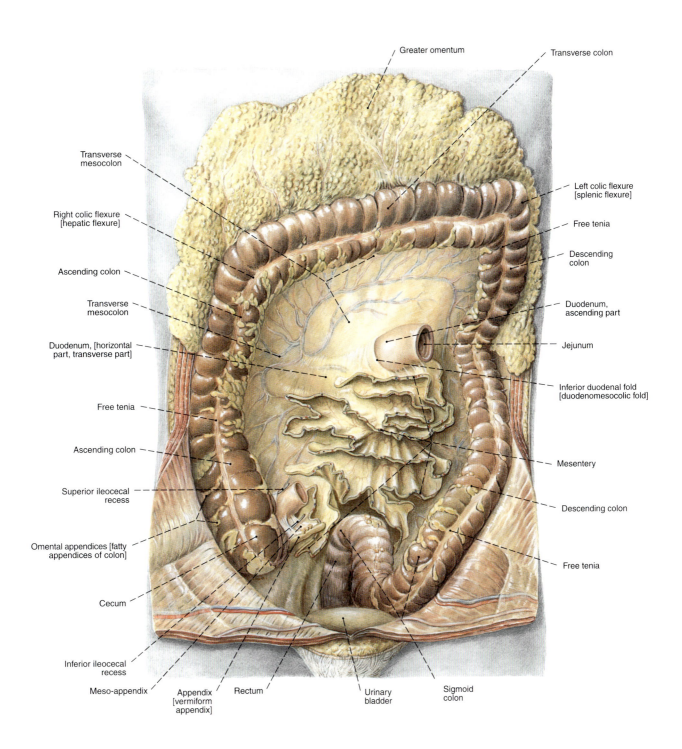

Greater omentum

Transverse colon

Transverse mesocolon

Left colic flexure [splenic flexure]

Right colic flexure [hepatic flexure]

Free tenia

Ascending colon

Descending colon

Transverse mesocolon

Duodenum, ascending part

Duodenum, [horizontal part, transverse part]

Jejunum

Inferior duodenal fold [duodenomesocolic fold]

Free tenia

Ascending colon

Mesentery

Superior ileocecal recess

Descending colon

Omental appendices [fatty appendices of colon]

Free tenia

Cecum

Inferior ileocecal recess

Meso-appendix

Appendix [vermiform appendix]

Rectum

Urinary bladder

Sigmoid colon

Fig. 1007   Mesentery; large intestine; greater omentum and transverse colon reflected cranially, small intestine severed next to the duodenojejunal flexure, at the terminal ileum and at the mesentery, and then removed; ventral aspect.

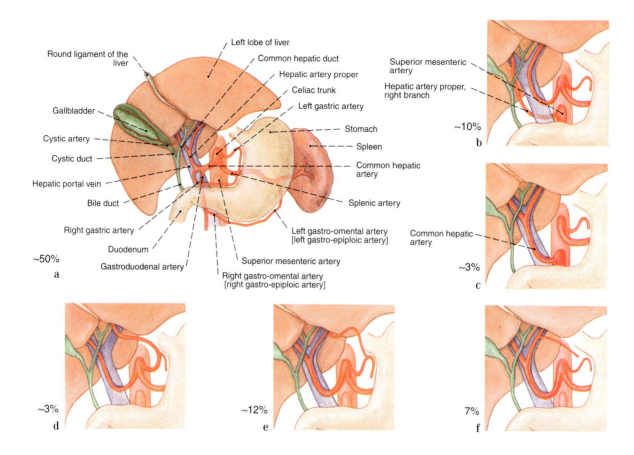

Fig. 1013 a-d   Variations in the blood supply of the liver.

a   "Normal textbook case"

b   Superior mesenteric artery, participating in the supply of the right lobe of liver

c   Common hepatic artery, originating from the superior mesenteric artery

d   Left gastric artery, supplying the left lobe of liver

e   Branch of left gastric artery, participating in the supply of the left lobe of liver, in addition to left branch of hepatic artery proper

f   Accessory branch of hepatic artery proper, supplying the lesser curvature of the stomach

In 25% the superior mesenteric artery participates in the arterial blood supply of the liver.

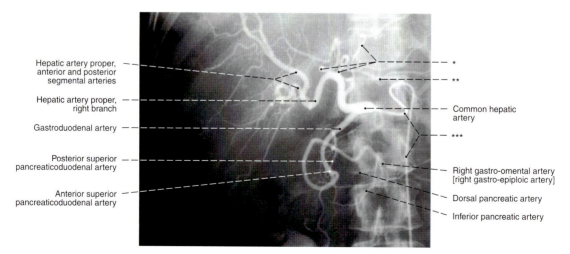

Fig. 1014   Common hepatic artery; AP radiograph after selective injection of contrast medium into the common hepatic artery; ventral aspect.

   * Branches to the left lobe of liver, replacing the left branch of hepatic artery proper.

   ** Accessory branch from the hepatic artery to the lesser curvature of the stomach.

   *** Catheter in aorta.

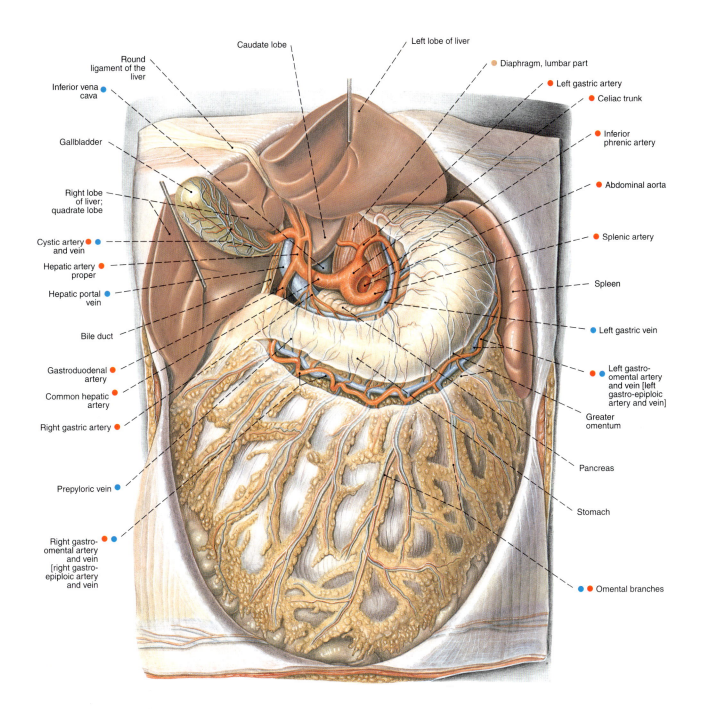

Caudate lobe

Left lobe of liver

Round ligament of the liver

Diaphragm, lumbar part

Inferior vena cava

Left gastric artery

Celiac trunk

Gallbladder

Inferior phrenic artery

Right lobe of liver; quadrate lobe

Abdominal aorta

Cystic artery and vein

Splenic artery

Hepatic artery proper

Spleen

Hepatic portal vein

Bile duct

Left gastric vein

Gastroduodenal artery

Left gastro-omental artery and vein [left gastro-epiploic artery and vein]

Common hepatic artery

Greater omentum

Right gastric artery

Pancreas

Prepyloric vein

Stomach

Right gastro-omental artery and vein [right gastro-epiploic artery and vein

Omental branches

Fig. 1015 Blood vessels of the upper abdomen; lesser omentum removed to expose celiac trunk and its branches; the gastrocolic ligament and the gastro-omental [gastro-epiploic] arteries and veins dissected at the greater curvature of the stomach; the vestibule of the omental bursa [lesser sac] opened; ventral aspect.

The distance of the arteries from the lesser and greater curvature is variable.

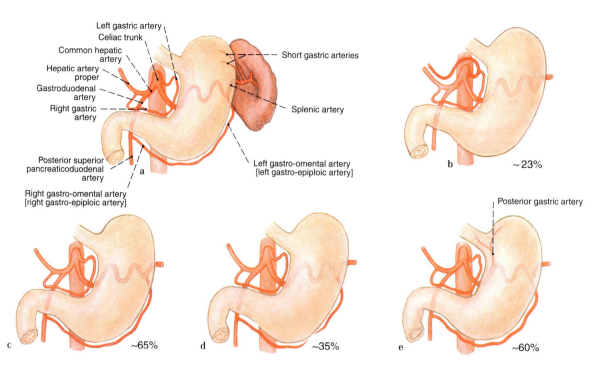

Fig. 1016 a-d   Variations in the arterial blood supply of the stomach.

  a   "Normal textbook case," closed arcade at the lesser and greater curvature

  b   Left gastric artery participating in the supply of the left lobe of liver

  c   Anastomosis between right and left gastro-omental

arteries [left gastro-epiploic arteries] at greater curvature (closed arcade)

  d   No anastomosis between right and left gastro-omental arteries [left gastro-epiploic arteries] at greater curvature (not closed arcade)

  e   Accessory posterior gastric artery branching off the splenic artery and supplying the posterior wall of stomach

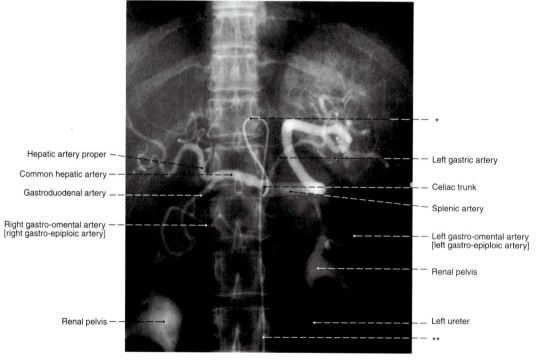

Fig. 1017   Arteries of stomach, spleen, and liver; AP radiograph after selective injection of contrast medium into the celiac trunk (celiac arteriography) and simultaneous visualization of the renal pelvis after intravenous injection of a renal-excreted contrast medium; ventral aspect.

  * Loop of catheter in aorta.

  * * Catheter in aorta.

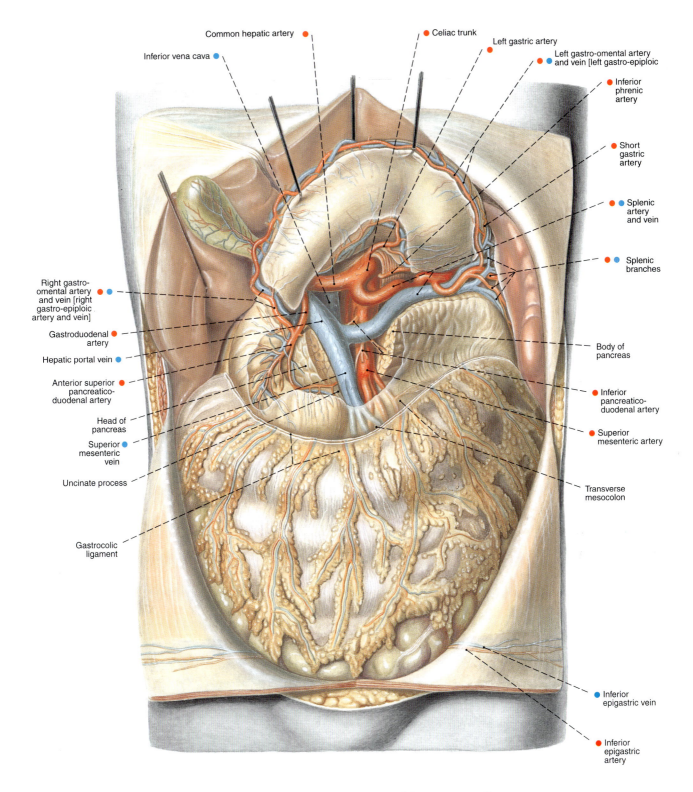

Common hepatic artery

Inferior vena cava

Celiac trunk

Left gastric artery

Left gastro-omental artery
and vein [left gastro-epiploic

Inferior
phrenic
artery

Short
gastric
artery

Splenic
artery
and vein

Splenic
branches

Right gastro-
omental artery
and vein [right
gastro-epiploic
artery and vein]

Gastroduodenal
artery

Hepatic portal vein

Anterior superior
pancreatico-
duodenal artery

Head of
pancreas

Superior
mesenteric
vein

Uncinate process

Gastrocolic
ligament

Body of
pancreas

Inferior
pancreatico-
duodenal artery

Superior
mesenteric artery

Transverse
mesocolon

Inferior
epigastric vein

Inferior
epigastric
artery

Fig. 1018   Blood vessels of the upper abdomen; gastrocolic
ligament severed; stomach retracted cranially by a hook to
expose celiac trunk; body of pancreas partially removed to
expose the junction of the splenic and superior mesenteric
veins; omental bursa [lesser sac] opened; ventral aspect.

The uncinate process of pancreas frequently pushes
far behind the mesenteric blood vessels.

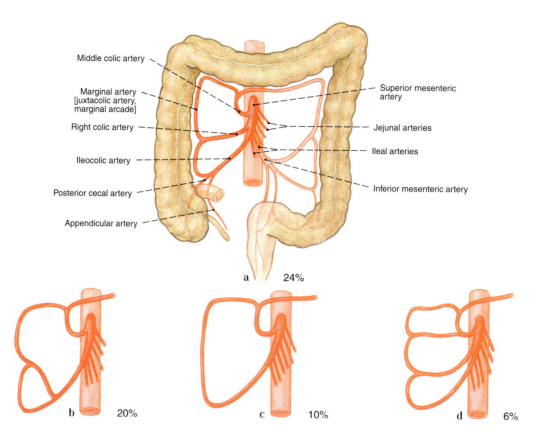

Middle colic artery

Marginal artery
[juxtacolic artery,
marginal arcade]

Right colic artery

Ileocolic artery

Posterior cecal artery

Appendicular artery

Superior mesenteric
artery

Jejunal arteries

Ileal arteries

Inferior mesenteric artery

a   24%

b   20%   c   10%   d   6%

Fig. 1019 a-d   Variations in the branches of the superior mesenteric artery to the large intestine.

a   "Normal textbook case," ascending and transverse colon supplied by three branches

b   Trunk-formation of ileocolic and right colic arteries
c   Two branches only with right colic artery absent
d   Double right colic artery

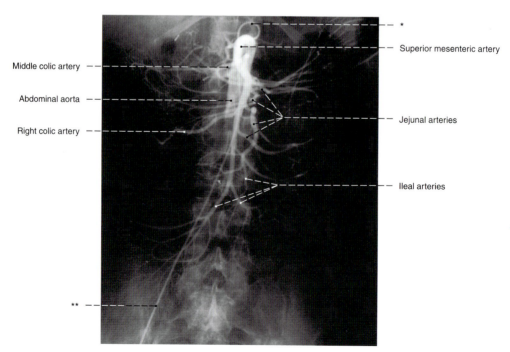

Middle colic artery

Abdominal aorta

Right colic artery

*

Superior mesenteric artery

Jejunal arteries

Ileal arteries

**

Fig. 1020   Superior mesenteric artery; AP radiograph after selective injection of contrast medium into the beginning of the superior mesenteric artery; ventral aspect.

* Catheter in aorta.
** Catheter in the common iliac artery.

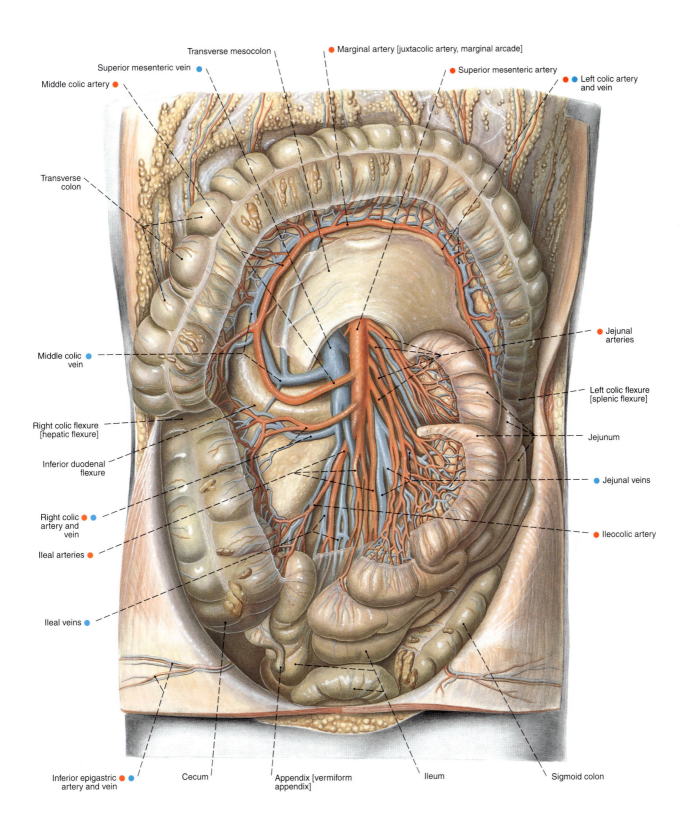

Transverse mesocolon

● Marginal artery [juxtacolic artery, marginal arcade]

Superior mesenteric vein ●

● Superior mesenteric artery

Middle colic artery ●

●● Left colic artery and vein

Transverse colon

●● Jejunal arteries

Middle colic vein ●

Left colic flexure [splenic flexure]

Right colic flexure [hepatic flexure]

Jejunum

Inferior duodenal flexure

●● Jejunal veins

Right colic artery and vein ●●

Ileal arteries ●

● Ileocolic artery

Ileal veins ●

Inferior epigastric artery and vein ●●

Cecum

Appendix [vermiform appendix]

Ileum

Sigmoid colon

Fig. 1021   Blood vessels of the lower abdomen; greater omentum and transverse colon retracted cranially; small intestine displaced to the left and visceral peritoneum partially removed to expose the blood vessels; ventral aspect. The arteries of the small intestine form arcades.

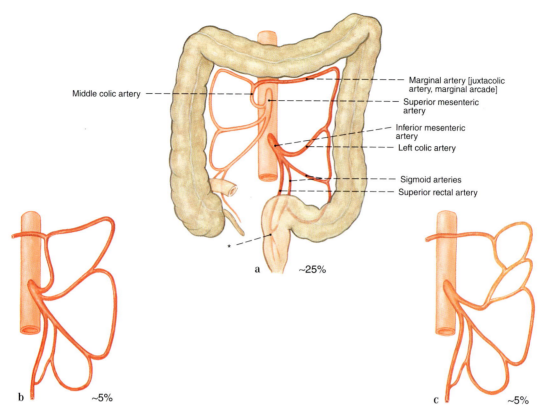

Middle colic artery

Marginal artery [juxtacolic artery, marginal arcade]

Superior mesenteric artery

Inferior mesenteric artery

Left colic artery

Sigmoid arteries

Superior rectal artery

a   ~25%

b   ~5%

c   ~5%

Fig. 1022 a-c   Variations in the branches of the inferior mesenteric artery.

a   Trifurcating trunk supplying the descending colon, the sigmoid colon, and the rectum

b   Accessory middle colic artery from the inferior mesenteric artery

c   Accessory middle colic artery from the left colic artery

* Clinically: critical point of SUDECK.

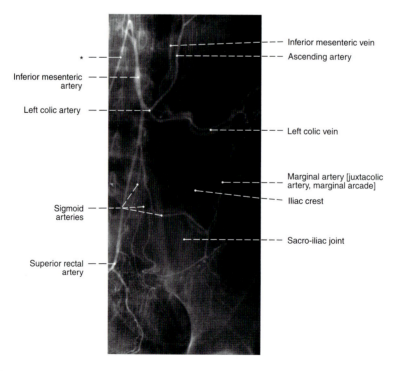

Inferior mesenteric vein

Ascending artery

*

Inferior mesenteric artery

Left colic artery

Left colic vein

Marginal artery [juxtacolic artery, marginal arcade]

Iliac crest

Sigmoid arteries

Sacro-iliac joint

Superior rectal artery

Fig. 1023   Inferior mesenteric artery; AP radiograph after selective injection of contrast medium into the beginning of the inferior mesenteric artery; ventral aspect.

The contrast medium partially runs off the colon already; therefore, the veins are also visible.

* Catheter in aorta.

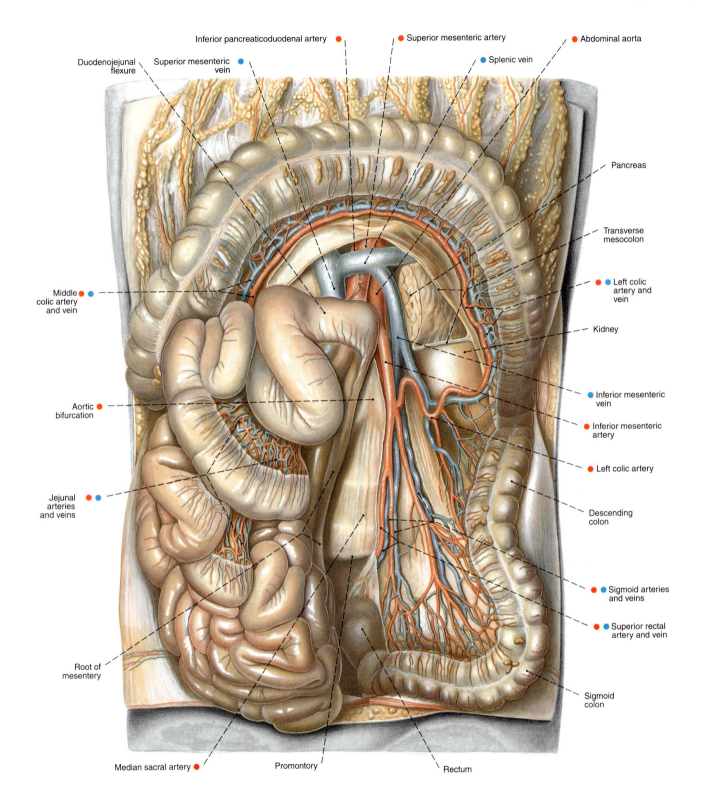

Inferior pancreaticoduodenal artery ●   ● Superior mesenteric artery   ● Abdominal aorta

Duodenojejunal flexure   Superior mesenteric vein ●   ● Splenic vein

Pancreas

Transverse mesocolon

● ● Left colic artery and vein

Kidney

Middle colic artery and vein ● ●

Inferior mesenteric vein ●

Inferior mesenteric artery ●

Aortic bifurcation ●

● Left colic artery

Descending colon

Jejunal arteries and veins ● ●

● ● Sigmoid arteries and veins

Root of mesentery

● ● Superior rectal artery and vein

Sigmoid colon

Median sacral artery ●   Promontory   Rectum

Fig. 1024   Inferior mesenteric artery and vein; small intestine displaced to the right; transverse colon retracted cranially; peritoneum removed to expose the blood vessels of descending and sigmoid colon; ventral aspect.

The connections of the left and middle colic arteries is accomplished by the marginal artery [juxtacolic artery, marginal arcade].

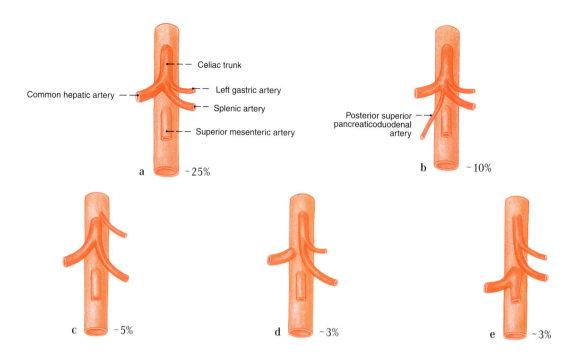

Fig. 1025 a-e   Variations of the celiac trunk.
a   "Normal textbook case", trifurcating trunk
b   Division into four branches
c   Formation of a hepatosplenic trunk
d   Formation of a gastrosplenic trunk
e   Formation of a gastrosplenic trunk and a hepatomesenteric trunk

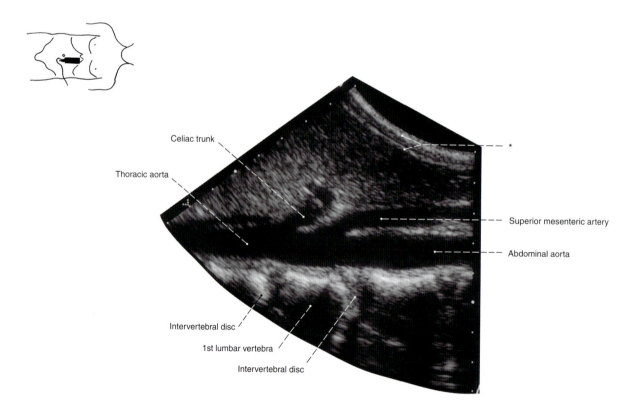

Fig. 1026   Abdominal aorta; ultrasound scan in nearly sagittal plane. Note the short distance between celiac trunk and superior mesenteric artery, which runs partially parallel to the abdominal aorta.
* Abdominal wall.

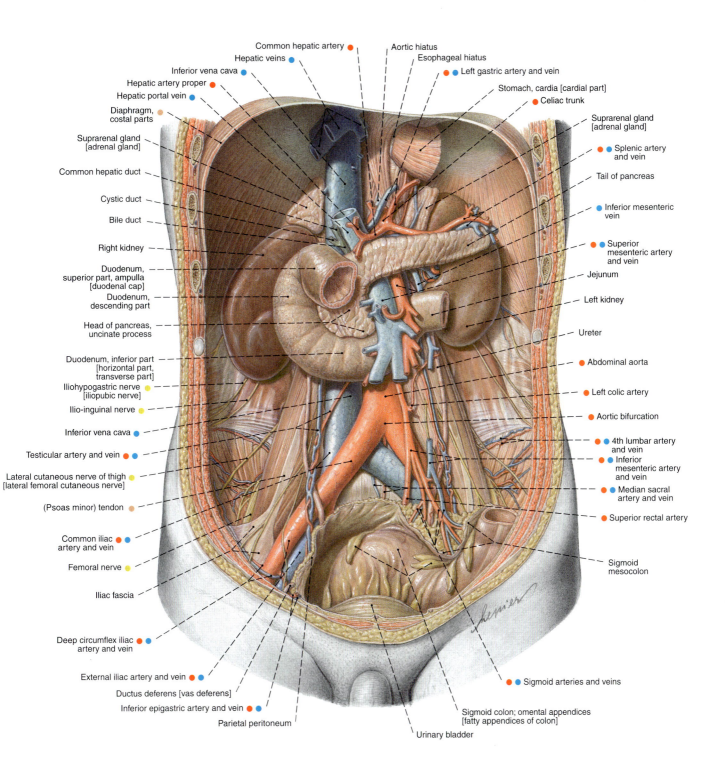

Common hepatic artery
Hepatic veins
Inferior vena cava
Hepatic artery proper
Hepatic portal vein
Diaphragm, costal parts
Suprarenal gland [adrenal gland]
Common hepatic duct
Cystic duct
Bile duct
Right kidney
Duodenum, superior part, ampulla [duodenal cap]
Duodenum, descending part
Head of pancreas, uncinate process
Duodenum, inferior part [horizontal part, transverse part]
Iliohypogastric nerve [iliopubic nerve]
Ilio-inguinal nerve
Inferior vena cava
Testicular artery and vein
Lateral cutaneous nerve of thigh [lateral femoral cutaneous nerve]
(Psoas minor) tendon
Common iliac artery and vein
Femoral nerve
Iliac fascia
Deep circumflex iliac artery and vein
External iliac artery and vein
Ductus deferens [vas deferens]
Inferior epigastric artery and vein
Parietal peritoneum

Aortic hiatus
Esophageal hiatus
Left gastric artery and vein
Stomach, cardia [cardial part]
Celiac trunk
Suprarenal gland [adrenal gland]
Splenic artery and vein
Tail of pancreas
Inferior mesenteric vein
Superior mesenteric artery and vein
Jejunum
Left kidney
Ureter
Abdominal aorta
Left colic artery
Aortic bifurcation
4th lumbar artery and vein
Inferior mesenteric artery and vein
Median sacral artery and vein
Superior rectal artery
Sigmoid mesocolon
Sigmoid arteries and veins
Sigmoid colon; omental appendices [fatty appendices of colon]
Urinary bladder

Fig. 1027 **Retroperitoneal space in the male; parietal** peritoneum extensively removed; ventral aspect.

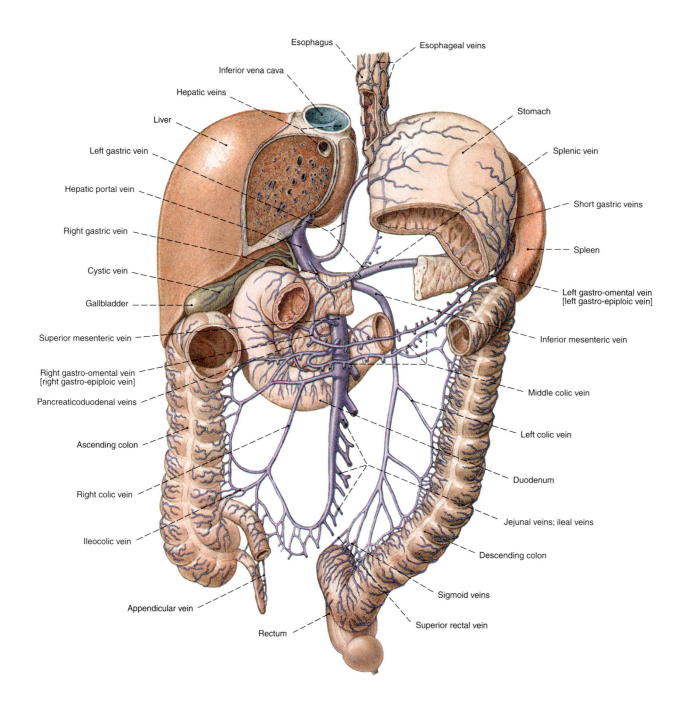

Esophagus

Esophageal veins

Inferior vena cava

Hepatic veins

Liver

Stomach

Left gastric vein

Splenic vein

Hepatic portal vein

Short gastric veins

Right gastric vein

Cystic vein

Spleen

Gallbladder

Left gastro-omental vein
[left gastro-epiploic vein]

Superior mesenteric vein

Inferior mesenteric vein

Right gastro-omental vein
[right gastro-epiploic vein]

Pancreaticoduodenal veins

Middle colic vein

Ascending colon

Left colic vein

Right colic vein

Duodenum

Ileocolic vein

Jejunal veins; ileal veins

Descending colon

Appendicular vein

Sigmoid veins

Rectum

Superior rectal vein

Fig. 1028   Tributaries of hepatic portal vein; parts
of stomach and transverse colon and also larger
parts of jejunum and ileum removed; ventral aspect.

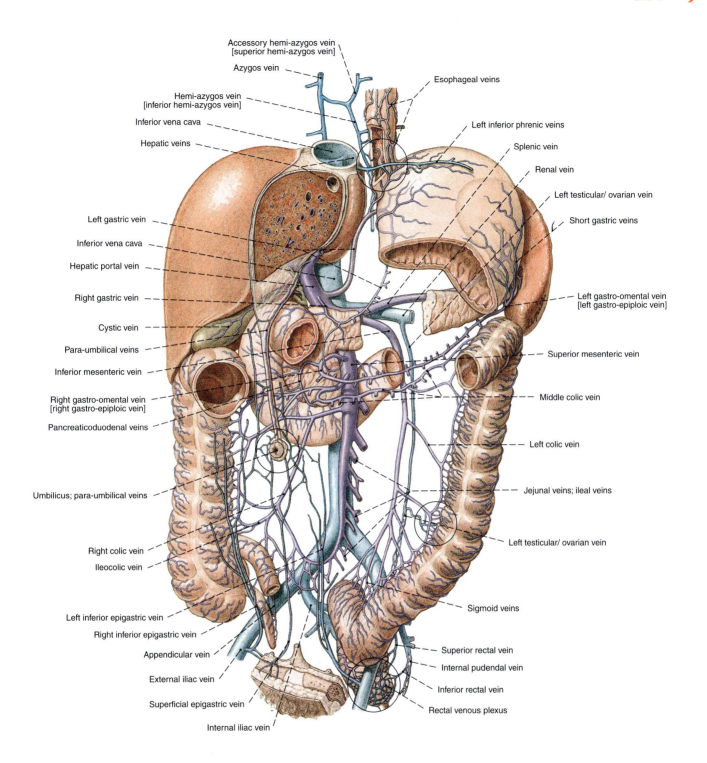

Accessory hemi-azygos vein [superior hemi-azygos vein]

Azygos vein

Hemi-azygos vein [inferior hemi-azygos vein]

Inferior vena cava

Hepatic veins

Left gastric vein

Inferior vena cava

Hepatic portal vein

Right gastric vein

Cystic vein

Para-umbilical veins

Inferior mesenteric vein

Right gastro-omental vein [right gastro-epiploic vein]

Pancreaticoduodenal veins

Umbilicus; para-umbilical veins

Right colic vein

Ileocolic vein

Left inferior epigastric vein

Right inferior epigastric vein

Appendicular vein

External iliac vein

Superficial epigastric vein

Internal iliac vein

Esophageal veins

Left inferior phrenic veins

Splenic vein

Renal vein

Left testicular/ ovarian vein

Short gastric veins

Left gastro-omental vein [left gastro-epiploic vein]

Superior mesenteric vein

Middle colic vein

Left colic vein

Jejunal veins; ileal veins

Left testicular/ ovarian vein

Sigmoid veins

Superior rectal vein

Internal pudendal vein

Inferior rectal vein

Rectal venous plexus

Fig. 1029   Connections between tributaries of hepatic portal vein and inferior vena cava; ventral aspect. These connections–indicated by circles–are called "portocaval anastomoses."

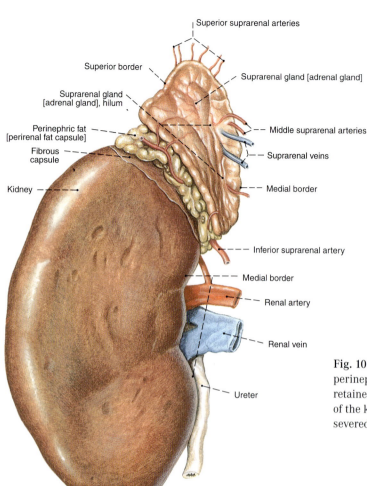

Superior suprarenal arteries

Superior border

Suprarenal gland [adrenal gland], hilum

Perinephric fat [perirenal fat capsule]

Fibrous capsule

Kidney

Suprarenal gland [adrenal gland]

Middle suprarenal arteries

Suprarenal veins

Medial border

Inferior suprarenal artery

Medial border

Renal artery

Renal vein

Ureter

Fig. 1030   Right kidney; suprarenal gland [adrenal gland]; perinephric fat [perirenal fat capsule] and fibrous capsule retained at the superior pole [superior extremity] of the kidney; renal artery and vein, as well as ureter, severed close to the hilum of kidney; ventral aspect.

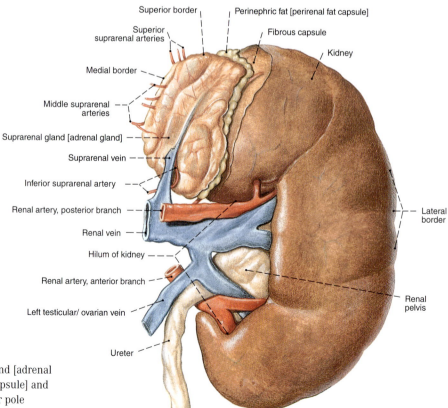

Superior border

Perinephric fat [perirenal fat capsule]

Superior suprarenal arteries

Fibrous capsule

Kidney

Medial border

Middle suprarenal arteries

Suprarenal gland [adrenal gland]

Suprarenal vein

Inferior suprarenal artery

Renal artery, posterior branch

Renal vein

Hilum of kidney

Renal artery, anterior branch

Left testicular/ ovarian vein

Ureter

Lateral border

Renal pelvis

Fig. 1031   Left kidney; suprarenal gland [adrenal gland]; perinephric fat [perirenal fat capsule] and fibrous capsule retained at the superior pole [superior extremity] of the kidney; ventral aspect.

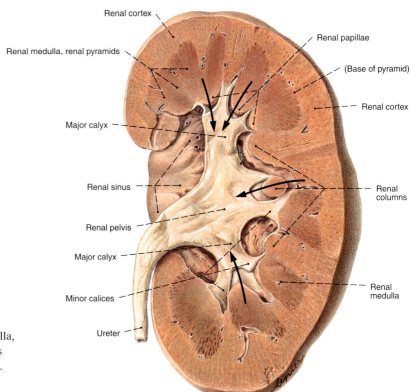

Renal cortex

Renal medulla, renal pyramids

Renal papillae

(Base of pyramid)

Renal cortex

Major calyx

Renal sinus

Renal columns

Renal pelvis

Major calyx

Renal medulla

Minor calices

Ureter

Fig. 1032   Left kidney; oblique vertical hemisection showing renal cortex, renal medulla, and renal pelvis after removal of blood vessels and fat body of the renal sinus; ventral aspect.

Arrows point from the renal pyramids toward the calices.

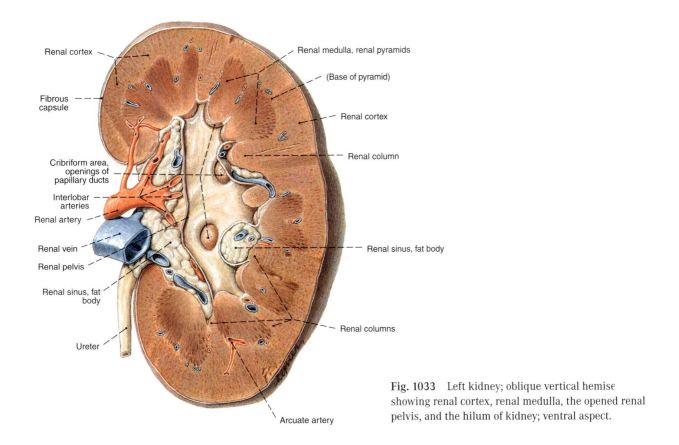

Renal cortex

Renal medulla, renal pyramids

(Base of pyramid)

Fibrous capsule

Renal cortex

Renal column

Cribriform area, openings of papillary ducts

Interlobar arteries

Renal artery

Renal vein

Renal sinus, fat body

Renal pelvis

Renal sinus, fat body

Ureter

Renal columns

Arcuate artery

Fig. 1033   Left kidney; oblique vertical hemise showing renal cortex, renal medulla, the opened renal pelvis, and the hilum of kidney; ventral aspect.

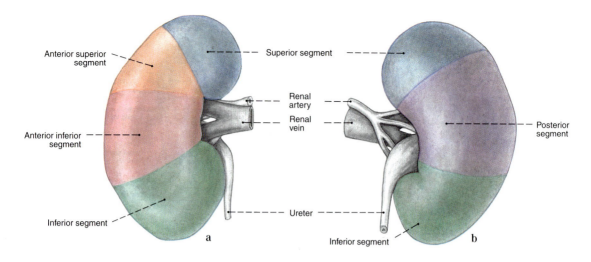

Fig. 1039 a, b   Renal segments of right kidney; individual
segments are indicated by same colors.

a   Ventral aspect
b   Dorsal aspect

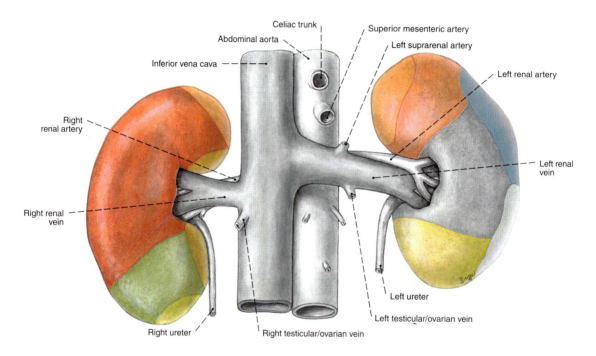

Fig. 1040   Kidney and neighboring organs on the
ventral surface; ventral aspect.

Contact areas of kidneys

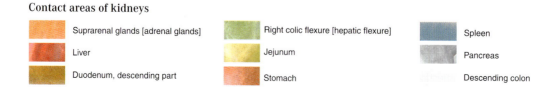

Suprarenal glands [adrenal glands]

Liver

Duodenum, descending part

Right colic flexure [hepatic flexure]

Jejunum

Stomach

Spleen

Pancreas

Descending colon

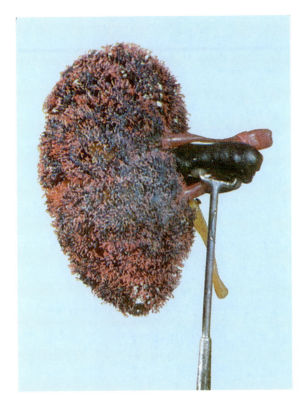

Fig. 1041 Right renal arteries and veins; renal pelvis; corrosion cast after injection of colored polymer into the renal blood vessels and into the renal pelvis (arteries: red, veins: blue, renal pelvis: yellow); ventral aspect.

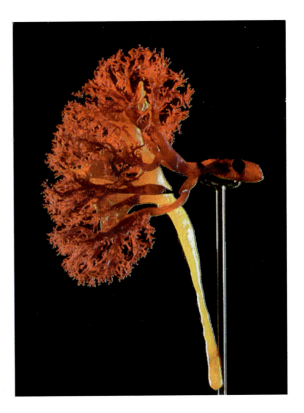

Fig. 1042 Right renal arteries and renal pelvis; corrosion cast after injection of red polymer into the renal arteries and yellow polymer into the ureter; ventral aspect.

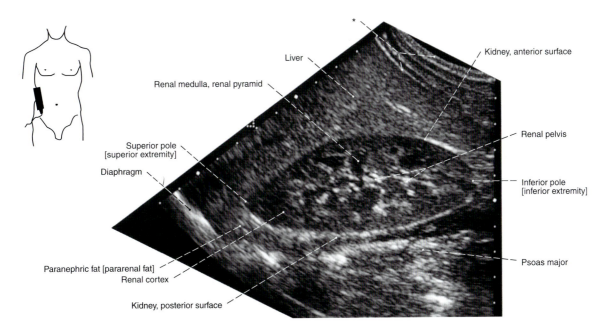

Fig. 1043 Right kidney; ultrasound scan; transducer directed from ventrocaudal to dorsocaudal; lateral aspect.

In addition to the renal pelvis, both the renal cortex and the renal medulla are distinguishable.

* Abdominal wall.

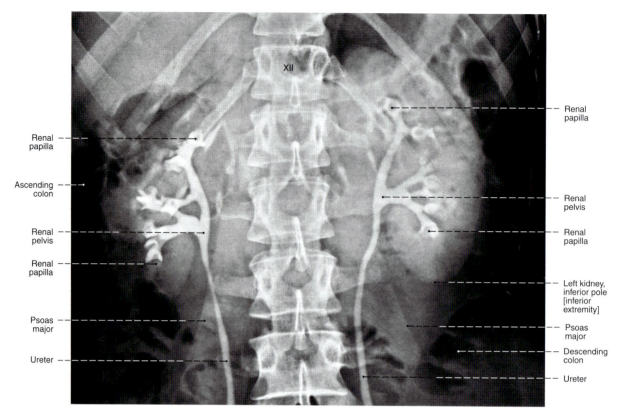

XII

Renal
papilla

Ascending
colon

Renal
pelvis

Renal
papilla

Psoas
major

Ureter

Renal
papilla

Renal
pelvis

Renal
papilla

Left kidney,
inferior pole
[inferior
extremity]

Psoas
major

Descending
colon

Ureter

Fig. 1044   Kidney; renal pelvis; ureter; AP radiograph after retrograde injection of contrast medium via both ureters, visualizing also the urine-draining systems within the kidneys; ventral aspect.

XII = 12th thoracic vertebra.

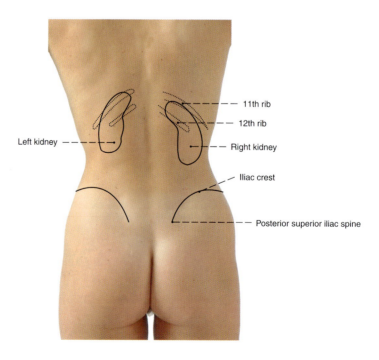

11th rib

12th rib

Left kidney

Right kidney

Iliac crest

Posterior superior iliac spine

Fig. 1045   Projection of kidneys onto the back. The longitudinal axes of the kidneys diverge caudolaterally. The right kidney is usually more caudal than the left.
Compare Fig. 1092.

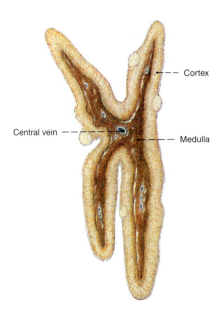

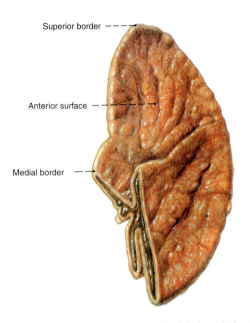

Fig. 1046   Right suprarenal gland [adrenal gland]; sagittal section; lateral aspect.

    The figure has been drawn from a fresh specimen. In fixed specimen color differentiation between cortex and medulla are less distinct.

Fig. 1047   Right suprarenal gland [adrenal gland]; the lower part sectioned sagittally; ventral aspect.
See also remarks for Fig. 1046.

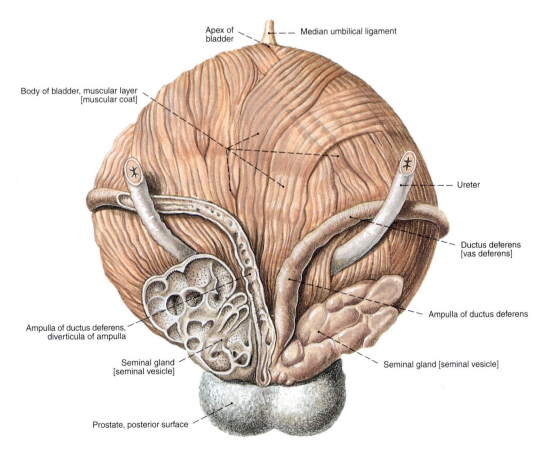

Fig. 1048   Urinary bladder; ductus deferentes [vasa deferentia]; seminal glands [seminal vesicles]; prostate; external muscular layer of urinary bladder dissected; left seminal gland [seminal vesicle] and ductus deferens [vas deferens] cut open.

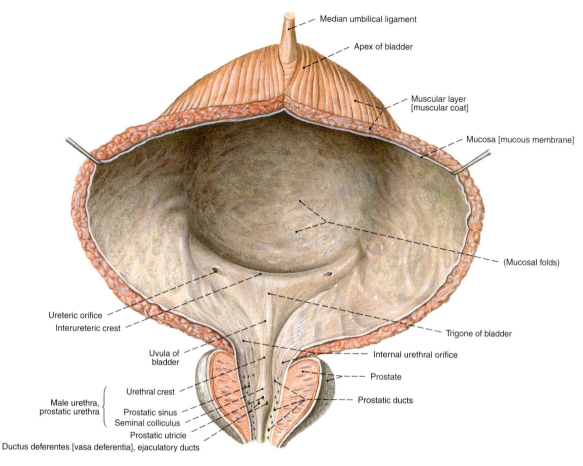

Median umbilical ligament

Apex of bladder

Muscular layer [muscular coat]

Mucosa [mucous membrane]

(Mucosal folds)

Ureteric orifice

Interureteric crest

Trigone of bladder

Uvula of bladder

Internal urethral orifice

Prostate

Prostatic ducts

Urethral crest

Male urethra, prostatic urethra

Prostatic sinus

Seminal colliculus

Prostatic utricle

Ductus deferentes [vasa deferentia], ejaculatory ducts

Fig. 1049 Urinary bladder; prostate; urethra; opened by a longitudinal median section; external muscular layer of urinary bladder dissected; ventral aspect.

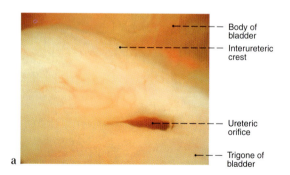

Body of bladder

Interureteric crest

Ureteric orifice

Trigone of bladder

a

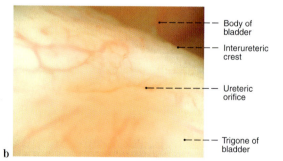

Body of bladder

Interureteric crest

Ureteric orifice

Trigone of bladder

b

Fig. 1050 a, b Urinary bladder; ureteric orifice visualized by an endoscope introduced through the urethra (cystoscopy).

a   ureteric orifice open, a peristaltic wave has transported urine into the urinary bladder

b   ureteric orifice closed

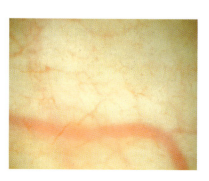

Fig. 1051 Urinary bladder; endoscopic view (cystoscopy) of mucosa [mucous membrane] of the body of bladder; inferior aspect.

In a full, healthy bladder no mucosal folds are visible.

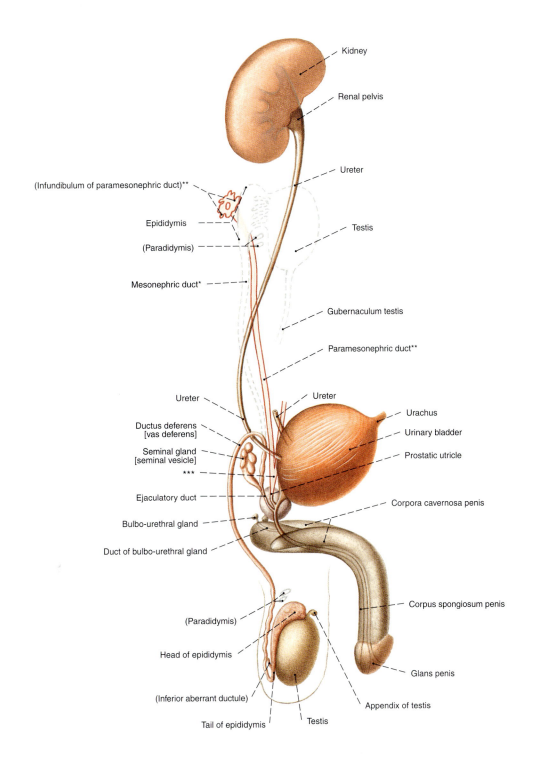

Kidney

Renal pelvis

Ureter

(Infundibulum of paramesonephric duct)**

Epididymis

(Paradidymis)

Mesonephric duct*

Testis

Gubernaculum testis

Paramesonephric duct**

Ureter

Ureter

Urachus

Ductus deferens [vas deferens]

Urinary bladder

Seminal gland [seminal vesicle]

Prostatic utricle

***

Ejaculatory duct

Corpora cavernosa penis

Bulbo-urethral gland

Duct of bulbo-urethral gland

Corpus spongiosum penis

(Paradidymis)

Head of epididymis

Glans penis

(Inferior aberrant ductule)

Appendix of testis

Tail of epididymis

Testis

Fig. 1052   Male urogenital organs; diagram of the development: degenerating parts: pale pink, positions before descensus testis in dotted lines; lateral aspect.

Epididymis = genital part of mesonephros
Paradidymis = renal part of mesonephros

* WOLFFIAN duct

** MUELLERIAN duct

*** junction of paramesonephric ducts (MUELLERIAN ducts)

Compare fig. 1062, development in the female.

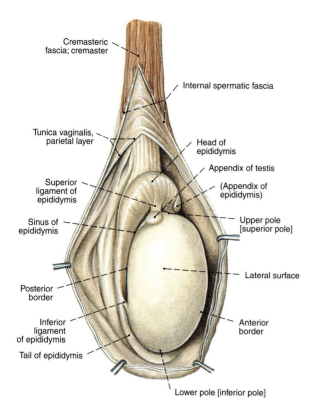

Cremasteric fascia; cremaster

Internal spermatic fascia

Tunica vaginalis, parietal layer

Head of epididymis

Appendix of testis

Superior ligament of epididymis

(Appendix of epididymis)

Sinus of epididymis

Upper pole [superior pole]

Lateral surface

Posterior border

Inferior ligament of epididymis

Anterior border

Tail of epididymis

Lower pole [inferior pole]

Fig. 1053 Right testis; epididymis; layers of scrotum opened stepwise; lateral aspect.

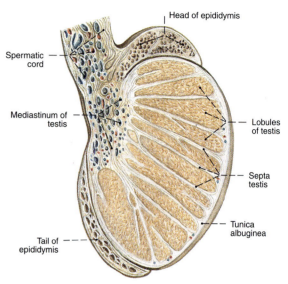

Head of epididymis

Spermatic cord

Mediastinum of testis

Lobules of testis

Septa testis

Tunica albuginea

Tail of epididymis

Fig. 1054 Right testis; epididymis; sagittal section; lateral aspect.

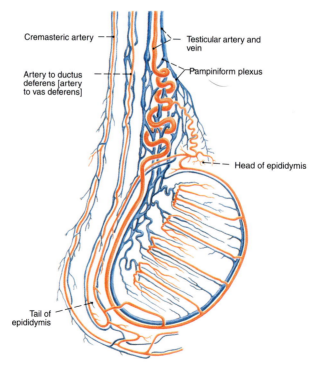

Cremasteric artery

Testicular artery and vein

Artery to ductus deferens [artery to vas deferens]

Pampiniform plexus

Head of epididymis

Tail of epididymis

Fig. 1055 Blood vessels of testis; epididymis, and spermatic cord; lateral aspect.
The arteries form anastomoses.

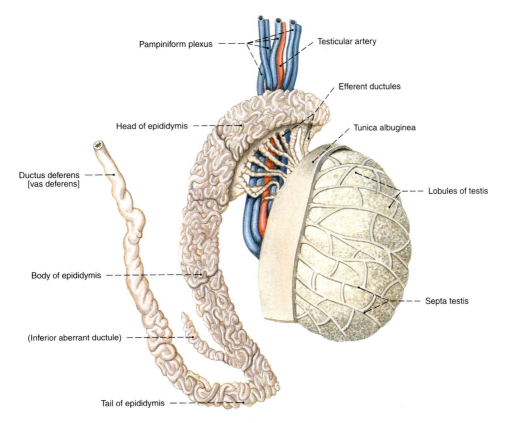

Pampiniform plexus

Testicular artery

Efferent ductules

Head of epididymis

Tunica albuginea

Ductus deferens [vas deferens]

Lobules of testis

Body of epididymis

Septa testis

(Inferior aberrant ductule)

Tail of epididymis

Fig. 1056   Testis; epididymis; ductus deferens [vas deferens]; tunica albuginea extensively removed to expose septa testis; epididymis retracted from testis and duct of epididymis dissected to show its tortuous course (length 5-6 m); lateral aspect.

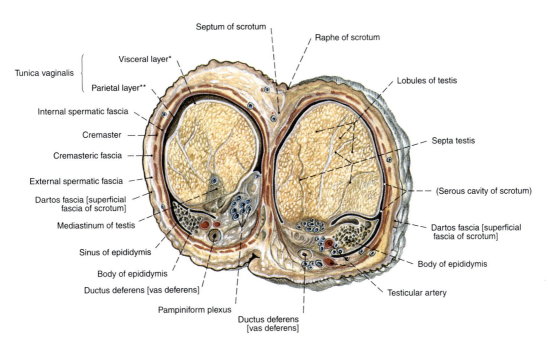

Septum of scrotum

Raphe of scrotum

Tunica vaginalis

Visceral layer*

Parietal layer**

Lobules of testis

Internal spermatic fascia

Cremaster

Septa testis

Cremasteric fascia

External spermatic fascia

(Serous cavity of scrotum)

Dartos fascia [superficial fascia of scrotum]

Mediastinum of testis

Dartos fascia [superficial fascia of scrotum]

Sinus of epididymis

Body of epididymis

Body of epididymis

Ductus deferens [vas deferens]

Testicular artery

Pampiniform plexus

Ductus deferens [vas deferens]

Fig. 1057   Testis; epididymis; scrotum; transverse section to expose the layers of scrotum and sheaths of testis; cranial aspect.
The cross sections are different in size because the testes generally do not lie at the same level in the scrotum.

* also: eporchium

** also: periorchiumAuch: Periorchium

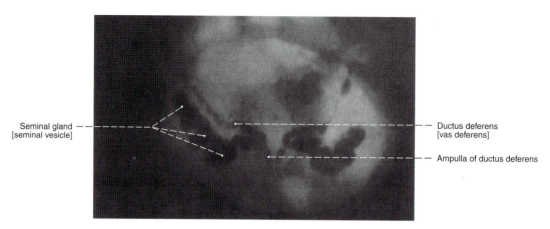

Seminal gland [seminal vesicle]

Ductus deferens [vas deferens]

Ampulla of ductus deferens

Fig. 1058   Ductus deferentes [vasa deferentia]; seminal glands [seminal vesicles]; AP radiograph after injection of contrast medium via the ejaculatory ducts; ventral aspect.

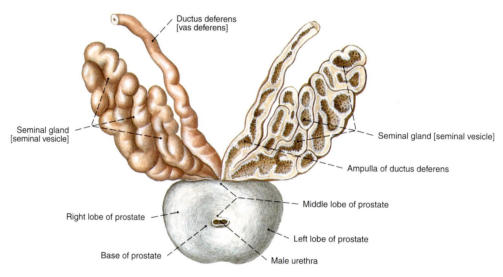

Ductus deferens [vas deferens]

Seminal gland [seminal vesicle]

Seminal gland [seminal vesicle]

Ampulla of ductus deferens

Middle lobe of prostate

Right lobe of prostate

Left lobe of prostate

Base of prostate

Male urethra

Fig. 1059   Ductus deferentes [vasa deferentia]; seminal glands [seminal vesicles]; prostate; exposure of prostate by sectioning the urethra below the urinary bladder; left ductus deferens [vas deferens] and seminal gland [seminal vesicle] opened with a longitudinal section; cranial aspect.

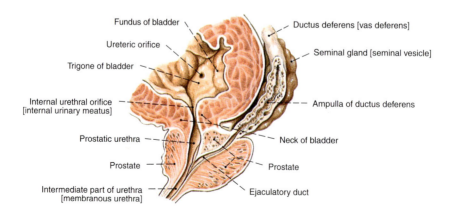

Fundus of bladder

Ureteric orifice

Trigone of bladder

Internal urethral orifice [internal urinary meatus]

Prostatic urethra

Prostate

Intermediate part of urethra [membranous urethra]

Ductus deferens [vas deferens]

Seminal gland [seminal vesicle]

Ampulla of ductus deferens

Neck of bladder

Prostate

Ejaculatory duct

Fig. 1060   Urinary bladder; prostate; ductus deferentes [vasa deferentia]; seminal glands [seminal vesicles]; oblique section to expose opening of left ejaculatory duct into the urethra; left lateral aspect.

The thickness of the muscular layer [muscular coat] of the bladder indicates a contracted empty bladder.

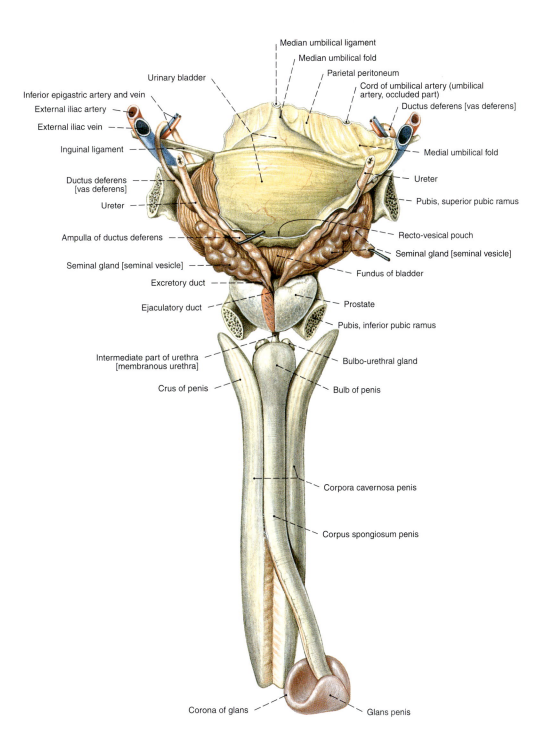

Median umbilical ligament

Median umbilical fold

Parietal peritoneum

Cord of umbilical artery (umbilical artery, occluded part)

Ductus deferens [vas deferens]

Urinary bladder

Inferior epigastric artery and vein

External iliac artery

External iliac vein

Inguinal ligament

Medial umbilical fold

Ductus deferens [vas deferens]

Ureter

Ampulla of ductus deferens

Seminal gland [seminal vesicle]

Excretory duct

Ejaculatory duct

Ureter

Pubis, superior pubic ramus

Recto-vesical pouch

Seminal gland [seminal vesicle]

Fundus of bladder

Prostate

Pubis, inferior pubic ramus

Intermediate part of urethra [membranous urethra]

Crus of penis

Bulbo-urethral gland

Bulb of penis

Corpora cavernosa penis

Corpus spongiosum penis

Corona of glans

Glans penis

Fig. 1061   Urinary bladder; ductus deferentes [vasa deferentia]; seminal glands [seminal vesicles]; prostate; male urethra; parts of pubis retained; a wedge-shaped part of the prostate removed to expose the left ejaculatory duct; distal part of corpus spongiosum penis retracted dorsally; dorsal aspect.

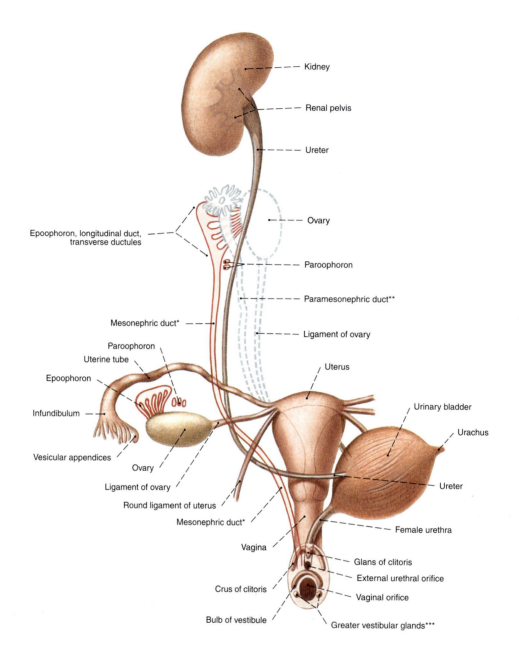

Kidney

Renal pelvis

Ureter

Ovary

Epoophoron, longitudinal duct, transverse ductules

Paroophoron

Paramesonephric duct**

Mesonephric duct*

Ligament of ovary

Paroophoron

Uterine tube

Epoophoron

Uterus

Infundibulum

Urinary bladder

Urachus

Vesicular appendices

Ovary

Ligament of ovary

Ureter

Round ligament of uterus

Mesonephric duct*

Female urethra

Vagina

Glans of clitoris

External urethral orifice

Crus of clitoris

Vaginal orifice

Bulb of vestibule

Greater vestibular glands***

Fig. 1062   Female urogenital organs; diagram of the development: degenerating parts: pale pink, positions before descensus ovarii in dotted lines; urinary bladder retracted laterally; ventral aspect.

Epoophoron = genital part of mesonephros.
Paroophoron = renal part of mesonephros.

* WOLFFIAN duct.
** MUELLERIAN duct.
*** BARTHOLIN's glands.

Compare Fig. 1052, development in the male.

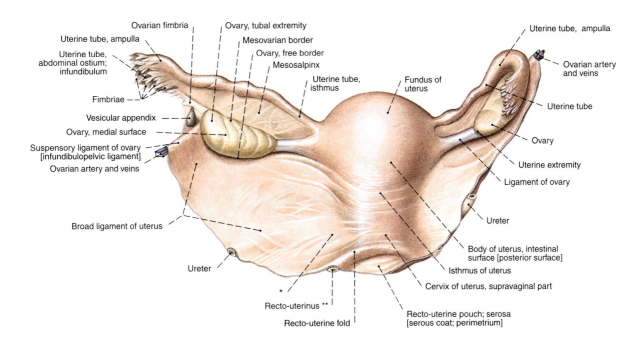

Ovarian fimbria
Ovary, tubal extremity
Mesovarian border
Uterine tube, ampulla
Ovary, free border
Uterine tube, abdominal ostium; infundibulum
Mesosalpinx
Uterine tube, ampulla
Uterine tube, isthmus
Fundus of uterus
Ovarian artery and veins
Fimbriae
Uterine tube
Vesicular appendix
Ovary, medial surface
Ovary
Suspensory ligament of ovary [infundibulopelvic ligament]
Uterine extremity
Ovarian artery and veins
Ligament of ovary
Ureter
Broad ligament of uterus
Body of uterus, intestinal surface [posterior surface]
Ureter
Isthmus of uterus
Cervix of uterus, supravaginal part
*
Recto-uterinus **
Recto-uterine pouch; serosa [serous coat; perimetrium]
Recto-uterine fold

Fig. 1063   Female internal genitalia; dorsal aspect.

* Clinically: cardinal ligament; see Fig. 1070.
** Clinically: uterosacral ligament.

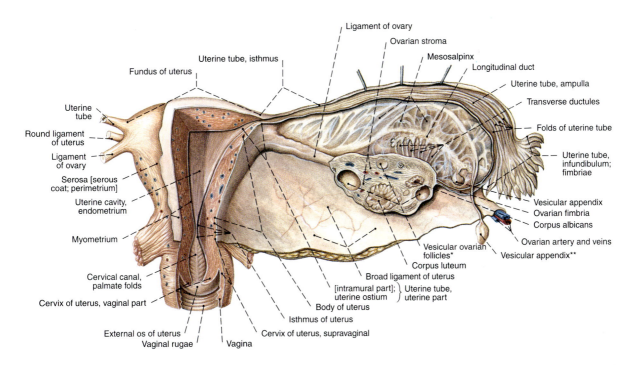

Ligament of ovary
Ovarian stroma
Mesosalpinx
Uterine tube, isthmus
Longitudinal duct
Fundus of uterus
Uterine tube, ampulla
Transverse ductules
Uterine tube
Folds of uterine tube
Round ligament of uterus
Ligament of ovary
Uterine tube, infundibulum; fimbriae
Serosa [serous coat; perimetrium]
Uterine cavity, endometrium
Vesicular appendix
Ovarian fimbria
Corpus albicans
Myometrium
Ovarian artery and veins
Vesicular appendix**
Cervical canal, palmate folds
Vesicular ovarian follicles*
Corpus luteum
Cervix of uterus, vaginal part
Broad ligament of uterus
[intramural part]; uterine ostium
Uterine tube, uterine part
External os of uterus
Body of uterus
Vaginal rugae
Vagina
Isthmus of uterus
Cervix of uterus, supravaginal

Fig. 1064   Female internal genitalia; female in reproductive age; image of lumen of vagina, uterus, and right uterine tube; ovary sectioned frontally and peritoneum removed from mesosalpinx; dorsal aspect.

* Clinically: GRAAFian follicle.
** Stalked hydatid.

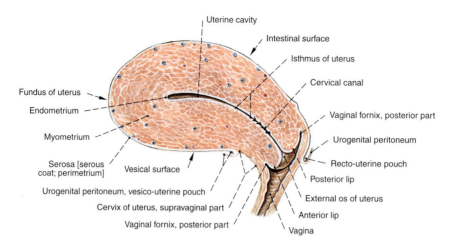

Fig. 1065 Uterus; vagina; female in reproductive age; median section exposing the lumen; lateral aspect.

Fig. 1066 Uterus; vagina; normal angles between vagina, cervix of uterus, and body of uterus; schematic median section; lateral aspect.

* Longitudinal axis of vagina.
** Longitudinal axis of cervix of uterus.
*** Longitudinal axis of body of uterus.

Angle between vagina and cervix of uterus = version
Angle between cervix and body of uterus = flexion
Normal relationships of uterus: anteversion, anteflexion
Position in relation to median plane = position
(compare Fig. 1067, uterus in dextroposition).

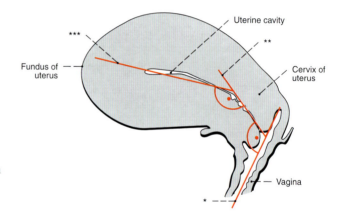

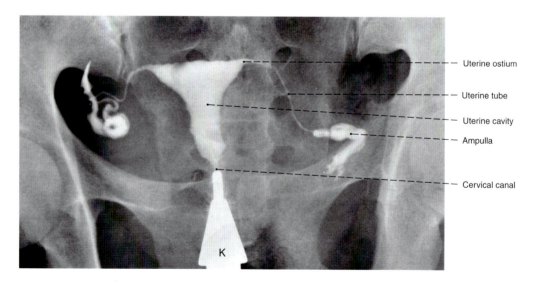

Fig. 1067 Uterus; uterine tube; AP radiograph after injection of contrast medium via the cervix of uterus (hysterosalpingography); ventral aspect.

This previously used clinical method enabled diagnosis of passage of uterine tube.
K = adapter for injection tube for contrast medium.

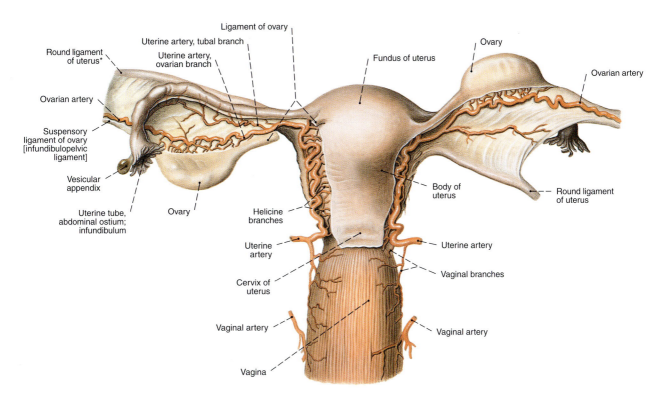

Fig. 1068   Arteries of female internal genitalia; broad ligament of uterus extensively and peritoneum partially removed; part of left ligament of ovary removed; dorsal aspect.

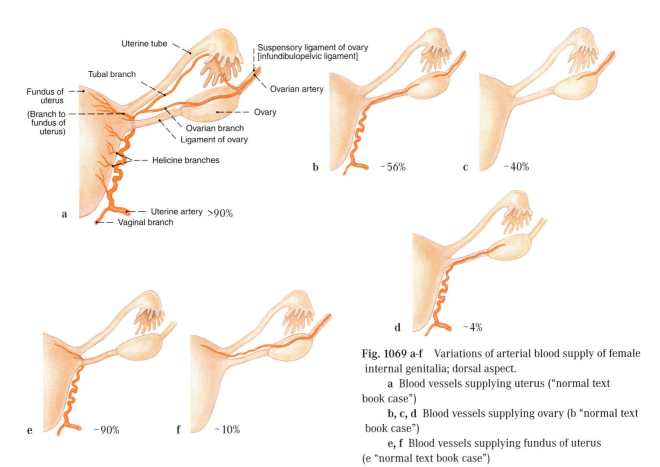

Fig. 1069 a-f   Variations of arterial blood supply of female internal genitalia; dorsal aspect.

    a Blood vessels supplying uterus ("normal text book case")

    b, c, d Blood vessels supplying ovary (b "normal text book case")

    e, f Blood vessels supplying fundus of uterus (e "normal text book case")

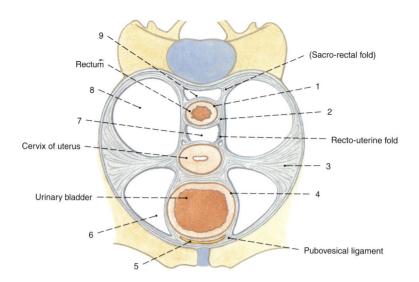

9
Rectum
8
7
Cervix of uterus
Urinary bladder
6
5
(Sacro-rectal fold)
1
2
Recto-uterine fold
3
4
Pubovesical ligament

Fig. 1070 Uterus; diagram of ligaments and fascial spaces in the lesser pelvis [true pelvis]; transverse section at level of cervix of uterus; superior aspect.

Recent anatomical studies raise the question about the existence of ligaments from the uterus to the lateral wall of the pelvis, which have been called cardinal ligament of uterus.

1 = rectal fascia
2 = uterosacral ligament
3 = cardinal ligament, parametrium
4 = vesical fascia
5 = retropubic space (prevesical cave of RETZIUS)
6 = paravesical space, paracystium
7 = recto-uterine pouch (pouch of DOUGLAS)
8 = pararectal space, paraproctium
9 = retrorectal space

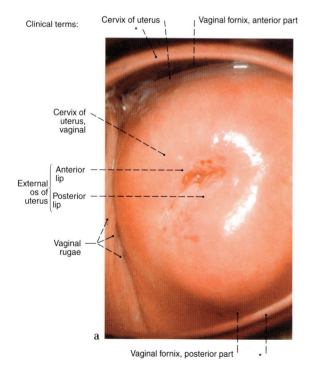

Clinical terms:
Cervix of uterus
*
Vaginal fornix, anterior part
Cervix of uterus, vaginal
Anterior lip
External os of uterus
Posterior lip
Vaginal rugae
a
Vaginal fornix, posterior part *

*
Vaginal fornix, anterior part
Cervix of uterus, vaginal part
Anterior lip
External os of uterus
Posterior lip
Vagina
b
*
Vaginal fornix, posterior part

Fig. 1071 a, b Cervix of uterus, vaginal part.
a Photo of a young female, who has not born a child before (nulliparous)
b Photo of a young female who has born two children

Inspection of the vaginal part of cervix is enabled by spreading the normally slit-like vagina with two specula (*); caudal aspect. The vaginal part of cervix projects clearly into the vagina.

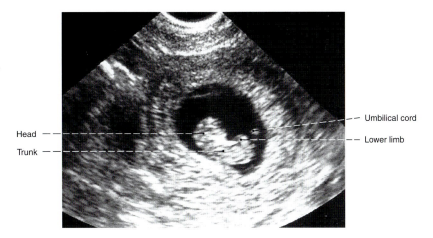

Head — — —

Trunk — — —

— — Umbilical cord

— — Lower limb

Fig. 1072 Uterus with embryo; ultrasound scan in the 10th week of pregnancy, scanned through the abdominal wall; right lateral aspect.

The embryo swims in the amniotic fluid of the chorionic cavity.

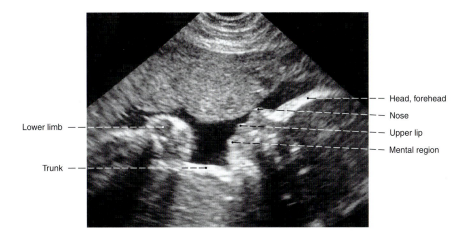

Lower limb — — —

Trunk — — —

— — Head, forehead

— — Nose

— — Upper lip

— — Mental region

Fig. 1073 Uterus with fetus; ultrasound scan in the 28th week of pregnancy, scanned through the abdominal wall; left lateral aspect.

During ultrasonography movements of the limbs and opening of the mouth can be examined.

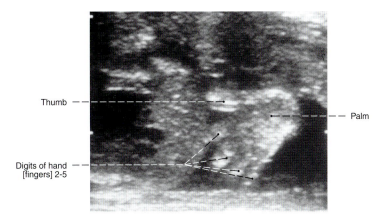

Thumb — — —

Digits of hand — — [fingers] 2-5

— — Palm

Fig. 1074 Hand of a fetus; ultrasound scan in the 24th week of pregnancy; details such as the fingers can be studied; lateral aspect.

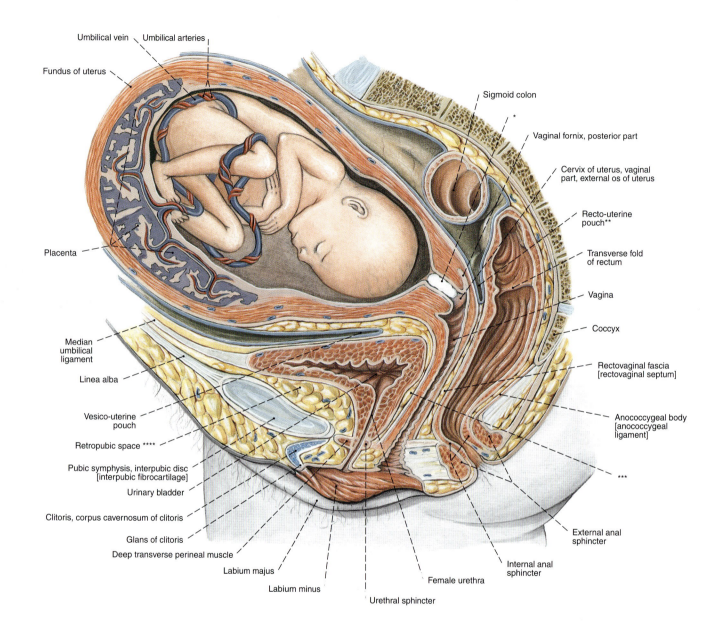

Umbilical vein

Umbilical arteries

Fundus of uterus

Sigmoid colon

Vaginal fornix, posterior part

Cervix of uterus, vaginal part, external os of uterus

Recto-uterine pouch**

Transverse fold of rectum

Placenta

Vagina

Coccyx

Median umbilical ligament

Rectovaginal fascia [rectovaginal septum]

Linea alba

Anococcygeal body [anococcygeal ligament]

Vesico-uterine pouch

Retropubic space ****

***

Pubic symphysis, interpubic disc [interpubic fibrocartilage]

Urinary bladder

External anal sphincter

Clitoris, corpus cavernosum of clitoris

Glans of clitoris

Internal anal sphincter

Deep transverse perineal muscle

Female urethra

Labium majus

Labium minus

Urethral sphincter

Fig. 1075 Uterus with fetus; pelvis sectioned in the median plane; left lateral aspect.
The wall of uterus becomes even thinner at the end of pregnancy.

* Mucous plug (of KRISTELLER) in the cervical canal of uterus.
** Pouch of DOUGLAS.
*** Vesicovaginal septum.
**** Cave of RETZIUS.

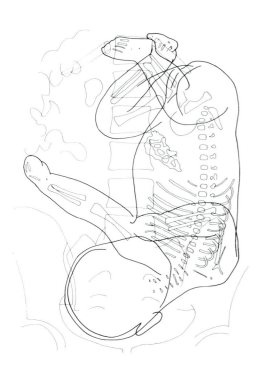

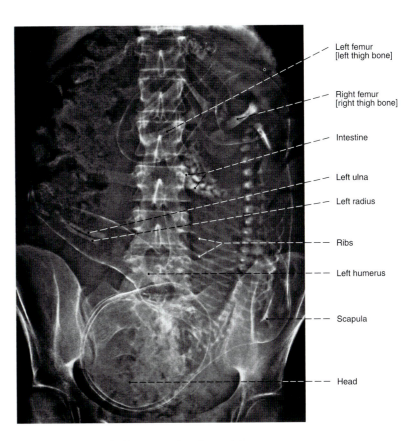

Left femur
[left thigh bone]

Right femur
[right thigh bone]

Intestine

Left ulna

Left radius

Ribs

Left humerus

Scapula

Head

Fig. 1076 Fetus; AP radiograph
shortly before birth; ventral aspect.

Previously this method was occasionally used to measure
the size of the head of the fetus in relation to the pelvis
of the female.

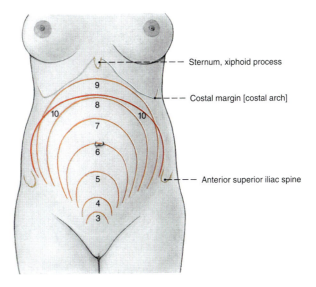

Sternum, xiphoid process

Costal margin [costal arch]

Anterior superior iliac spine

Fig. 1077 Uterus; sizes during pregnancy;
numerals indicate the end of the respective month
of pregnancy (28 days); in the last month the fundus
of uterus goes down again.

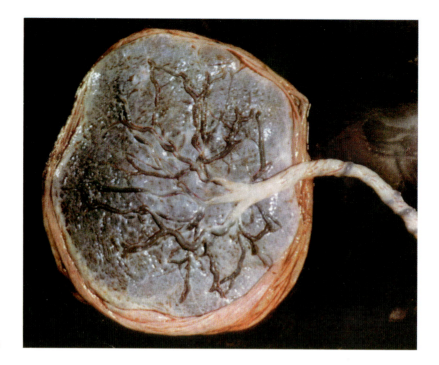

a

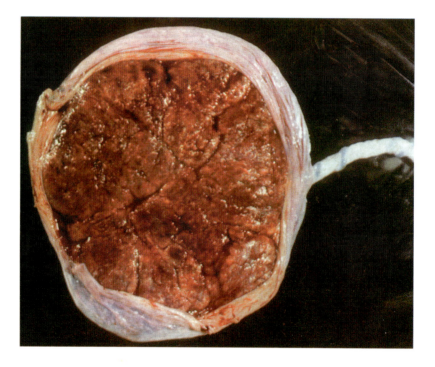

b

Fig. 1078 a, b   Placenta; umbilical cord.
a   View of fetal surface
b   View of maternal surface of a parturient placenta

The fetal surface is shiny and smooth because of the amnion;
the maternal surface is divided into lobes (= cotyledons) by
deep grooves and colored blood red.

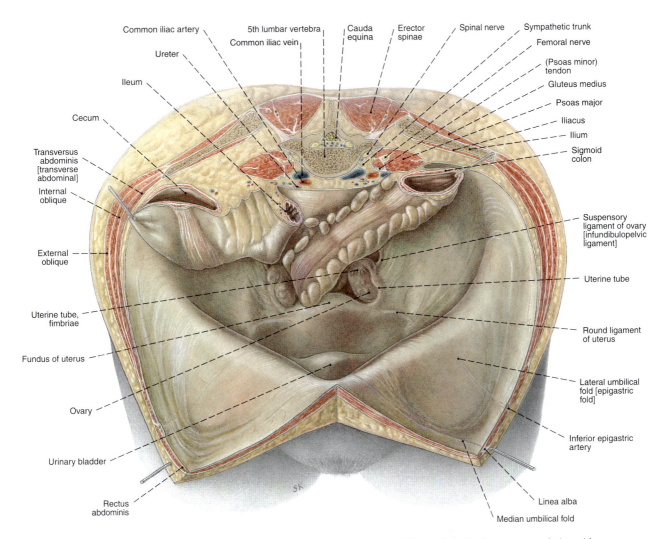

Common iliac artery
Ureter
Ileum
Cecum
Transversus abdominis [transverse abdominal]
Internal oblique
External oblique
Uterine tube, fimbriae
Fundus of uterus
Ovary
Urinary bladder
Rectus abdominis

5th lumbar vertebra
Common iliac vein
Cauda equina
Erector spinae
Spinal nerve
Sympathetic trunk
Femoral nerve
(Psoas minor) tendon
Gluteus medius
Psoas major
Iliacus
Ilium
Sigmoid colon
Suspensory ligament of ovary [infundibulopelvic ligament]
Uterine tube
Round ligament of uterus
Lateral umbilical fold [epigastric fold]
Inferior epigastric artery
Linea alba
Median umbilical fold

Fig. 1079 Female internal genitalia; horizontal section at level of 5th lumbar vertebra; anterior abdomina wall sectionedlongitudinally in the right rectus abdominis and retracted laterally by hooks; cecum and sigmoid colon retracted cranially by a hook; ventral superior aspect.

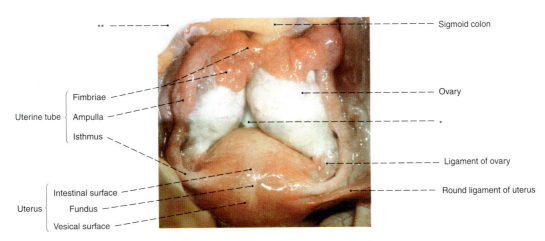

**
Uterine tube { Fimbriae, Ampulla, Isthmus }
Uterus { Intestinal surface, Fundus, Vesical surface }

Sigmoid colon
Ovary
*
Ligament of ovary
Round ligament of uterus

Fig. 1080 Female internal genitalia; surgical exposure of a young female; ovaries are displaced superomedially by compresses (*) in the pouch of DOUGLAS; ventral superior aspect.

** Swab.

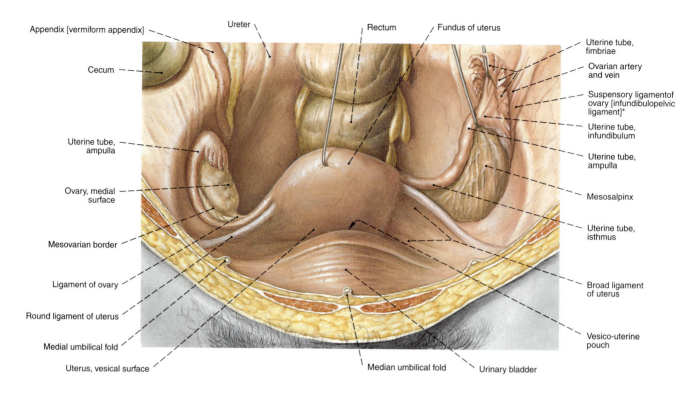

Appendix [vermiform appendix]
Cecum
Uterine tube, ampulla
Ovary, medial surface
Mesovarian border
Ligament of ovary
Round ligament of uterus
Medial umbilical fold
Uterus, vesical surface
Ureter
Rectum
Fundus of uterus
Median umbilical fold
Urinary bladder
Uterine tube, fimbriae
Ovarian artery and vein
Suspensory ligament of ovary [infundibulopelvic ligament]*
Uterine tube, infundibulum
Uterine tube, ampulla
Mesosalpinx
Uterine tube, isthmus
Broad ligament of uterus
Vesico-uterine pouch

Fig. 1081   Female internal genitalia; uterus retracted by a hook to expose vesico-uterine pouch and broad ligament of uterus; left uterine tube retracted cranially to expose mesosalpinx; ventral aspect.

The close relationship of the appendages (ovary and uterine tube) with the appendix [vermiform appendix] may cause differential diagnostic problems in the case of inflammations.

*Clinically: infundibulopelvic ligament.

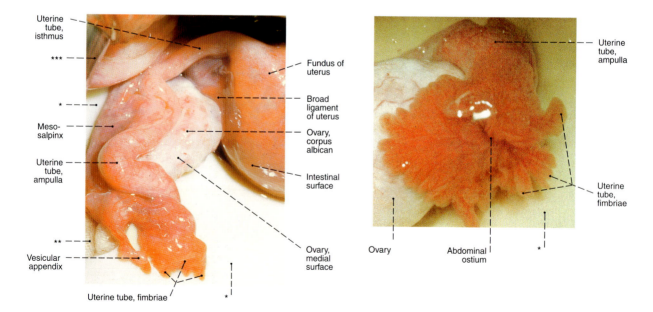

Uterine tube, isthmus
***
*
Meso-salpinx
Uterine tube, ampulla
**
Vesicular appendix
Uterine tube, fimbriae
*
Fundus of uterus
Broad ligament of uterus
Ovary, corpus albican
Intestinal surface
Ovary, medial surface
Uterine tube, ampulla
Uterine tube, fimbriae
Ovary
Abdominal ostium
*

Fig. 1082   Uterine tube, ovary; surgical exposure in a young female; dorsal superior aspect.

* Plastic tray to elevate ovary and uterine tube.

** Swab.

*** Surgical hook.

Fig. 1083   Abdominal ostium of uterine tube, ovary; surgical exposure in a young female; the pelvic cavity filled with saline to expose the fimbriae; dorsal superior aspect.

* Plastic tray to elevate uterine tube.

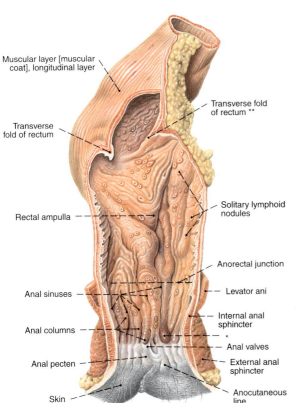

Muscular layer [muscular coat], longitudinal layer

Transverse fold of rectum

Transverse fold of rectum **

Rectal ampulla

Solitary lymphoid nodules

Anorectal junction

Anal sinuses

Levator ani

Anal columns

Internal anal sphincter

*

Anal valves

Anal pecten

External anal sphincter

Skin

Anocutaneous line

Fig. 1084 Rectum; anus; frontal section exposing mucosa [mucous membrane] and sphincters; ventral aspect.

* Hemorrhoidal node.
** KOHLRAUSCH's fold.

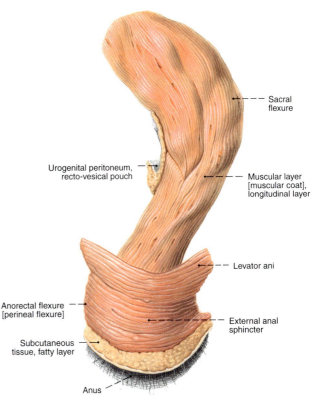

Sacral flexure

Urogenital peritoneum, recto-vesical pouch

Muscular layer [muscular coat], longitudinal layer

Levator ani

Anorectal flexure [perineal flexure]

External anal sphincter

Subcutaneous tissue, fatty layer

Anus

Fig. 1085 Rectum; anus; surrounding tissue extensively removed to expose muscular layer [muscular coat]; right lateral aspect.

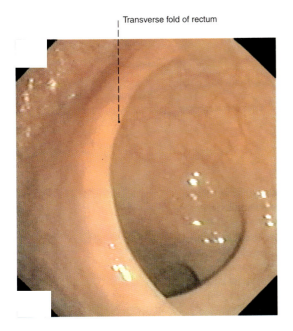

Transverse fold of rectum

Fig. 1086 Rectum; anus; rectoscopic view of rectal ampulla by an endoscope inserted through the anal canal to examine the mucosa [mucous membrane]; inferior aspect.

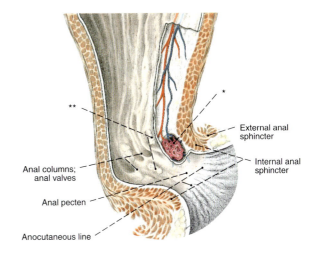

**

External anal sphincter

*

Internal anal sphincter

Anal columns; anal valves

Anal pecten

Anocutaneous line

Fig. 1087 Rectum; anus; median section exposing arteriovenous anastomoses in the anal columns; mucosa [mucous membrane] partially removed; left lateral aspect. Closure of the anus is achieved by muscles (internal and external anal sphincters, levator ani), mucosal folds, and erectile-type arteriovenous anastomoses.

* Rectal glomerulus, numerous arteriovenous anastomoses in the anal columns.
** Clinically: hemorrhoidal zone.

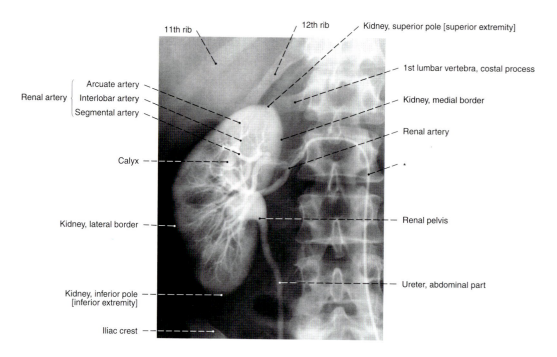

11th rib

12th rib

Kidney, superior pole [superior extremity]

Arcuate artery

Renal artery   Interlobar artery

Segmental artery

1st lumbar vertebra, costal process

Kidney, medial border

Renal artery

Calyx

*

Kidney, lateral border

Renal pelvis

Kidney, inferior pole [inferior extremity]

Ureter, abdominal part

Iliac crest

Fig. 1090   Kidney; AP radiograph after intravenous injection of contrast medium, which is excreted via the kidney (i.v. pyelography) to visualize renal pelvis and ureter; simultaneous visualization of arteries by injection of contrast medium into the renal artery through a catheter* introduced via the aorta (arteriography).

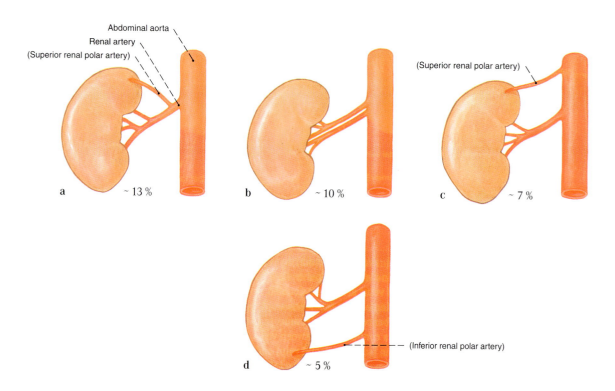

Abdominal aorta

Renal artery

(Superior renal polar artery)

a   ~ 13 %

b   ~ 10 %

(Superior renal polar artery)

c   ~ 7 %

d   ~ 5 %

(Inferior renal polar artery)

Fig. 1091 a-d   Variations in the arterial blood supply of the kidney.

a   Renal artery with a branch to the superior pole [superior extremity]
b   Two renal arteries to hilum of kidney
c   Accessory artery to the superior pole [superior extremity]
d   Accessory artery to the inferior pole [inferior extremity]

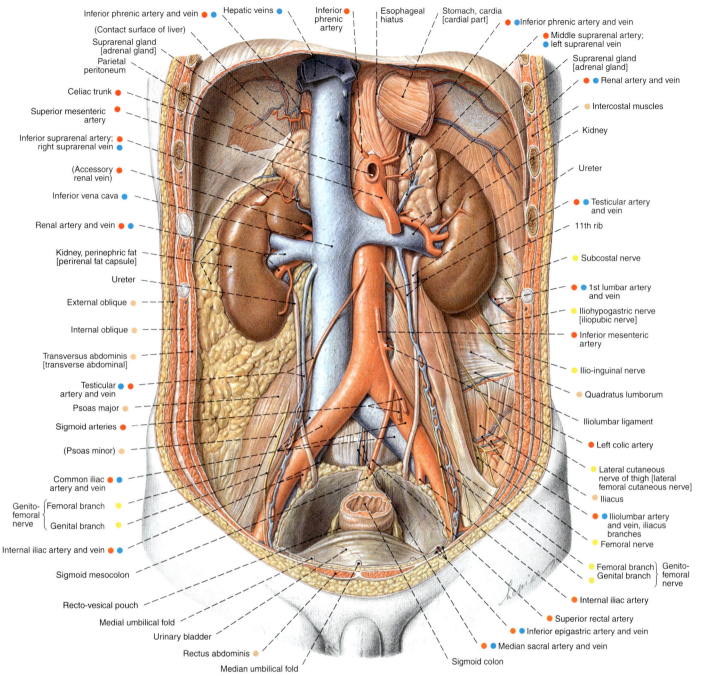

Inferior phrenic artery and vein ● ● — Hepatic veins ● — Inferior phrenic artery — Esophageal hiatus — Stomach, cardia [cardial part] — ● ● Inferior phrenic artery and vein

● Middle suprarenal artery; ● left suprarenal vein

(Contact surface of liver)

Suprarenal gland [adrenal gland]

Parietal peritoneum

Celiac trunk ●

Superior mesenteric artery ●

Inferior suprarenal artery; ● right suprarenal vein ●

(Accessory renal vein) ●

Inferior vena cava ●

Renal artery and vein ● ● ●

Kidney, perinephric fat [perirenal fat capsule]

Ureter

External oblique ●

Internal oblique ●

Transversus abdominis [transverse abdominal] ●

Testicular ● ● artery and vein

Psoas major ●

Sigmoid arteries ●

(Psoas minor) ●

Common iliac ● ● artery and vein

Genito-femoral nerve { Femoral branch ● — Genital branch ● }

Internal iliac artery and vein ● ● ●

Sigmoid mesocolon

Recto-vesical pouch

Medial umbilical fold

Urinary bladder

Rectus abdominis ●

Median umbilical fold

Suprarenal gland [adrenal gland]

● ● Renal artery and vein

● Intercostal muscles

Kidney

Ureter

● ● Testicular artery and vein

11th rib

● Subcostal nerve

● ● 1st lumbar artery and vein

● Iliohypogastric nerve [iliopubic nerve]

● Inferior mesenteric artery

● Ilio-inguinal nerve

● Quadratus lumborum

Iliolumbar ligament

● Left colic artery

● Lateral cutaneous nerve of thigh [lateral femoral cutaneous nerve]

● Iliacus

● ● Iliolumbar artery and vein, iliacus branches

● Femoral nerve

Femoral branch ● — Genital branch ● } Genito-femoral nerve

● Internal iliac artery

● Superior rectal artery

● ● Inferior epigastric artery and vein

● ● Median sacral artery and vein

Sigmoid colon

Fig. 1092   Position of retroperitoneal organs in the male; intestine, liver, pancreas, and spleen removed; ventral aspect. While the left testicular vein drains into the left renal vein, the right testicular artery drains directly into the inferior vena cava. Similar relationships apply for the ovarian veins.

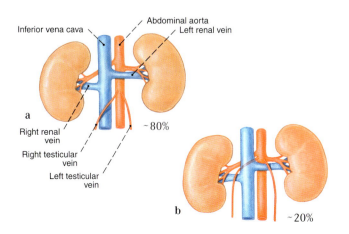

Inferior vena cava — Abdominal aorta — Left renal vein

a

Right renal vein

Right testicular vein

Left testicular vein

~ 80%

b   ~ 20%

Fig. 1093 a, b   Variations of the course of the testicular arteries.

a   "Normal textbook case"

b   Both testicular arteries originating superior to the renal veins; right testicular artery dorsal to inferior vena cava, left testicular artery ventral to renal vein

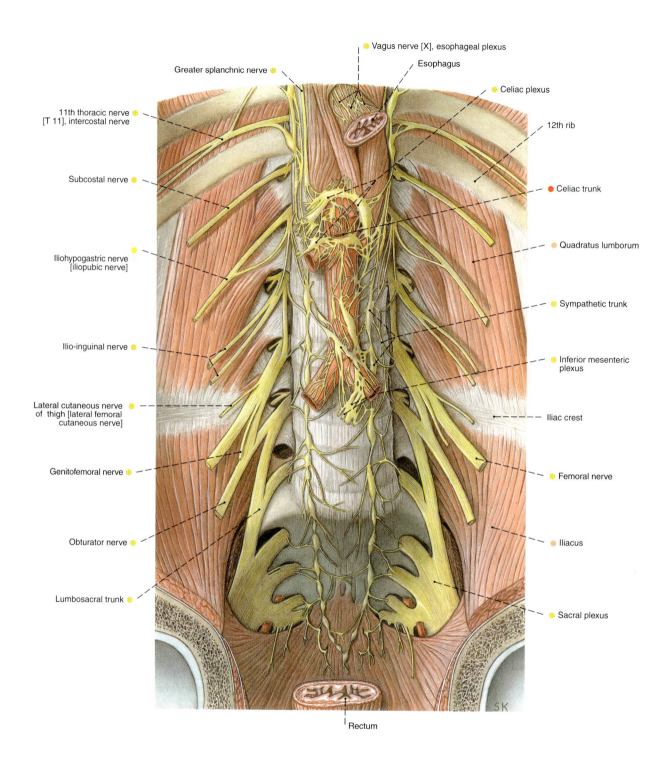

Fig. 1096 Nerves of the posterior abdominal wall, lumbosacral plexus, and abdominal part of autonomic division [autonomic part of peripheral nervous system]; viscera, blood vessels, and psoas major removed; ventral aspect.

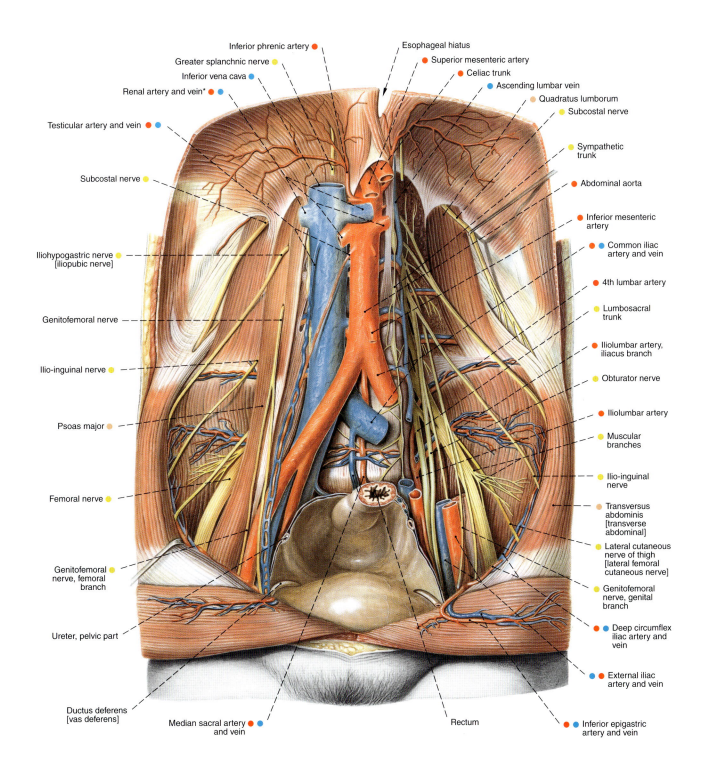

Inferior phrenic artery ●
Greater splanchnic nerve ●
Inferior vena cava ●
Renal artery and vein* ● ●
Testicular artery and vein ● ●
Subcostal nerve ●
Iliohypogastric nerve ●
[iliopubic nerve]
Genitofemoral nerve
Ilio-inguinal nerve ●
Psoas major ●
Femoral nerve ●
Genitofemoral
nerve, femoral
branch ●
Ureter, pelvic part
Ductus deferens
[vas deferens]
Median sacral artery ● ●
and vein

Esophageal hiatus
Superior mesenteric artery ●
Celiac trunk ●
Ascending lumbar vein ●
Quadratus lumborum ●
Subcostal nerve ●
Sympathetic trunk ●
Abdominal aorta ●
Inferior mesenteric artery ●
Common iliac artery and vein ● ●
4th lumbar artery ●
Lumbosacral trunk ●
Iliolumbar artery, iliacus branch ●
Obturator nerve ●
Iliolumbar artery ●
Muscular branches ●
Ilio-inguinal nerve ●
Transversus abdominis [transverse abdominal] ●
Lateral cutaneous nerve of thigh [lateral femoral cutaneous nerve] ●
Genitofemoral nerve, genital branch ●
Deep circumflex iliac artery and vein ● ●
External iliac artery and vein ● ●
Inferior epigastric artery and vein ● ●
Rectum

Fig. 1097   Blood vessels and nerves of the posterior
abdominal wall in the male; left psoas major and iliac
artery and vein extensively removed to expose lumbar
plexus; ventral aspect.

* In approximately 10% the left renal vein passes dorsal to the aorta.

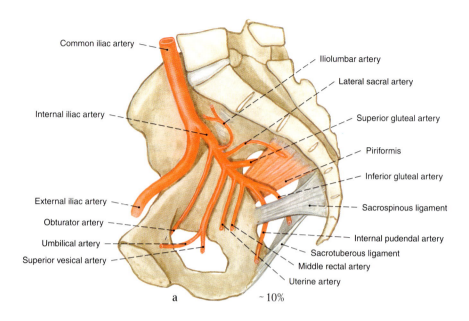

Common iliac artery

Internal iliac artery

External iliac artery

Obturator artery

Umbilical artery

Superior vesical artery

Iliolumbar artery

Lateral sacral artery

Superior gluteal artery

Piriformis

Inferior gluteal artery

Sacrospinous ligament

Internal pudendal artery

Sacrotuberous ligament

Middle rectal artery

Uterine artery

a ~ 10%

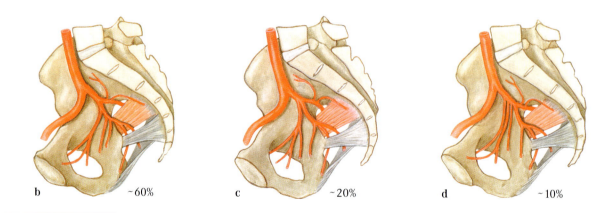

b ~ 60%   c ~ 20%   d ~ 10%

Fig. 1100 a-d   Variations of branching pattern of internal iliac artery;
right lateral aspect.

a Origin of all branches from the trunk of the internal iliac artery
b Division of the internal iliac artery into two main branches ("normal textbook case")
c Division of the internal iliac artery into three main branches
d Division of the internal iliac artery into more than three main branches

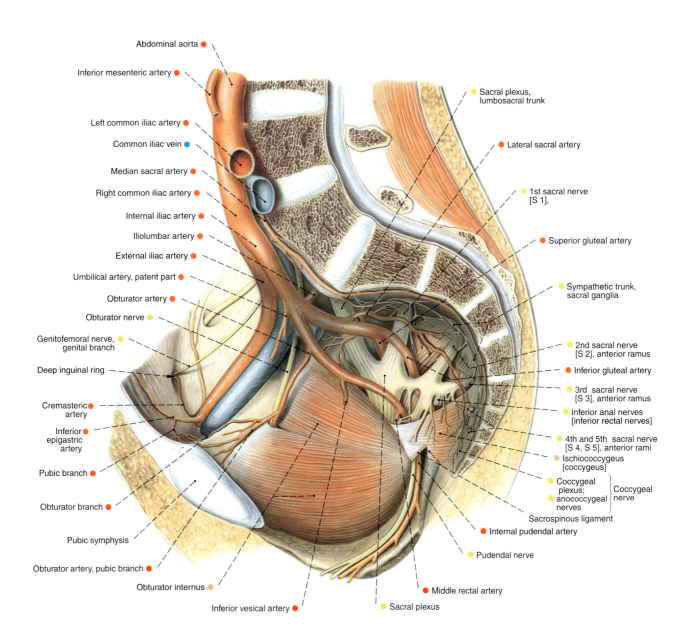

Abdominal aorta ●

Inferior mesenteric artery ●

Left common iliac artery ●

Common iliac vein ●

Median sacral artery ●

Right common iliac artery ●

Internal iliac artery ●

Iliolumbar artery ●

External iliac artery ●

Umbilical artery, patent part ●

Obturator artery ●

Obturator nerve ●

Genitofemoral nerve, genital branch ●

Deep inguinal ring

Cremasteric ● artery

Inferior ● epigastric artery

Pubic branch ●

Obturator branch ●

Pubic symphysis

Obturator artery, pubic branch ●

Obturator internus ●

Inferior vesical artery ●

Sacral plexus, lumbosacral trunk ●

● Lateral sacral artery

1st sacral nerve ● [S 1],

● Superior gluteal artery

Sympathetic trunk, ● sacral ganglia

2nd sacral nerve ● [S 2], anterior ramus

● Inferior gluteal artery

3rd sacral nerve ● [S 3], anterior ramus

Inferior anal nerves ● [inferior rectal nerves]

4th and 5th sacral nerve ● [S 4, S 5], anterior rami

● Ischiococcygeus [coccygeus]

Coccygeal ● plexus; ┐ Coccygeal anococcygeal ● │ nerve nerves ┘

Sacrospinous ligament

● Internal pudendal artery

Pudendal nerve ●

Middle rectal artery ●

Sacral plexus ●

Fig. 1101 Internal iliac artery; sacral plexus; demonstration of the branches after removal of all pelvic viscera and fascias in a median sectioned pelvis: sacrospinous ligament incised to demonstrate the course of the internal pudendal artery; right lateral aspect. Compare Fig. 1100.

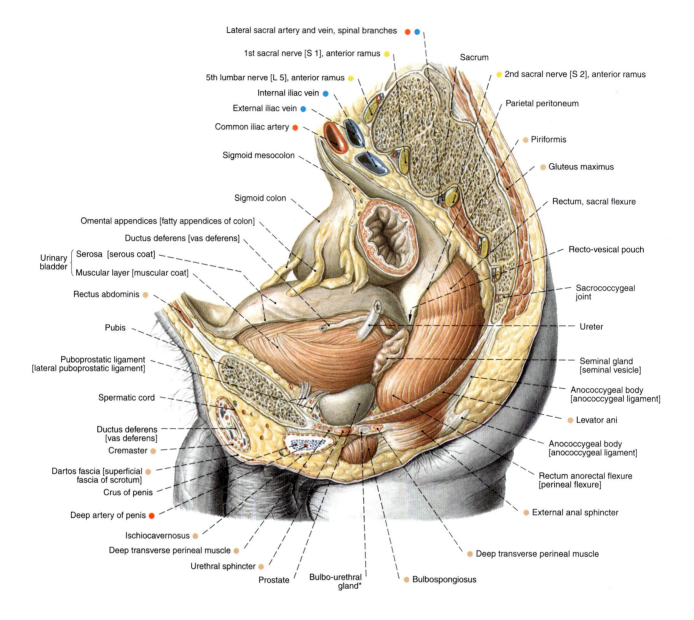

Lateral sacral artery and vein, spinal branches

1st sacral nerve [S 1], anterior ramus

5th lumbar nerve [L 5], anterior ramus

Internal iliac vein

External iliac vein

Common iliac artery

Sigmoid mesocolon

Sigmoid colon

Omental appendices [fatty appendices of colon]

Ductus deferens [vas deferens]

Urinary bladder { Serosa [serous coat]
Muscular layer [muscular coat]

Rectus abdominis

Pubis

Puboprostatic ligament [lateral puboprostatic ligament]

Spermatic cord

Ductus deferens [vas deferens]

Cremaster

Dartos fascia [superficial fascia of scrotum]

Crus of penis

Deep artery of penis

Ischiocavernosus

Deep transverse perineal muscle

Urethral sphincter

Prostate

Bulbo-urethral gland*

Bulbospongiosus

Sacrum

2nd sacral nerve [S 2], anterior ramus

Parietal peritoneum

Piriformis

Gluteus maximus

Rectum, sacral flexure

Recto-vesical pouch

Sacrococcygeal joint

Ureter

Seminal gland [seminal vesicle]

Anococcygeal body [anococcygeal ligament]

Levator ani

Anococcygeal body [anococcygeal ligament]

Rectum anorectal flexure [perineal flexure]

External anal sphincter

Deep transverse perineal muscle

Fig. 1102   Male pelvic viscera; left paramedian section
of the pelvis; peritoneum of lateral surface of urinary
bladder partially removed to expose the course of ureter
and ductus deferens [vas deferens]; right lateral aspect.

* Clinically also COWPER's gland.

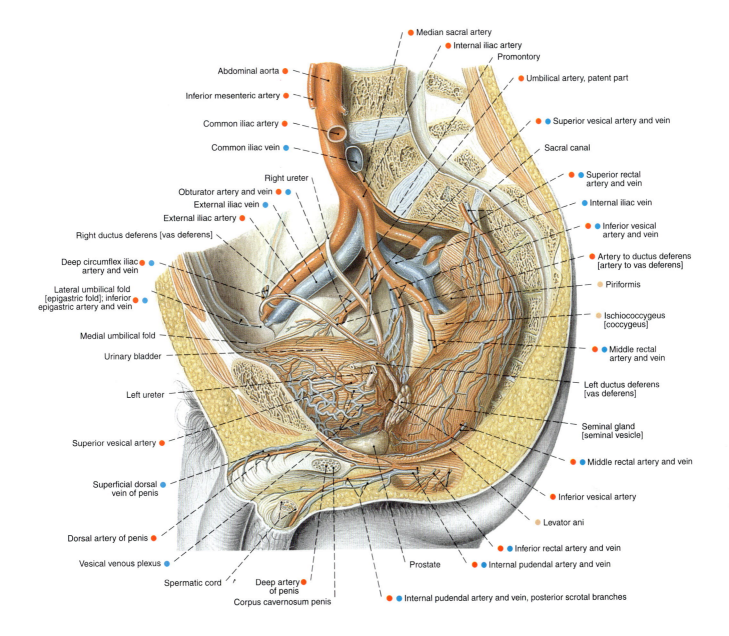

● Median sacral artery

● Internal iliac artery

Promontory

Abdominal aorta ●

● Umbilical artery, patent part

Inferior mesenteric artery ●

● ● Superior vesical artery and vein

Common iliac artery ●

Sacral canal

Common iliac vein ●

● ● Superior rectal artery and vein

Right ureter

● Internal iliac vein

Obturator artery and vein ● ●

External iliac vein ●

● Inferior vesical artery and vein

External iliac artery ●

Right ductus deferens [vas deferens]

● Artery to ductus deferens [artery to vas deferens]

Deep circumflex iliac ● ● artery and vein

● Piriformis

Lateral umbilical fold [epigastric fold]; inferior ● ● epigastric artery and vein

● Ischiococcygeus [coccygeus]

Medial umbilical fold

● ● Middle rectal artery and vein

Urinary bladder

Left ductus deferens [vas deferens]

Left ureter

Seminal gland [seminal vesicle]

Superior vesical artery ●

● ● Middle rectal artery and vein

Superficial dorsal ● vein of penis

● Inferior vesical artery

● Levator ani

Dorsal artery of penis ●

● ● Inferior rectal artery and vein

Vesical venous plexus ●

● ● Internal pudendal artery and vein

Spermatic cord

Prostate

Deep artery ● of penis

● ● Internal pudendal artery and vein, posterior scrotal branches

Corpus cavernosum penis

Fig. 1103 Blood supply of the male pelvic viscera; left paramedian section of the pelvis; peritoneum extensively removed; right lateral aspect.

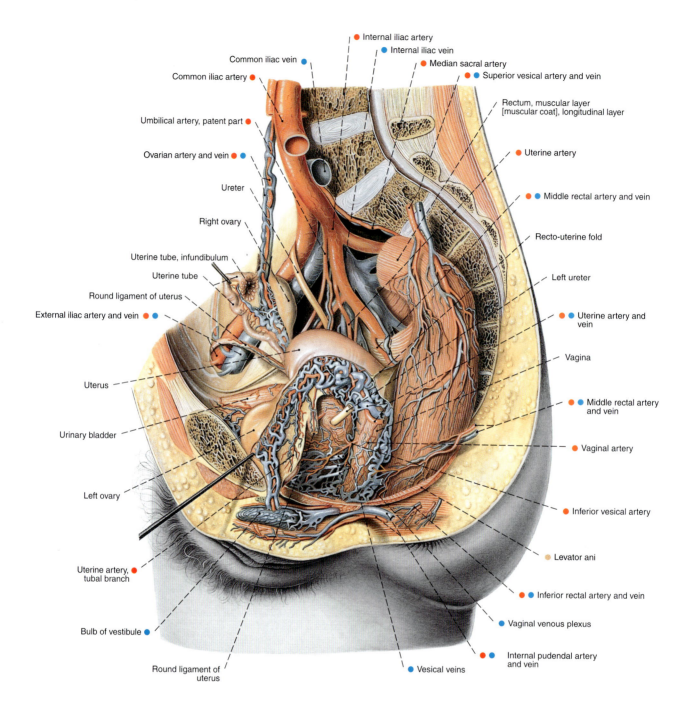

Internal iliac artery

Internal iliac vein

Common iliac vein

Median sacral artery

Common iliac artery

Superior vesical artery and vein

Umbilical artery, patent part

Rectum, muscular layer
[muscular coat], longitudinal layer

Ovarian artery and vein

Uterine artery

Ureter

Middle rectal artery and vein

Right ovary

Recto-uterine fold

Uterine tube, infundibulum

Left ureter

Uterine tube

Round ligament of uterus

Uterine artery and vein

External iliac artery and vein

Vagina

Uterus

Middle rectal artery and vein

Urinary bladder

Vaginal artery

Left ovary

Inferior vesical artery

Levator ani

Uterine artery, tubal branch

Inferior rectal artery and vein

Vaginal venous plexus

Bulb of vestibule

Internal pudendal artery and vein

Round ligament of uterus

Vesical veins

Fig. 1104   Blood supply of the female pelvic viscera; left
paramedian section of the pelvis; intestine extensively
and peritoneum partially removed; right ovary retracted
cranially and left ovary retracted ventrocaudally to
expose the blood vessels; right lateral aspect.

Well-developed venous plexuses surround the
pelvic viscera. In elderly females the ovarian artery is
frequently atrophic and, thus, difficult to dissect.

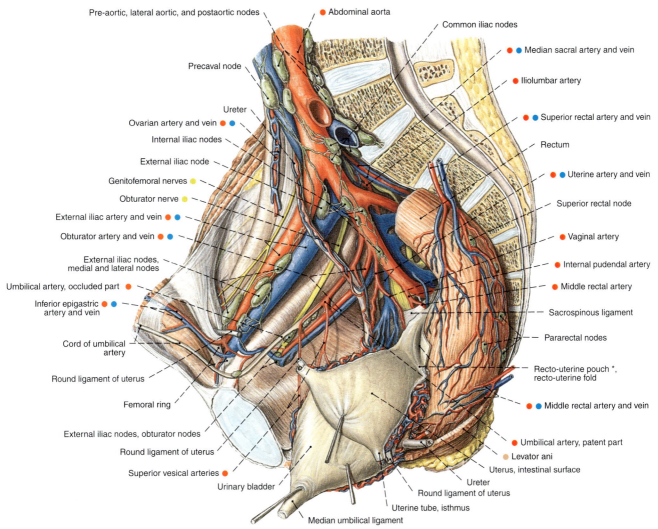

Pre-aortic, lateral aortic, and postaortic nodes — ● Abdominal aorta

Common iliac nodes

● ● Median sacral artery and vein

Precaval node

● Iliolumbar artery

Ureter

● ● Superior rectal artery and vein

Ovarian artery and vein ● ●

Internal iliac nodes

Rectum

External iliac node

● ● Uterine artery and vein

Genitofemoral nerves ●

Obturator nerve ●

Superior rectal node

External iliac artery and vein ● ●

● Vaginal artery

Obturator artery and vein ● ●

● Internal pudendal artery

External iliac nodes, medial and lateral nodes

● Middle rectal artery

Umbilical artery, occluded part ●

Sacrospinous ligament

Inferior epigastric artery and vein ● ●

Pararectal nodes

Cord of umbilical artery

Recto-uterine pouch *, recto-uterine fold

Round ligament of uterus

● ● Middle rectal artery and vein

Femoral ring

External iliac nodes, obturator nodes

● Umbilical artery, patent part

Round ligament of uterus

● Levator ani

Superior vesical arteries ●

Uterus, intestinal surface

Urinary bladder

Ureter

Round ligament of uterus

Uterine tube, isthmus

Median umbilical ligament

Fig. 1105 Lymphatic vessels and lymph nodes of the right pelvic wall in the female; median section of the pelvis; uterus retracted anteriorly to the left and peritoneum extensively removed; lateral aspect.

The lymph nodes are generally much smaller than shown, but always present. Via lymphatic vessels of the round ligament of uterus tumor cells may invade from the uterus to the inguinal lymph nodes.

* Clinically: pouch of DOUGLAS.

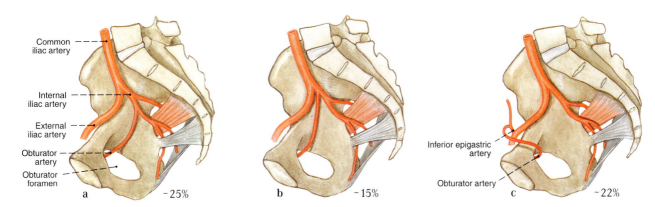

Common iliac artery

Internal iliac artery

External iliac artery

Obturator artery

Obturator foramen

Inferior epigastric artery

Obturator artery

a ~25% **b** ~15% **c** ~22%

Fig. 1106 a-c Variations in the origin of obturator artery; right lateral aspect.
a Origin from ventral branch of internal iliac artery ("normal textbook case")

b Separate origin from internal iliac artery
c Origin from external iliac artery
Only in 75% the obturator artery is a branch of the trunk of the internal iliac artery.

Pelvic diaphragm [pelvic floor] and urogenital diaphragm [superficial and deep perineal spaces] (Figs. 1107, 1108, 1115-1118, 1126, 1128)

The pelvic floor comprises two muscles that overlie each other partially. The pelvic diaphragm includes the levator ani and the ischiococcygeus [coccygeus].

Between both inferior pubic rami stretches a triangular plate, the urogenital diaphragm. Its fibers are directed transversally and they close the urogenital hiatus. Amongst others it comprises the deep transverse perineal muscle, the urethral sphincter (both together also called urethral compressor), and the superficial transverse perineal muscle. In the male only the urethra, in the female both urethra and vagina penetrate the urogenital diaphragm.

Muscle / *innervation*	Origin	Insertion	Function
1. Levator ani *Branches of sacral nerve (S 3 and S 4)* Comprises: Pubococcygeus, puboprostaticus [levator prostatae], pubovaginalis puborectalis, iliococcygeus	**Pubococcygeus:** pubis (inner surface nest to pubic symphysis), tendinous arch of levator ani, ischial spine **Iliococcygeus:** tendinous arch of levator ani (posterior third)	Perineal body (prerectal fibers), in the male into the prostatic fascia (levator prostatae), in the female into the vaginal wall (pubovaginalis), merges with the external anal sphincter, surrounds the anus (puborectalis), anococcygeal body, coccyx	Surrounds the rectum dorsally; the medial free border forms the urogenital hiatus, in the male for passing of the urethra, in the female for passing of urethra and vagina; suspension band for the pelvic floor
2. Ischiococcygeus [coccygeus] *Branches of sacral nerve (S 4 and S 5)*	Ischial spine (inner surface; blends with the sacrospinous ligament)	Sacrum (lateral border of lower segments), coccyx	Supports pelvic floor
3. External anal sphincter *Pudendal nerve (sacral plexus)*	**Subcutaneous part:** dermis [corium] and subcutaneous tissue surrounding anus **Superficial part:** Perineal body **Deep part:** Ring-like fibers up to levator ani	Dermis [corium] and subcutaneous tissue surrounding anus, anococcygeal ligament	External sphincter of anus
4. Deep transverse perineal muscle *Pudendal nerve (sacral plexus)*	Ramus of ischium, adventitia of internal pudendal vessels (obliquely over pubic arch, resp. subpubic angel, completed by inferior pubic ligament and transverse perineal ligament)	Trapezoid muscle plate with openings for urethra in the male, respectively urethra and vagina in the female	Secures urogenital hiatus
5. Superficial transverse perineal muscle *Pudendal nerve (sacral plexus) (inconstant muscle)*	Superficial part of deep perineal transverse muscle	Blends with perineal body	Supports deep perineal transverse muscle
6. Urethral sphincter *Pudendal nerve (sacral plexus) embraces the intermediate part of urethra [membranous urethra]*	Ring muscle	Ring muscle	Secures urogenital hiatus; assists urinary continence; closes urinary bladder during ejaculation
7. Ischiocavernosus *Pudendal nerve (sacral plexus)*	Ramus of ischium	Tunica albuginea of corpus spongiosum	Fixes crura of penis in the male, respectively crura of clitoris in the female to the ischiopubic ramus and to the urogenital diaphragm; assist ejaculation respectively orgasm
8. Bulbospongiosus *Pudendal nerve (sacral plexus)* Embraces the bulb of penis in the male and the bulb of vestibule in the female	Perineal body, in the male also from the inferior surface of the corpus spongiosum penis (raphe of penis)	In the male it courses laterally to the corpus spongiosum of penis to the inferior urogenital fascia and to the dorsum of penis; in the female the fibers are attached to the corpus cavernosum of clitoris and to the inferior urogenital fascia	Fixes bulb of penis in the male, respectively bulb of vestibule in the female to the urogenital diaphragm; assists ejaculation in the male, respectively orgasm in the female

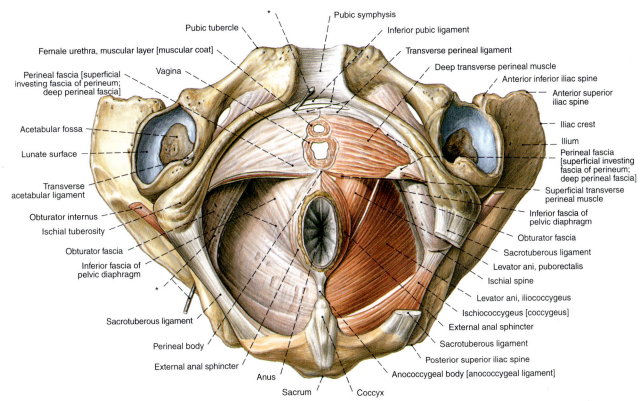

Pubic symphysis
*
Pubic tubercle
Inferior pubic ligament
Female urethra, muscular layer [muscular coat]
Transverse perineal ligament
Perineal fascia [superficial investing fascia of perineum; deep perineal fascia]
Vagina
Deep transverse perineal muscle
Anterior inferior iliac spine
Acetabular fossa
Anterior superior iliac spine
Lunate surface
Iliac crest
Transverse acetabular ligament
Ilium
Perineal fascia [superficial investing fascia of perineum; deep perineal fascia]
Obturator internus
Superficial transverse perineal muscle
Ischial tuberosity
Inferior fascia of pelvic diaphragm
Obturator fascia
Obturator fascia
Inferior fascia of pelvic diaphragm
Sacrotuberous ligament
Levator ani, puborectalis
Ischial spine
Levator ani, iliococcygeus
Sacrotuberous ligament
Ischiococcygeus [coccygeus]
Perineal body
External anal sphincter
External anal sphincter
Sacrotuberous ligament
Anus
Posterior superior iliac spine
Sacrum
Anococcygeal body [anococcygeal ligament]
Coccyx

Fig. 1107 Perineal muscles and pelvic diaphragm [pelvic floor] in the female; left sacrotuberous ligament partially removed to expose ischiococcygeus [coccygeus]; caudal aspect.

In the elderly female the superficial transverse perineal muscle frequently contains only a few muscle fibers.

* Probe in pudendal canal (ALCOCK's canal).

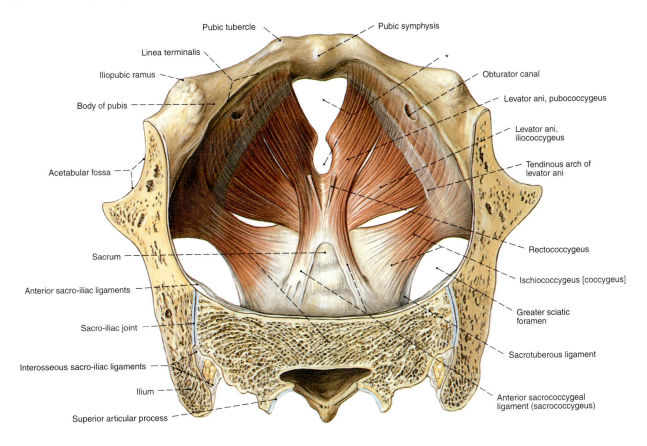

Pubic tubercle
Pubic symphysis
Linea terminalis
*
Iliopubic ramus
Obturator canal
Body of pubis
Levator ani, pubococcygeus
Levator ani, iliococcygeus
Acetabular fossa
Tendinous arch of levator ani
Sacrum
Rectococcygeus
Anterior sacro-iliac ligaments
Ischiococcygeus [coccygeus]
Sacro-iliac joint
Greater sciatic foramen
Interosseous sacro-iliac ligaments
Sacrotuberous ligament
Ilium
Anterior sacrococcygeal ligament (sacrococcygeus)
Superior articular process

Fig. 1108 Pelvic diaphragm [pelvic floor] in the female; upper part of pelvic girdle sectioned in the transverse plane; cranial aspect.

Ischiococcygeus [coccygeus] and sacrococcygeus frequently contain only a few muscle fibers which cover the corresponding ligaments.

* Clinically: urogenital hiatus.

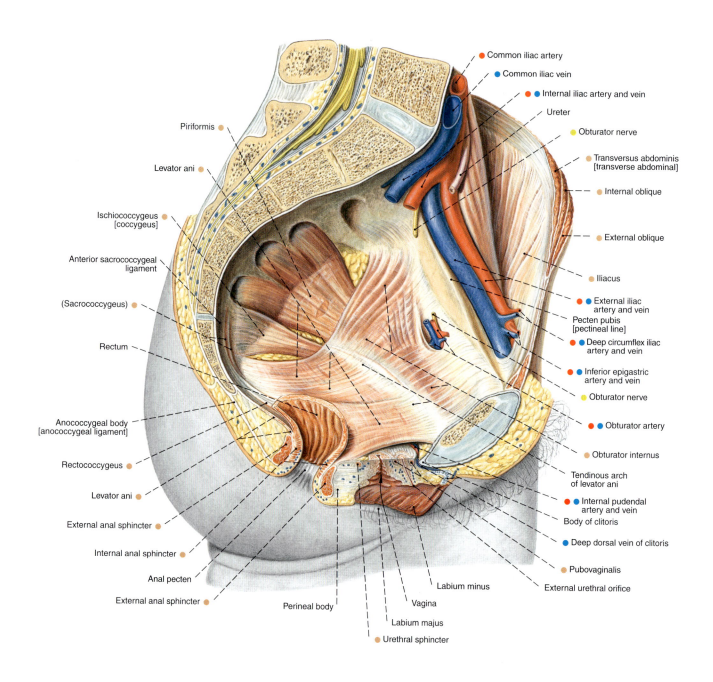

Piriformis

Levator ani

Ischiococcygeus
[coccygeus]

Anterior sacrococcygeal
ligament

(Sacrococcygeus)

Rectum

Anococcygeal body
[anococcygeal ligament]

Rectococcygeus

Levator ani

External anal sphincter

Internal anal sphincter

Anal pecten

External anal sphincter

Common iliac artery

Common iliac vein

Internal iliac artery and vein

Ureter

Obturator nerve

Transversus abdominis
[transverse abdominal]

Internal oblique

External oblique

Iliacus

External iliac
artery and vein

Pecten pubis
[pectineal line]

Deep circumflex iliac
artery and vein

Inferior epigastric
artery and vein

Obturator nerve

Obturator artery

Obturator internus

Tendinous arch
of levator ani

Internal pudendal
artery and vein

Body of clitoris

Deep dorsal vein of clitoris

Pubovaginalis

External urethral orifice

Labium minus

Vagina

Labium majus

Urethral sphincter

Perineal body

Fig. 1109 Muscles of pelvic diaphragm [pelvic
floor] in the female; median section of the pelvis;
organs entirely and most of the nerves and blood
vessels removed to expose musculature; left
lateral aspect.

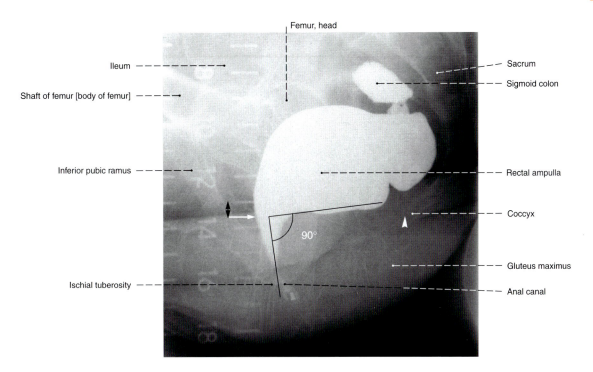

Femur, head

Ileum

Shaft of femur [body of femur]

Inferior pubic ramus

Ischial tuberosity

Sacrum

Sigmoid colon

Rectal ampulla

Coccyx

Gluteus maximus

Anal canal

90°

Fig. 1110 Rectum; lateral radiograph after filling with contrast medium and voluntary closure of anus (defecography) . The junction between anus and rectum (arrow) is located at the tip of the coccyx (white arrowhead). The angle between anal and rectal axes is 90°. This angle is caused by the loop of levator ani (puborectalis). Scale in cm.

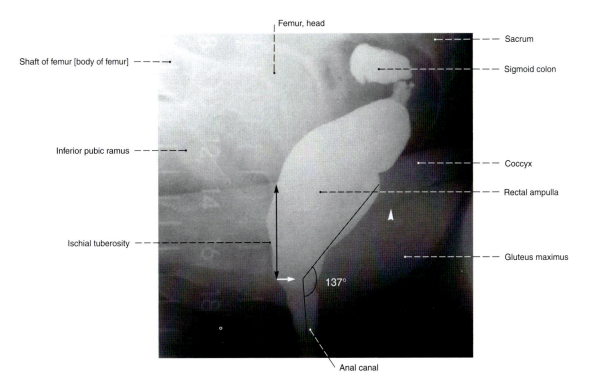

Femur, head

Shaft of femur [body of femur]

Inferior pubic ramus

Ischial tuberosity

Sacrum

Sigmoid colon

Coccyx

Rectal ampulla

Gluteus maximus

137°

Anal canal

Fig. 1111 Rectum; lateral radiograph after filling with contrast medium during defecation (defecography). Compared to Fig. 1110 the anorectal junction has descended, and the angle has increased to 137° due to relaxation of the loop of levator ani. The bend that acts like a valve is now straightened, and the column of feces presses directly upon the anal canal for defecation.

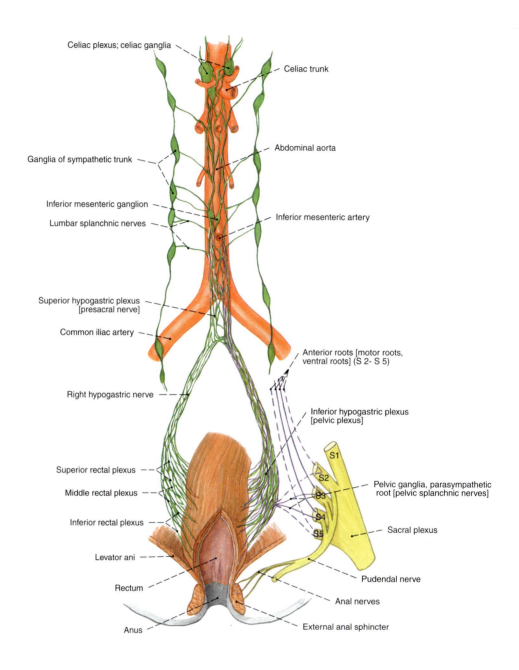

Celiac plexus; celiac ganglia

Celiac trunk

Ganglia of sympathetic trunk

Abdominal aorta

Inferior mesenteric ganglion

Lumbar splanchnic nerves

Inferior mesenteric artery

Superior hypogastric plexus [presacral nerve]

Common iliac artery

Anterior roots [motor roots, ventral roots] (S 2- S 5)

Right hypogastric nerve

Inferior hypogastric plexus [pelvic plexus]

S1

Superior rectal plexus

S2

Middle rectal plexus

S3

Pelvic ganglia, parasympathetic root [pelvic splanchnic nerves]

S4

Inferior rectal plexus

S5

Sacral plexus

Levator ani

Rectum

Pudendal nerve

Anal nerves

Anus

External anal sphincter

Fig. 1112 Rectum; diagram of innervation; ventral aspect.
green = sympathetic part
purple = parasympathetic part

Parasympathetic fibers course through the hypogastric plexus [presacral nerve] to the pelvic viscera and also cranially via the hypogastric nerve. The inferior hypogastric plexus [pelvic plexus] contains both sympathetic and parasympathetic fibers and ganglia (pelvic ganglia).

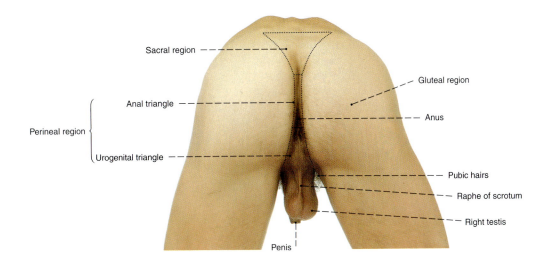

Sacral region —

Gluteal region

Anal triangle —

Anus

Perineal region {

Urogenital triangle —

Pubic hairs

Raphe of scrotum

Right testis

Penis

Fig. 1113 Gluteal and perineal region
in the male; dorsal aspect.
In the cold the cremaster pulls the
scrotum toward the perineum.

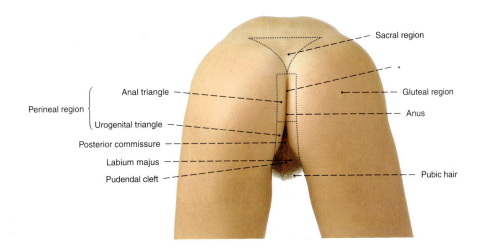

Sacral region

Anal triangle —

Gluteal region

Perineal region {

Anus

Urogenital triangle —

Posterior commissure —

Labium majus —

Pudendal cleft —

Pubic hair

Fig. 1114 Gluteal and perineal
region in the female; dorsal
aspect.
*Clinically: anal cleft.

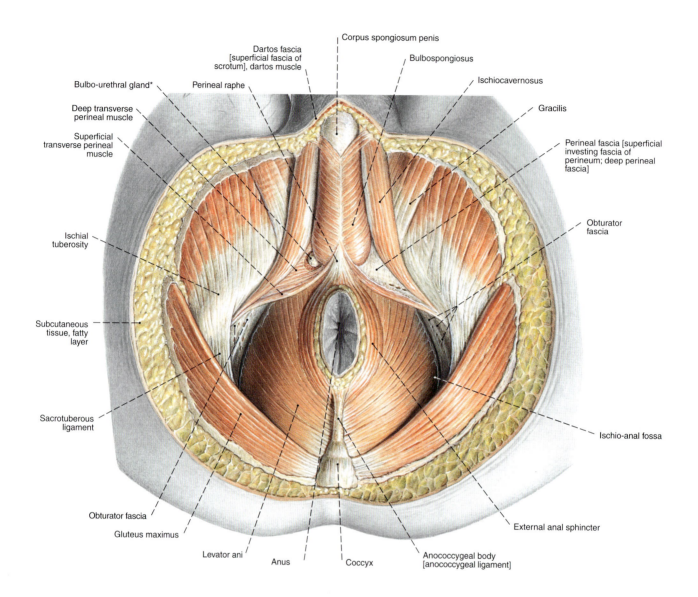

Fig. 1115   Perineum and pelvic diaphragm [pelvic floor] in the male; fat body of ischio-anal fossa removed; inferior fascia of urogenital diaphragm removed on the right and bulbo-urethral gland exposed; caudal aspect.

* Also COWPER's gland.

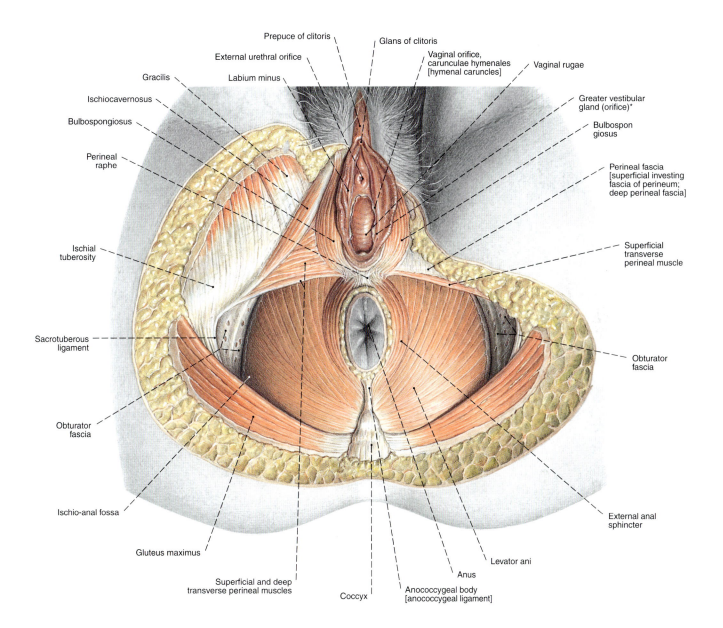

Prepuce of clitoris

Glans of clitoris

External urethral orifice

Vaginal orifice, carunculae hymenales [hymenal caruncles]

Vaginal rugae

Gracilis

Labium minus

Ischiocavernosus

Greater vestibular gland (orifice)*

Bulbospongiosus

Bulbospon giosus

Perineal raphe

Perineal fascia [superficial investing fascia of perineum; deep perineal fascia]

Ischial tuberosity

Superficial transverse perineal muscle

Sacrotuberous ligament

Obturator fascia

Obturator fascia

External anal sphincter

Ischio-anal fossa

Gluteus maximus

Levator ani

Superficial and deep transverse perineal muscles

Anus

Coccyx

Anococcygeal body [anococcygeal ligament]

Fig. 1116 Perineum; pelvic diaphragm [pelvic floor]; female external genitalia; fat body of ischio-anal fossa removed; caudal aspect.

* Also BARTHOLIN's gland.

Vaginal orifice and anus are situated close to each other. During parturition both skin and muscles of the perineum may be lacerated up to the anal sphincter muscles (1st–3rd grade perineal lacerations). These can be avoided by a prior lateral or median incision (lateral or median episiotomy).

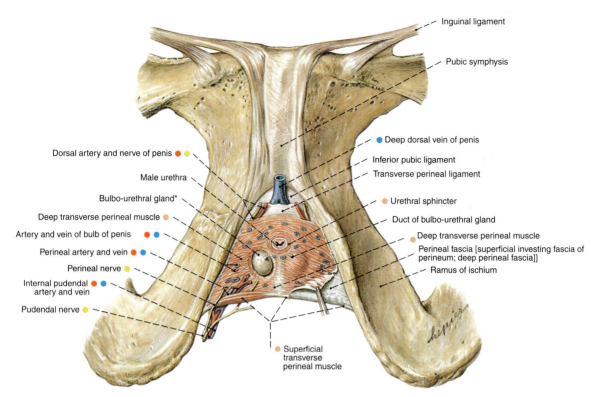

Inguinal ligament

Pubic symphysis

Deep dorsal vein of penis

Inferior pubic ligament

Transverse perineal ligament

Urethral sphincter

Duct of bulbo-urethral gland

Deep transverse perineal muscle

Perineal fascia [superficial investing fascia of perineum; deep perineal fascia]]

Ramus of ischium

Dorsal artery and nerve of penis

Male urethra

Bulbo-urethral gland*

Deep transverse perineal muscle

Artery and vein of bulb of penis

Perineal artery and vein

Perineal nerve

Internal pudendal artery and vein

Pudendal nerve

Superficial transverse perineal muscle

Fig. 1117 Urogenital diaphragm in the male; inferior fascia extensively removed; right bulbo-urethral gland dissected; caudal aspect. Compare Fig. 1118.

* Clinically: COWPER's gland.

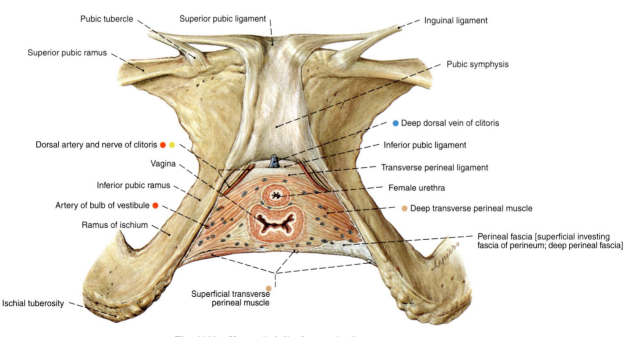

Pubic tubercle

Superior pubic ligament

Inguinal ligament

Superior pubic ramus

Pubic symphysis

Deep dorsal vein of clitoris

Inferior pubic ligament

Dorsal artery and nerve of clitoris

Vagina

Transverse perineal ligament

Inferior pubic ramus

Female urethra

Artery of bulb of vestibule

Deep transverse perineal muscle

Ramus of ischium

Perineal fascia [superficial investing fascia of perineum; deep perineal fascia]

Ischial tuberosity

Superficial transverse perineal muscle

Fig. 1118 Urogenital diaphragm in the female; inferior fascia extensively removed; caudal aspect. Compare Fig. 1117.

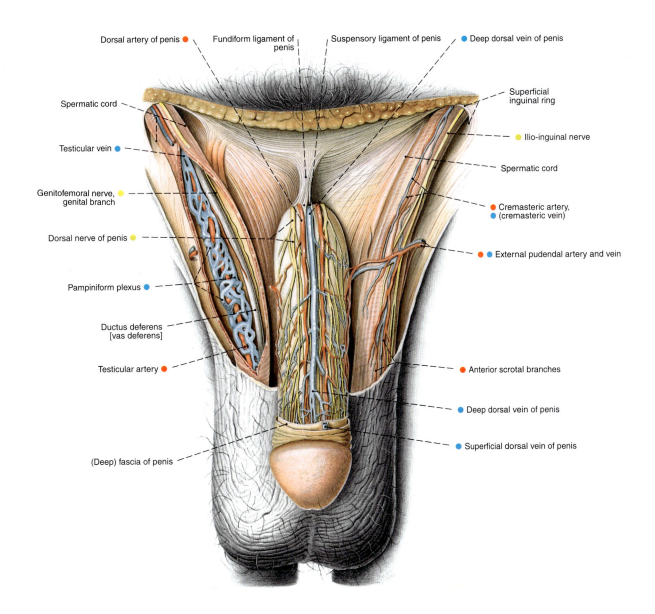

Dorsal artery of penis ●

Fundiform ligament of penis

Suspensory ligament of penis

Deep dorsal vein of penis ●

Spermatic cord

Superficial inguinal ring

Testicular vein ●

● Ilio-inguinal nerve

Spermatic cord

Genitofemoral nerve, ● genital branch

● Cremasteric artery, ● (cremasteric vein)

Dorsal nerve of penis ●

● ● External pudendal artery and vein

Pampiniform plexus ●

Ductus deferens [vas deferens]

Testicular artery ●

● Anterior scrotal branches

● Deep dorsal vein of penis

● Superficial dorsal vein of penis

(Deep) fascia of penis

Fig. 1119 External male genitalia; demonstration of nerves and blood vessels by extensive removal of skin and superficial fascia of penis; layers of spermatic cord incised on the right; ventral aspect.

The venous plexus (pampiniform plexus) surrounding the testicular artery is constantly well-developed.

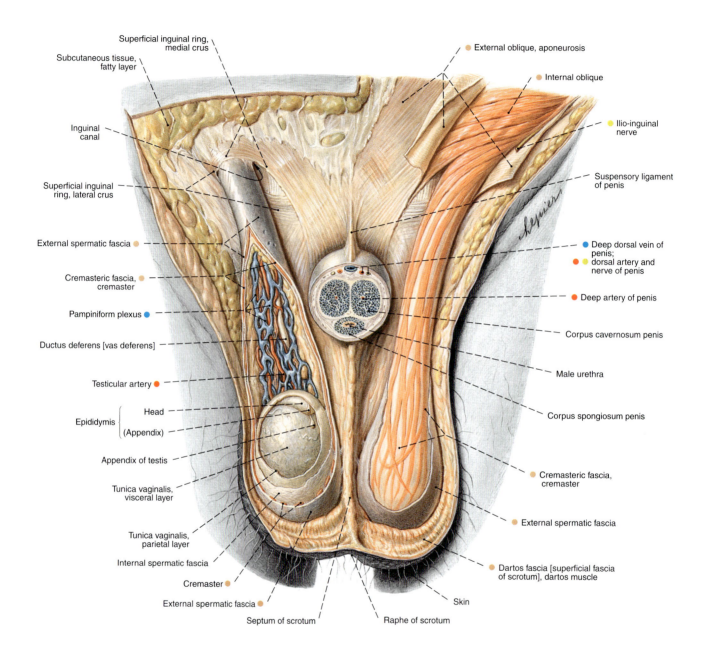

Superficial inguinal ring, medial crus

Subcutaneous tissue, fatty layer

Inguinal canal

Superficial inguinal ring, lateral crus

External spermatic fascia

Cremasteric fascia, cremaster

Pampiniform plexus

Ductus deferens [vas deferens]

Testicular artery

Epididymis { Head (Appendix)

Appendix of testis

Tunica vaginalis, visceral layer

Tunica vaginalis, parietal layer

Internal spermatic fascia

Cremaster

External spermatic fascia

Septum of scrotum

External oblique, aponeurosis

Internal oblique

Ilio-inguinal nerve

Suspensory ligament of penis

Deep dorsal vein of penis; dorsal artery and nerve of penis

Deep artery of penis

Corpus cavernosum penis

Male urethra

Corpus spongiosum penis

Cremasteric fascia, cremaster

External spermatic fascia

Dartos fascia [superficial fascia of scrotum], dartos muscle

Skin

Raphe of scrotum

Fig. 1120   Male genitalia; skin of abdomen and parts of skin of scrotum removed; body of penis severed; layers of spermatic cord dissected on the right; ventral aspect.
Compare Figs. 824 and 827, origin of cremaster and fascias from the muscles of the abdominal wall.

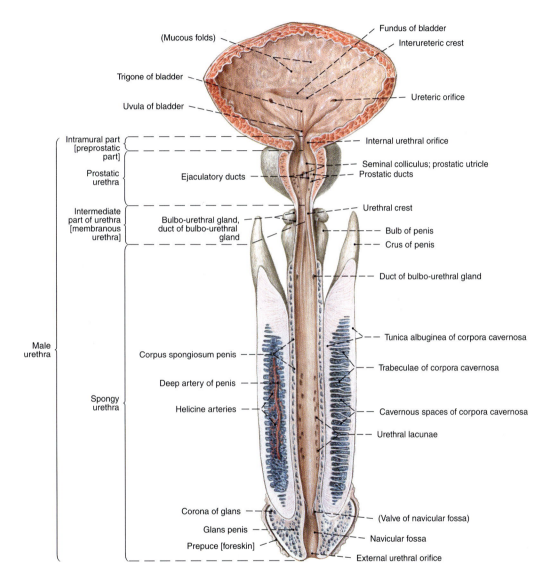

(Mucous folds)

Fundus of bladder

Interureteric crest

Trigone of bladder

Uvula of bladder

Ureteric orifice

Intramural part [preprostatic part]

Internal urethral orifice

Seminal colliculus; prostatic utricle

Prostatic urethra

Ejaculatory ducts

Prostatic ducts

Intermediate part of urethra [membranous urethra]

Bulbo-urethral gland, duct of bulbo-urethral gland

Urethral crest

Bulb of penis

Crus of penis

Duct of bulbo-urethral gland

Tunica albuginea of corpora cavernosa

Male urethra

Corpus spongiosum penis

Trabeculae of corpora cavernosa

Deep artery of penis

Helicine arteries

Cavernous spaces of corpora cavernosa

Spongy urethra

Urethral lacunae

Corona of glans

(Valve of navicular fossa)

Glans penis

Navicular fossa

Prepuce [foreskin]

External urethral orifice

Fig. 1121 Urinary bladder; prostate; male urethra; urinary bladder and urethra opened to expose the lumen; skin of penis extensively removed; ventral aspect.
In its normal position the urethra has an arched course (compare Fig. 1145).

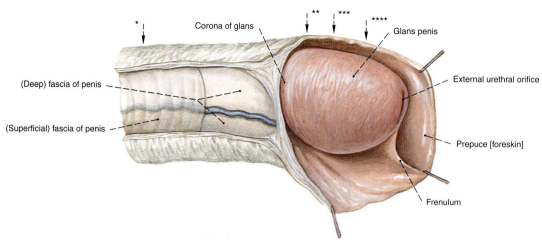

Fig. 1122   Penis with glans and prepuce [foreskin].
Skin and superficial fascia of penis removed layer by layer;
lateral aspect.

* Level of cross-section in Fig. 1123a.
** Level of cross-section in Fig. 1123b.
*** Level of cross-section in Fig. 1123c.
**** Level of cross-section in Fig. 1123d.

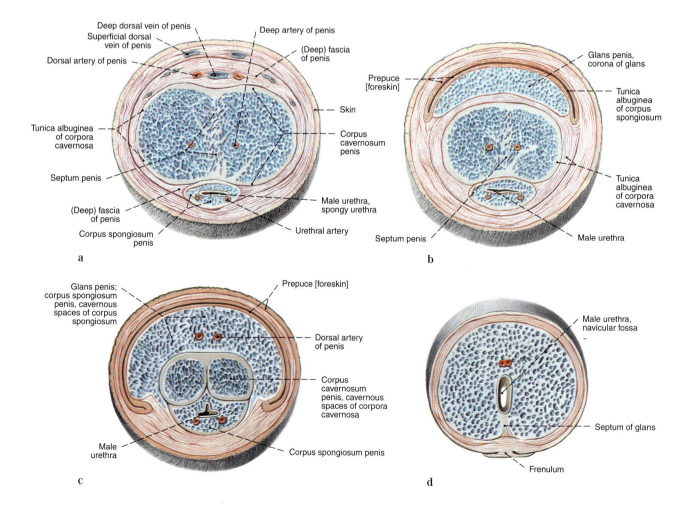

Fig. 1123 a-d   Penis; cross-sections; levels of section
indicated in Fig. 1122; ventral aspect.

a   Cross-section through the middle of body. Both corpora
cavernosa are incompletely separated by the septum
penis.

b   Cross-section at level of proximal circumference
of glans penis.

c   Cross-section through the middle of glans penis.

d   Cross-section at level of distal end of glans penis.

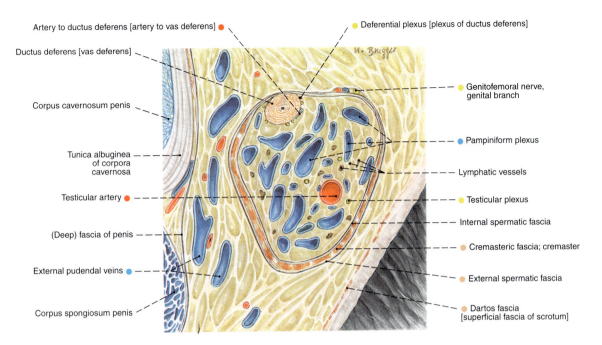

Artery to ductus deferens [artery to vas deferens] ●

Ductus deferens [vas deferens]

Corpus cavernosum penis

Tunica albuginea of corpora cavernosa

Testicular artery ●

(Deep) fascia of penis

External pudendal veins ●

Corpus spongiosum penis

Deferential plexus [plexus of ductus deferens] ●

Genitofemoral nerve, genital branch ●

Pampiniform plexus ●

Lymphatic vessels

Testicular plexus ●

Internal spermatic fascia

Cremasteric fascia; cremaster ●

External spermatic fascia ●

Dartos fascia [superficial fascia of scrotum] ●

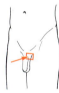

Fig. 1124 Left spermatic cord; frontal section; ventral aspect (250%).
Development of cremaster, pampiniform plexus , and the position of ductus deferens [vas deferens] are highly variable.

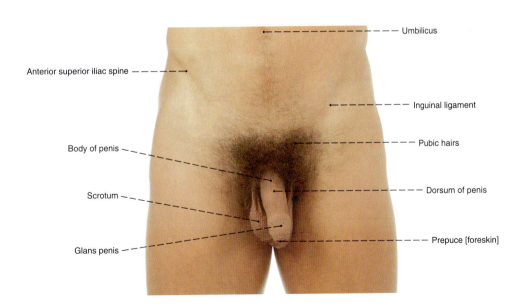

Umbilicus

Anterior superior iliac spine

Inguinal ligament

Pubic hairs

Body of penis

Dorsum of penis

Scrotum

Prepuce [foreskin]

Glans penis

Fig. 1125 External male genitalia; ventral aspect.

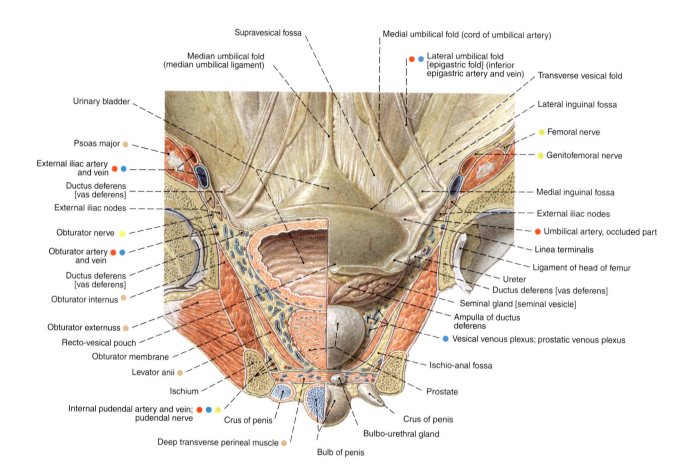

Supravesical fossa

Median umbilical fold
(median umbilical ligament)

Medial umbilical fold (cord of umbilical artery)

Lateral umbilical fold
[epigastric fold] (inferior
epigastric artery and vein)

Transverse vesical fold

Urinary bladder

Psoas major

External iliac artery
and vein

Ductus deferens
[vas deferens]

External iliac nodes

Obturator nerve

Obturator artery
and vein

Ductus deferens
[vas deferens]

Obturator internus

Obturator externuss

Recto-vesical pouch

Obturator membrane

Levator anii

Ischium

Internal pudendal artery and vein;
pudendal nerve

Crus of penis

Deep transverse perineal muscle

Bulb of penis

Lateral inguinal fossa

Femoral nerve

Genitofemoral nerve

Medial inguinal fossa

External iliac nodes

Umbilical artery, occluded part

Linea terminalis

Ligament of head of femur

Ureter

Ductus deferens [vas deferens]

Seminal gland [seminal vesicle]

Ampulla of ductus
deferens

Vesical venous plexus; prostatic venous plexus

Ischio-anal fossa

Prostate

Crus of penis

Bulbo-urethral gland

Fig. 1126 Pelvic diaphragm [pelvic floor]; pelvic
viscera and anterior abdominal wall in the male;
frontal section through the head of femur on the left;
urinary bladder and prostate not sectioned on the
right; dorsal aspect.

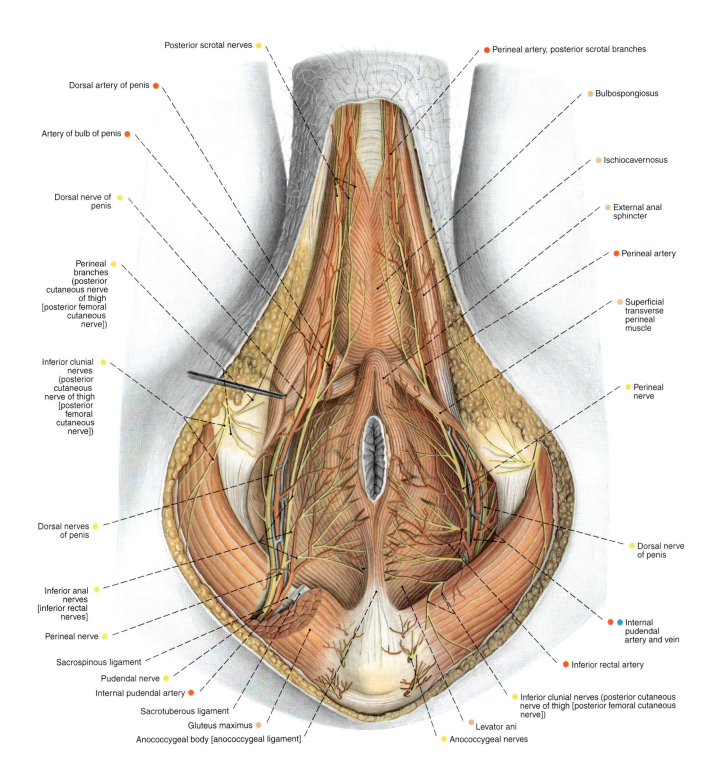

Posterior scrotal nerves

Dorsal artery of penis

Artery of bulb of penis

Dorsal nerve of penis

Perineal branches (posterior cutaneous nerve of thigh [posterior femoral cutaneous nerve])

Inferior clunial nerves (posterior cutaneous nerve of thigh [posterior femoral cutaneous nerve])

Dorsal nerves of penis

Inferior anal nerves [inferior rectal nerves]

Perineal nerve

Sacrospinous ligament

Pudendal nerve

Internal pudendal artery

Sacrotuberous ligament

Gluteus maximus

Anococcygeal body [anococcygeal ligament]

Perineal artery, posterior scrotal branches

Bulbospongiosus

Ischiocavernosus

External anal sphincter

Perineal artery

Superficial transverse perineal muscle

Perineal nerve

Dorsal nerve of penis

Internal pudendal artery and vein

Inferior rectal artery

Inferior clunial nerves (posterior cutaneous nerve of thigh [posterior femoral cutaneous nerve])

Levator ani

Anococcygeal nerves

Fig. 1127   Blood vessels and nerves of perineal region and external male genitalia; fat body of ischio-anal fossa removed and gluteus maximus incised to expose the course of pudendal nerve and internal pudendal artery; caudal aspect.

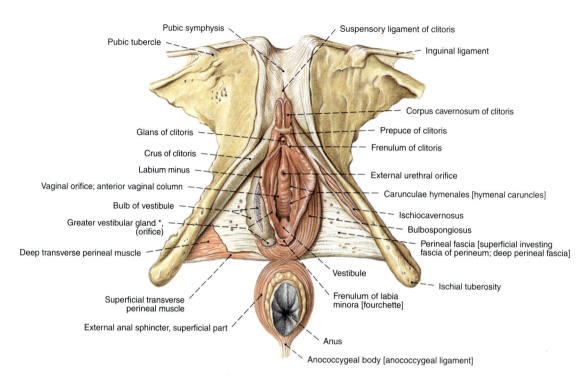

Pubic symphysis
Pubic tubercle
Suspensory ligament of clitoris
Inguinal ligament
Corpus cavernosum of clitoris
Glans of clitoris
Prepuce of clitoris
Crus of clitoris
Frenulum of clitoris
Labium minus
External urethral orifice
Vaginal orifice; anterior vaginal column
Carunculae hymenales [hymenal caruncles]
Bulb of vestibule
Ischiocavernosus
Greater vestibular gland *, (orifice)
Bulbospongiosus
Deep transverse perineal muscle
Perineal fascia [superficial investing fascia of perineum; deep perineal fascia]
Vestibule
Ischial tuberosity
Superficial transverse perineal muscle
Frenulum of labia minora [fourchette]
External anal sphincter, superficial part
Anus
Anococcygeal body [anococcygeal ligament]

Fig. 1128   External female genitalia; urogenital diaphragm; inferior fascia of urogenital diaphragm extensively removed, ischiocavernosus dissected on the left, bulbospongiosus removed to expose erectile tissue of bulb of vestibule; caudal ventral aspect.
* Clinically: BARTHOLIN's gland.

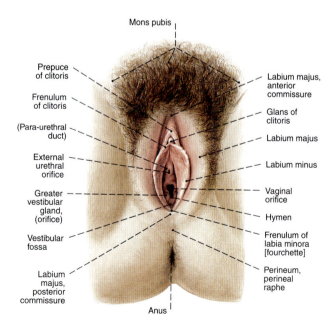

Mons pubis
Prepuce of clitoris
Frenulum of clitoris
(Para-urethral duct)
External urethral orifice
Greater vestibular gland, (orifice)
Vestibular fossa
Labium majus, posterior commissure
Anus
Labium majus, anterior commissure
Glans of clitoris
Labium majus
Labium minus
Vaginal orifice
Hymen
Frenulum of labia minora [fourchette]
Perineum, perineal raphe

Fig. 1129   External female genitalia; caudal aspect.
View of the vestibule is only possible when labia majora et minora are spread open with specula or the examiner's fingers (not shown).

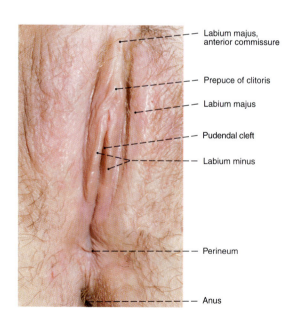

Labium majus, anterior commissure
Prepuce of clitoris
Labium majus
Pudendal cleft
Labium minus
Perineum
Anus

Fig. 1130   External female genitalia; caudal aspect.
Even when the legs are spread apart, the labia minora close the vaginal orifice as shown in this 26-year-old female.

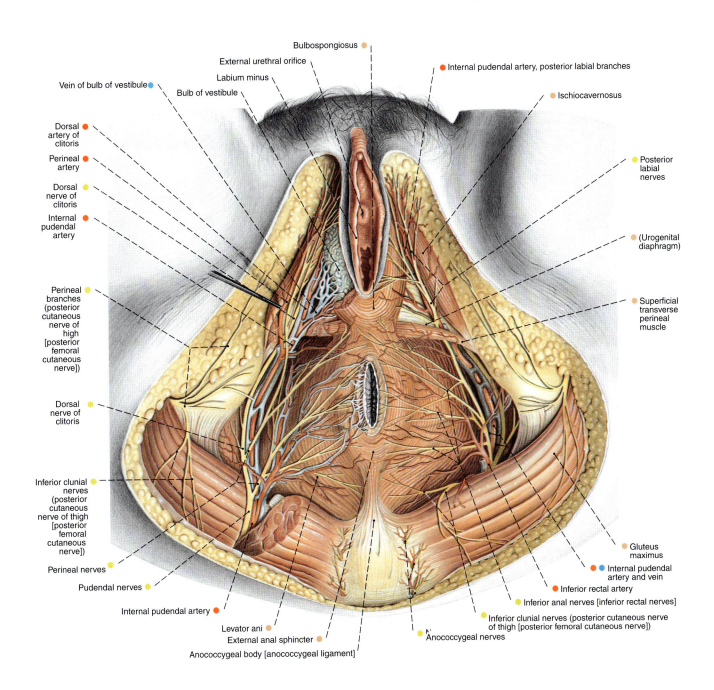

Bulbospongiosus

External urethral orifice

Labium minus

Internal pudendal artery, posterior labial branches

Ischiocavernosus

Vein of bulb of vestibule

Bulb of vestibule

Dorsal artery of clitoris

Perineal artery

Posterior labial nerves

Dorsal nerve of clitoris

Internal pudendal artery

(Urogenital diaphragm)

Perineal branches (posterior cutaneous nerve of high [posterior femoral cutaneous nerve])

Superficial transverse perineal muscle

Dorsal nerve of clitoris

Inferior clunial nerves (posterior cutaneous nerve of thigh [posterior femoral cutaneous nerve])

Gluteus maximus

Internal pudendal artery and vein

Inferior rectal artery

Perineal nerves

Pudendal nerves

Inferior anal nerves [inferior rectal nerves]

Internal pudendal artery

Inferior clunial nerves (posterior cutaneous nerve of thigh [posterior femoral cutaneous nerve])

Levator ani

Anococcygeal nerves

External anal sphincter

Anococcygeal body [anococcygeal ligament]

Fig. 1131 Blood vessels and nerves of perineal region and external female genitalia; subcutaneous tissue and fat body of ischio-anal fossa removed and gluteus maximus and deep transverse perineal muscle incised on the right to expose the course nerves and blood vessels; bulbospongiosus removed on the right to expose erectile tissue of bulb of vestibule; caudal aspect.

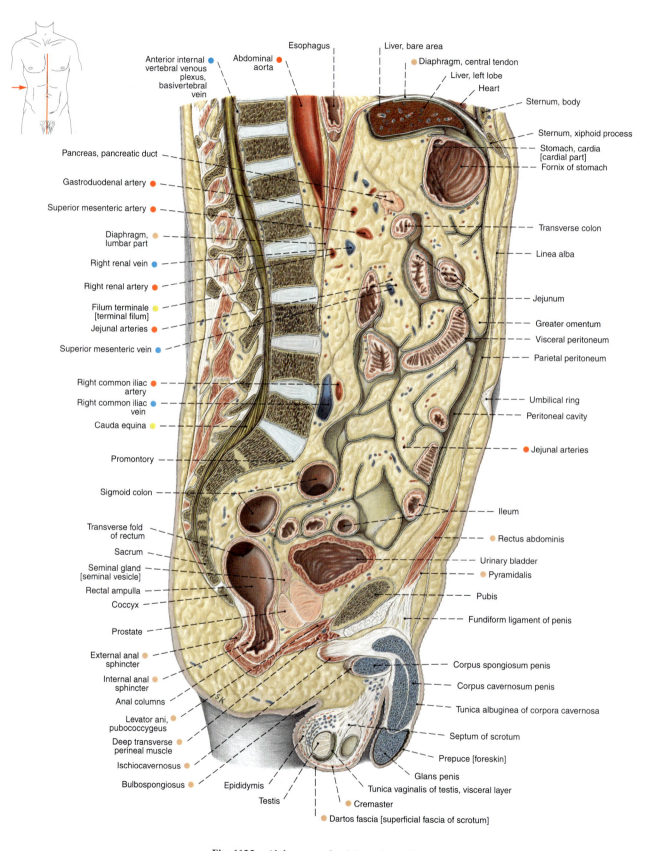

Anterior internal vertebral venous plexus, basivertebral vein

Abdominal aorta

Esophagus

Liver, bare area

Diaphragm, central tendon

Liver, left lobe

Heart

Sternum, body

Sternum, xiphoid process

Stomach, cardia [cardial part]

Fornix of stomach

Pancreas, pancreatic duct

Gastroduodenal artery

Superior mesenteric artery

Diaphragm, lumbar part

Right renal vein

Right renal artery

Filum terminale [terminal filum]

Jejunal arteries

Superior mesenteric vein

Right common iliac artery

Right common iliac vein

Cauda equina

Promontory

Sigmoid colon

Transverse fold of rectum

Sacrum

Seminal gland [seminal vesicle]

Rectal ampulla

Coccyx

Prostate

External anal sphincter

Internal anal sphincter

Anal columns

Levator ani, pubococcygeus

Deep transverse perineal muscle

Ischiocavernosus

Bulbospongiosus

Epididymis

Testis

Cremaster

Dartos fascia [superficial fascia of scrotum]

Tunica vaginalis of testis, visceral layer

Glans penis

Prepuce [foreskin]

Septum of scrotum

Tunica albuginea of corpora cavernosa

Corpus cavernosum penis

Corpus spongiosum penis

Fundiform ligament of penis

Pubis

Pyramidalis

Urinary bladder

Rectus abdominis

Ileum

Jejunal arteries

Peritoneal cavity

Umbilical ring

Parietal peritoneum

Visceral peritoneum

Greater omentum

Jejunum

Linea alba

Transverse colon

Fig. 1132   Abdomen and pelvis in the male;
median section; lateral aspect.
The external male genitalia and the ventral
parts of the pelvis are sectioned left to the median plane.

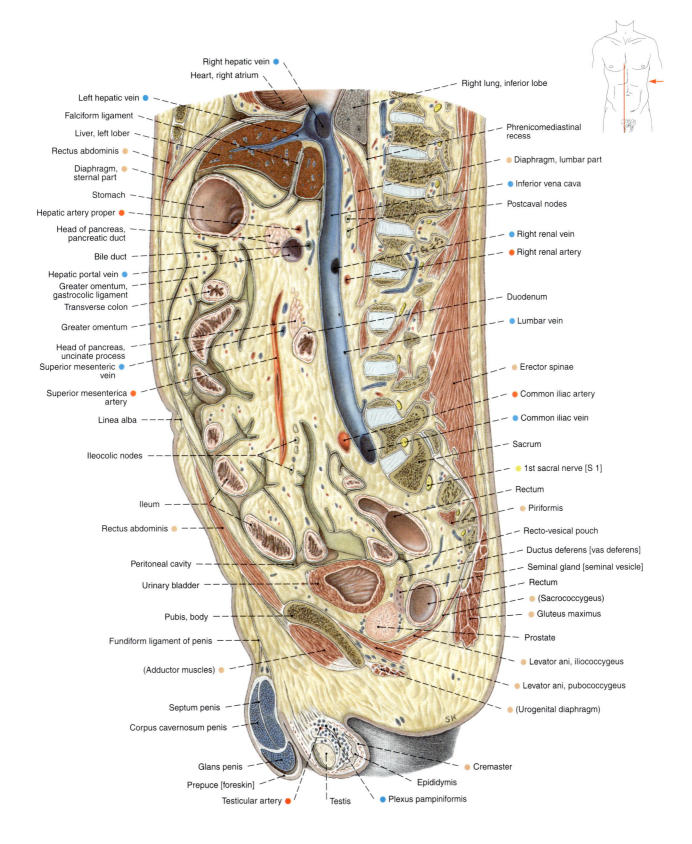

Right hepatic vein ●
Heart, right atrium
Left hepatic vein ●
Falciform ligament
Liver, left lober
Rectus abdominis ●
Diaphragm, sternal part ●
Stomach
Hepatic artery proper ●
Head of pancreas, pancreatic duct
Bile duct
Hepatic portal vein ●
Greater omentum, gastrocolic ligament
Transverse colon
Greater omentum
Head of pancreas, uncinate process
Superior mesenteric vein ●
Superior mesenterica artery ●
Linea alba
Ileocolic nodes
Ileum
Rectus abdominis ●
Peritoneal cavity
Urinary bladder
Pubis, body
Fundiform ligament of penis
(Adductor muscles) ●
Septum penis
Corpus cavernosum penis
Glans penis
Prepuce [foreskin]
Testicular artery ●
Testis

Right lung, inferior lobe
Phrenicomediastinal recess
Diaphragm, lumbar part ●
Inferior vena cava ●
Postcaval nodes
Right renal vein ●
Right renal artery ●
Duodenum
Lumbar vein ●
Erector spinae ●
Common iliac artery ●
Common iliac vein ●
Sacrum
1st sacral nerve [S 1] ●
Rectum
Piriformis ●
Recto-vesical pouch
Ductus deferens [vas deferens]
Seminal gland [seminal vesicle]
Rectum
(Sacrococcygeus) ●
Gluteus maximus ●
Prostate
Levator ani, iliococcygeus ●
Levator ani, pubococcygeus ●
(Urogenital diaphragm) ●
Cremaster ●
Epididymis
Plexus pampiniformis ●

Fig. 1133 Abdomen and pelvis in the male; right paramedian section; right medial aspect.
Due to a lateral curvature (scoliosis) of the lumbar vertebral column, it is sectioned further lateral than the thoracic vertebral column. Compared to the subcutaneous fat more fat is found in the greater omentum.

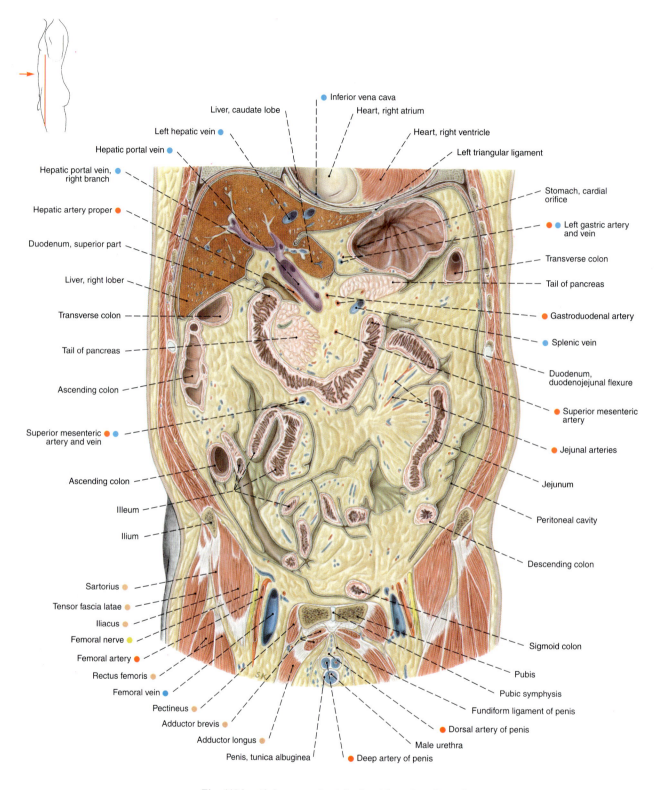

Inferior vena cava

Liver, caudate lobe

Heart, right atrium

Heart, right ventricle

Left hepatic vein

Left triangular ligament

Hepatic portal vein

Hepatic portal vein, right branch

Stomach, cardial orifice

Hepatic artery proper

Left gastric artery and vein

Duodenum, superior part

Transverse colon

Liver, right lober

Tail of pancreas

Transverse colon

Gastroduodenal artery

Tail of pancreas

Splenic vein

Ascending colon

Duodenum, duodenojejunal flexure

Superior mesenteric artery

Superior mesenteric artery and vein

Jejunal arteries

Ascending colon

Jejunum

Illeum

Peritoneal cavity

Ilium

Descending colon

Sartorius

Tensor fascia latae

Iliacus

Femoral nerve

Sigmoid colon

Femoral artery

Pubis

Rectus femoris

Pubic symphysis

Femoral vein

Fundiform ligament of penis

Pectineus

Dorsal artery of penis

Adductor brevis

Male urethra

Adductor longus

Penis, tunica albuginea

Deep artery of penis

Fig. 1134   Abdomen and pelvis; frontal section through most anterior part of peritoneal cavity; ventral aspect. Muscles, blood vessels, and nerves are labeled in Fig. 837.

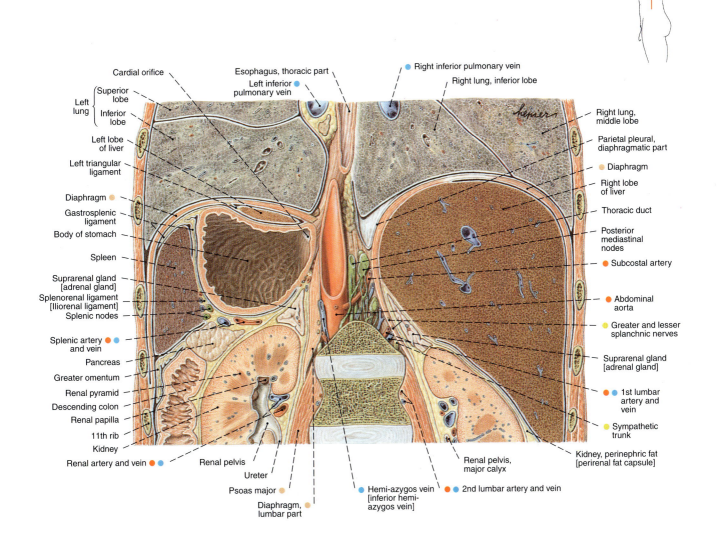

Cardial orifice

Esophagus, thoracic part

Right inferior pulmonary vein

Left inferior pulmonary vein

Right lung, inferior lobe

Left lung { Superior lobe / Inferior lobe }

Left lobe of liver

Right lung, middle lobe

Left triangular ligament

Parietal pleural, diaphragmatic part

Diaphragm

Diaphragm

Gastrosplenic ligament

Right lobe of liver

Body of stomach

Thoracic duct

Spleen

Posterior mediastinal nodes

Suprarenal gland [adrenal gland]

Subcostal artery

Splenorenal ligament [Iliorenal ligament]

Abdominal aorta

Splenic nodes

Greater and lesser splanchnic nerves

Splenic artery and vein

Suprarenal gland [adrenal gland]

Pancreas

Greater omentum

1st lumbar artery and vein

Renal pyramid

Descending colon

Sympathetic trunk

Renal papilla

11th rib

Kidney

Kidney, perinephric fat [perirenal fat capsule]

Renal artery and vein

Renal pelvis

Renal pelvis, major calyx

Ureter

Psoas major

Hemi-azygos vein [inferior hemi-azygos vein]

2nd lumbar artery and vein

Diaphragm, lumbar part

Fig. 1135 Abdomen; frontal section exposing diaphragm, upper abdominal organs and kidneys; dorsal aspect.
Due to the lumbar lordosis the 1st and 2nd lumbar vertebrae are sectioned.

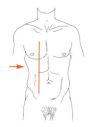

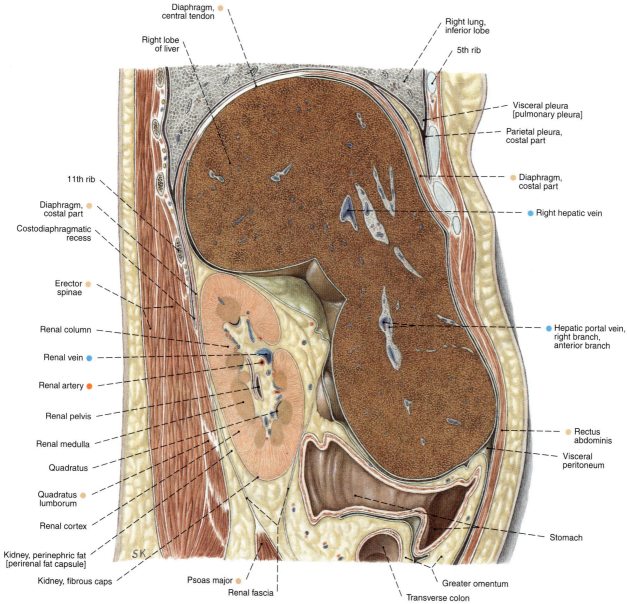

Diaphragm, central tendon

Right lobe of liver

Right lung, inferior lobe

5th rib

Visceral pleura [pulmonary pleura]

Parietal pleura, costal part

Diaphragm, costal part

Right hepatic vein

11th rib

Diaphragm, costal part

Costodiaphragmatic recess

Erector spinae

Renal column

Renal vein

Renal artery

Renal pelvis

Renal medulla

Quadratus

Quadratus lumborum

Renal cortex

Kidney, perinephric fat [perirenal fat capsule]

Kidney, fibrous caps

Psoas major

Renal fascia

Hepatic portal vein, right branch, anterior branch

Rectus abdominis

Visceral peritoneum

Stomach

Greater omentum

Transverse colon

SK

Fig. 1136 Abdomen; sagittal section through the upper abdomen at the level of the right kidney; viewed from the right.

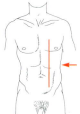

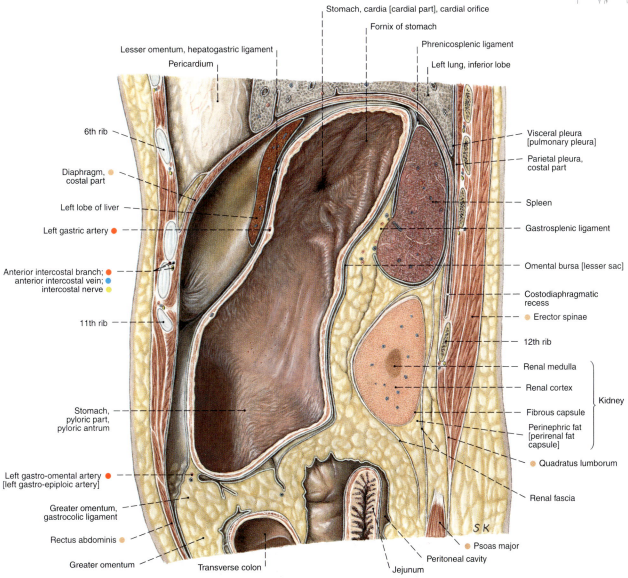

Stomach, cardia [cardial part], cardial orifice

Fornix of stomach

Lesser omentum, hepatogastric ligament

Phrenicosplenic ligament

Pericardium

Left lung, inferior lobe

6th rib

Visceral pleura [pulmonary pleura]

Diaphragm, ● costal part

Parietal pleura, costal part

Left lobe of liver

Spleen

Left gastric artery ●

Gastrosplenic ligament

Anterior intercostal branch; ●
anterior intercostal vein; ●
intercostal nerve ●

Omental bursa [lesser sac]

Costodiaphragmatic recess

11th rib

● Erector spinae

12th rib

Renal medulla

Renal cortex

Kidney

Stomach, pyloric part, pyloric antrum

Fibrous capsule

Perinephric fat [perirenal fat capsule]

● Quadratus lumborum

Left gastro-omental artery ●
[left gastro-epiploic artery]

Renal fascia

Greater omentum, gastrocolic ligament

Rectus abdominis ●

● Psoas major

Peritoneal cavity

Greater omentum

Transverse colon

Jejunum

SK

Fig. 1137   Abdomen; sagittal section through the upper abdomen at the level of the spleen; viewed from the left. The capsule of the liver is pathologically thickened.

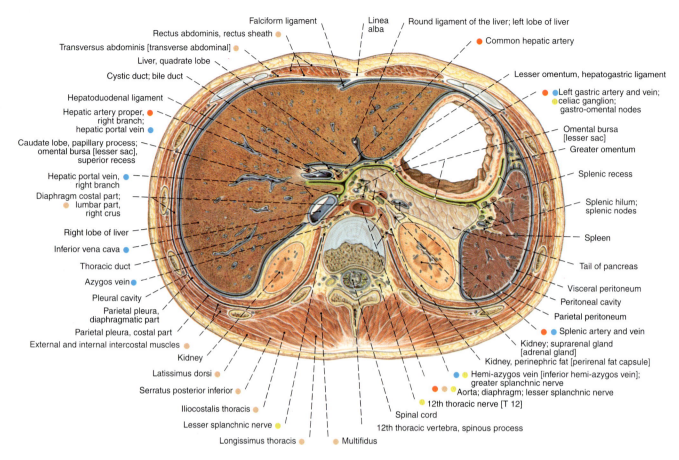

Falciform ligament
Rectus abdominis, rectus sheath
Transversus abdominis [transverse abdominal]
Liver, quadrate lobe
Cystic duct; bile duct
Hepatoduodenal ligament
Hepatic artery proper, right branch; hepatic portal vein
Caudate lobe, papillary process; omental bursa [lesser sac], superior recess
Hepatic portal vein, right branch
Diaphragm costal part; lumbar part, right crus
Right lobe of liver
Inferior vena cava
Thoracic duct
Azygos vein
Pleural cavity
Parietal pleura, diaphragmatic part
Parietal pleura, costal part
External and internal intercostal muscles
Kidney
Latissimus dorsi
Serratus posterior inferior
Iliocostalis thoracis
Lesser splanchnic nerve
Longissimus thoracis
Multifidus

Linea alba
Round ligament of the liver; left lobe of liver
Common hepatic artery
Lesser omentum, hepatogastric ligament
Left gastric artery and vein; celiac ganglion; gastro-omental nodes
Omental bursa [lesser sac]
Greater omentum
Splenic recess
Splenic hilum; splenic nodes
Spleen
Tail of pancreas
Visceral peritoneum
Peritoneal cavity
Parietal peritoneum
Splenic artery and vein
Kidney; suprarenal gland [adrenal gland]
Kidney, perinephric fat [perirenal fat capsule]
Hemi-azygos vein [inferior hemi-azygos vein]; greater splanchnic nerve
Aorta; diaphragm; lesser splanchnic nerve
12th thoracic nerve [T 12]
Spinal cord
12th thoracic vertebra, spinous process

Fig. 1138 Abdomen; transverse section at level of intervertebral disc between 12th thoracic and 1st lumbar vertebra; peritoneum in blue, in the area of the omental bursa [lesser sac] in yellow green; caudal aspect. In this specimen the subcutaneous tissue was poorly developed.

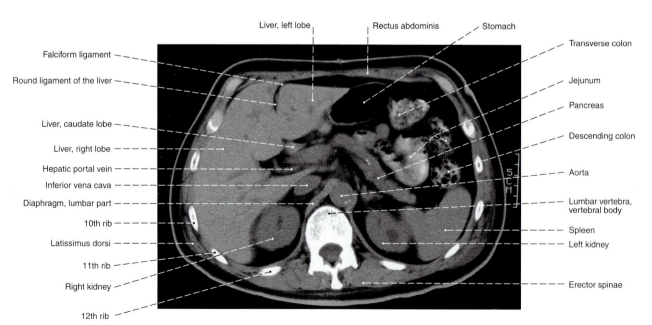

Liver, left lobe
Rectus abdominis
Stomach
Falciform ligament
Round ligament of the liver
Liver, caudate lobe
Liver, right lobe
Hepatic portal vein
Inferior vena cava
Diaphragm, lumbar part
10th rib
Latissimus dorsi
11th rib
Right kidney
12th rib

Transverse colon
Jejunum
Pancreas
Descending colon
Aorta
Lumbar vertebra, vertebral body
Spleen
Left kidney
Erector spinae

Fig. 1139 Abdomen; computer tomographic transverse section at level of 1st lumbar vertebrae; caudal aspect. Intestine is partially filled with contrast medium.

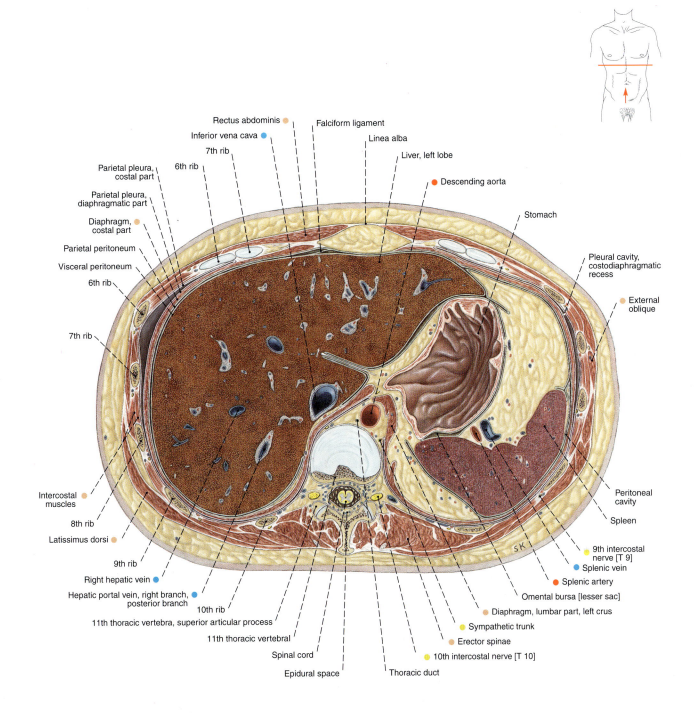

Rectus abdominis
Inferior vena cava
7th rib
6th rib
Parietal pleura, costal part
Parietal pleura, diaphragmatic part
Diaphragm, costal part
Parietal peritoneum
Visceral peritoneum
6th rib
7th rib
Intercostal muscles
8th rib
Latissimus dorsi
9th rib
Right hepatic vein
Hepatic portal vein, right branch, posterior branch
10th rib
11th thoracic vertebra, superior articular process
11th thoracic vertebral
Spinal cord
Epidural space

Falciform ligament
Linea alba
Liver, left lobe
Descending aorta
Stomach
Pleural cavity, costodiaphragmatic recess
External oblique
Peritoneal cavity
Spleen
9th intercostal nerve [T 9]
Splenic vein
Splenic artery
Omental bursa [lesser sac]
Diaphragm, lumbar part, left crus
Sympathetic trunk
Erector spinae
10th intercostal nerve [T 10]
Thoracic duct

S K

Fig. 1140 Abdomen; transverse section
through upper abdomen at level of 11t
thoracic vertebra; caudal aspect.

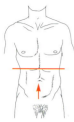

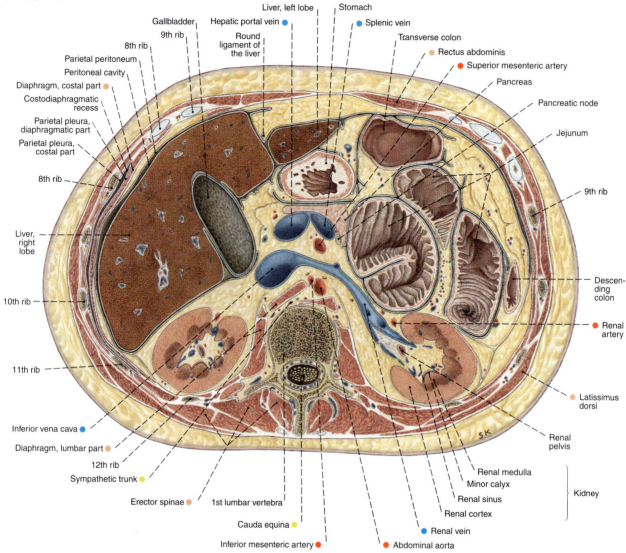

Liver, left lobe

Stomach

Gallbladder

Hepatic portal vein ●

Splenic vein ●

9th rib

Round ligament of the liver

Transverse colon

8th rib

Rectus abdominis ●

Parietal peritoneum

Superior mesenteric artery ●

Peritoneal cavity

Pancreas

Diaphragm, costal part ●

Pancreatic node

Costodiaphragmatic recess

Jejunum

Parietal pleura, diaphragmatic part

Parietal pleura, costal part

8th rib

9th rib

Liver, right lobe

Descending colon

10th rib

Renal artery ●

11th rib

Latissimus dorsi ●

Inferior vena cava ●

Renal pelvis

Diaphragm, lumbar part ●

Renal medulla

12th rib

Minor calyx

Sympathetic trunk ●

Renal sinus

Kidney

Erector spinae ●

1st lumbar vertebra

Renal cortex

Cauda equina ●

Renal vein ●

Inferior mesenteric artery ●

Abdominal aorta ●

Fig. 1141   Abdomen; transverse section through upper abdomen at level of 1st lumbar vertebra; caudal aspect.
The spinal cord has already become the cauda equina in this case. The stomach is contracted and thus the mucosa [mucous membrane] looks thickened.

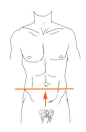

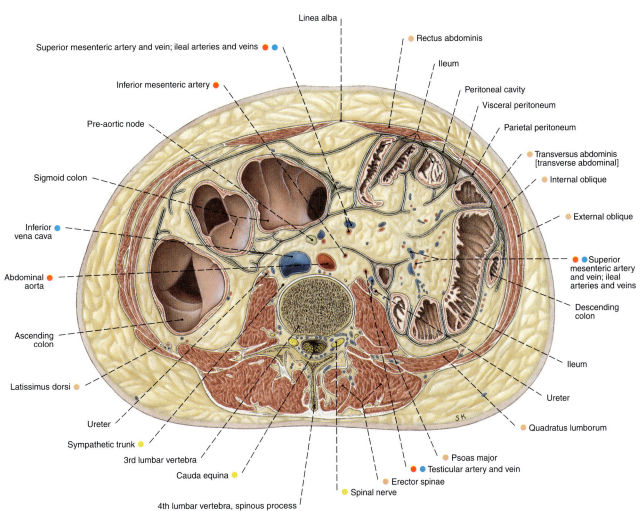

Linea alba

Superior mesenteric artery and vein; ileal arteries and veins ● ●

Inferior mesenteric artery ●

Pre-aortic node

Sigmoid colon

Inferior
vena cava ●

Abdominal ●
aorta

Ascending
colon

Latissimus dorsi ●

Ureter

Sympathetic trunk ●

3rd lumbar vertebra

Cauda equina ●

4th lumbar vertebra, spinous process

Rectus abdominis ●

Ileum

Peritoneal cavity

Visceral peritoneum

Parietal peritoneum

Transversus abdominis ●
[transverse abdominal]

Internal oblique ●

External oblique ●

● ● Superior
mesenteric artery
and vein; ileal
arteries and veins

Descending
colon

Ileum

Ureter

Quadratus lumborum ●

Psoas major ●

● ● Testicular artery and vein

Erector spinae ●

Spinal nerve ●

SK

Fig. 1142   Abdomen; transverse section through lower
abdomen at level of 3rd lumbar vertebra; caudal aspect.
In this case a far cranial extending loop of the sigmoid
colon was present, of which both the ascending and
descending parts have been sectioned.

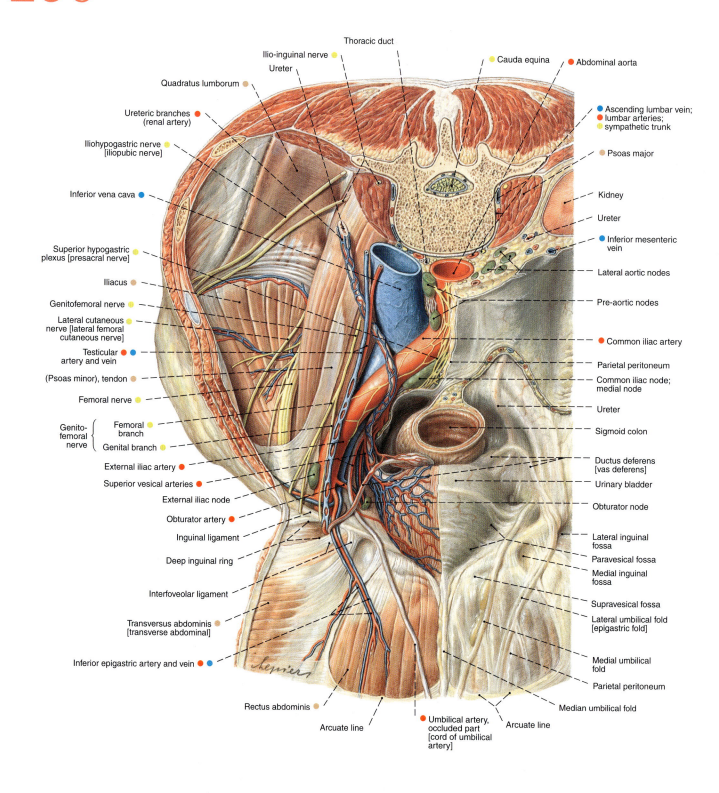

Fig. 1143 Abdominal wall and pelvic viscera in a male; posterior abdominal wall sectioned in the transverse plane; anterior abdominal wall reflected anteriorly; on the right peritoneum removed to expose blood vessels and nerves; cranial aspect.

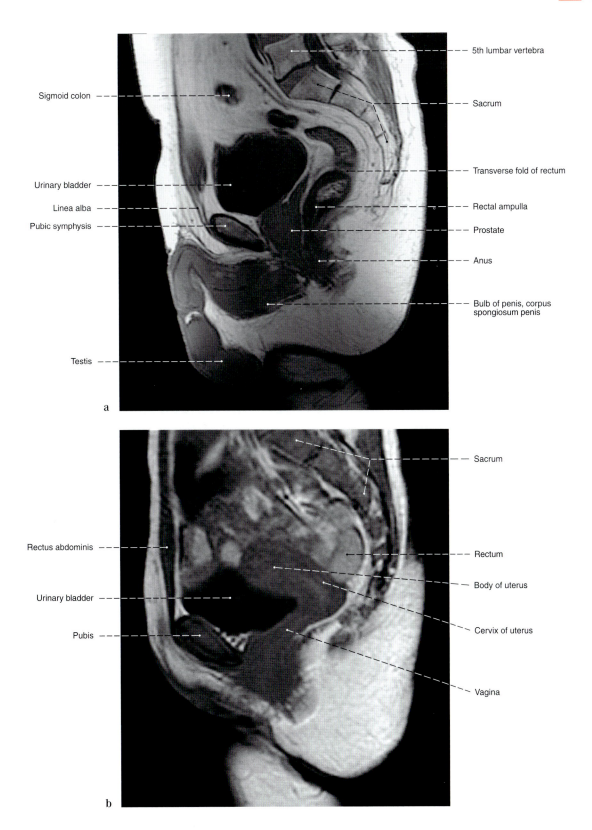

Sigmoid colon

Urinary bladder

Linea alba

Pubic symphysis

Testis

5th lumbar vertebra

Sacrum

Transverse fold of rectum

Rectal ampulla

Prostate

Anus

Bulb of penis, corpus spongiosum penis

a

Rectus abdominis

Urinary bladder

Pubis

Sacrum

Rectum

Body of uterus

Cervix of uterus

Vagina

b

Fig. 1144 a, b   Pelvis; magnetic resonance
image; paramedian section; viewed from the left.
a In the male
b In the female
Compare to Figs. 1145 and 1146.

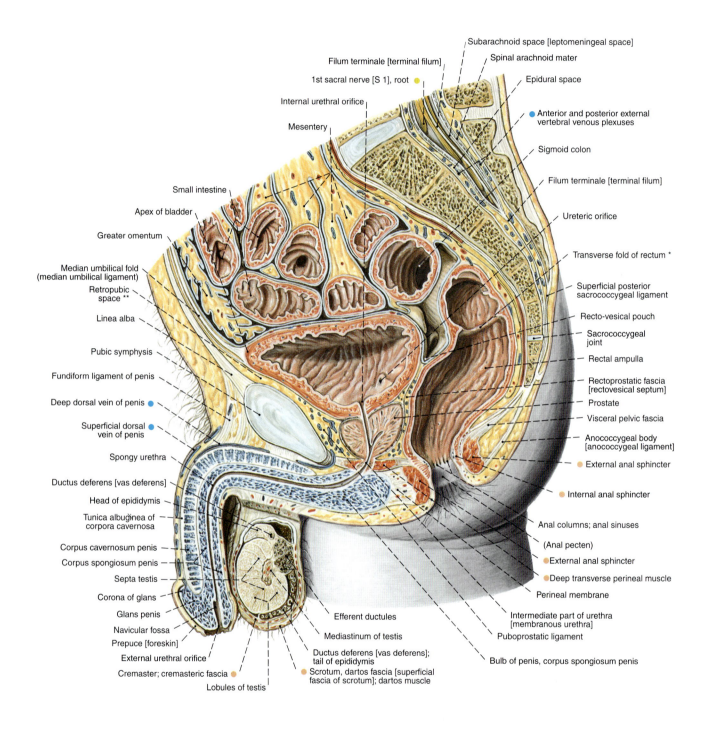

Subarachnoid space [leptomeningeal space]

Spinal arachnoid mater

Filum terminale [terminal filum]

Epidural space

1st sacral nerve [S 1], root

Internal urethral orifice

Anterior and posterior external
vertebral venous plexuses

Mesentery

Sigmoid colon

Filum terminale [terminal filum]

Small intestine

Ureteric orifice

Apex of bladder

Greater omentum

Transverse fold of rectum *

Median umbilical fold
(median umbilical ligament)

Superficial posterior
sacrococcygeal ligament

Retropubic
space **

Recto-vesical pouch

Linea alba

Sacrococcygeal
joint

Pubic symphysis

Rectal ampulla

Fundiform ligament of penis

Rectoprostatic fascia
[rectovesical septum]

Deep dorsal vein of penis

Prostate

Superficial dorsal
vein of penis

Visceral pelvic fascia

Anococcygeal body
[anococcygeal ligament]

Spongy urethra

External anal sphincter

Ductus deferens [vas deferens]

Internal anal sphincter

Head of epididymis

Tunica albuginea of
corpora cavernosa

Anal columns; anal sinuses

Corpus cavernosum penis

(Anal pecten)

Corpus spongiosum penis

External anal sphincter

Septa testis

Deep transverse perineal muscle

Corona of glans

Perineal membrane

Glans penis

Navicular fossa

Intermediate part of urethra
[membranous urethra]

Prepuce [foreskin]

Efferent ductules

Puboprostatic ligament

External urethral orifice

Mediastinum of testis

Cremaster; cremasteric fascia

Ductus deferens [vas deferens];
tail of epididymis

Bulb of penis, corpus spongiosum penis

Lobules of testis

Scrotum, dartos fascia [superficial
fascia of scrotum]; dartos muscle

Fig. 1145   Pelvis in the male; median
section; right lateral aspect.

*   Clinically : KOHLRAUSCH's fold.
**   Clinically: cave of RETZIUS.

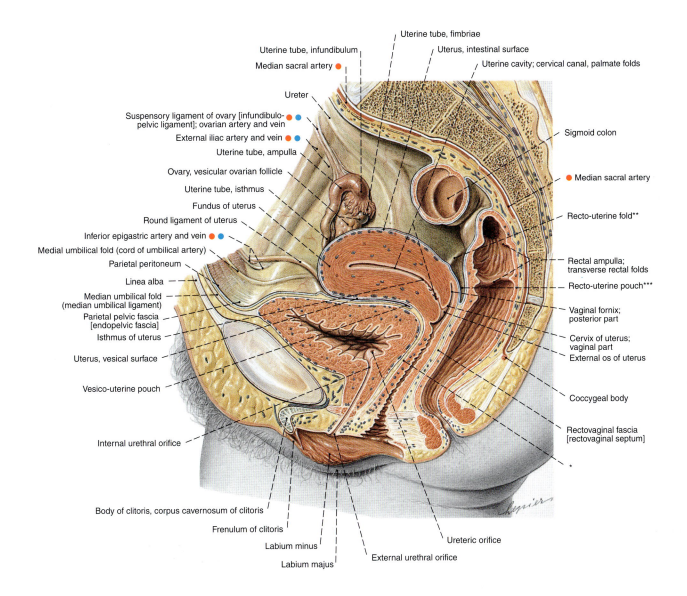

Uterine tube, infundibulum
Median sacral artery ●
Uterine tube, fimbriae
Uterus, intestinal surface
Uterine cavity; cervical canal, palmate folds
Ureter
Suspensory ligament of ovary [infundibulo- ● ● pelvic ligament]; ovarian artery and vein
External iliac artery and vein ● ●
Uterine tube, ampulla
Ovary, vesicular ovarian follicle
Uterine tube, isthmus
Fundus of uterus
Round ligament of uterus
Inferior epigastric artery and vein ● ●
Medial umbilical fold (cord of umbilical artery)
Parietal peritoneum
Linea alba
Median umbilical fold (median umbilical ligament)
Parietal pelvic fascia [endopelvic fascia]
Isthmus of uterus
Uterus, vesical surface
Vesico-uterine pouch
Internal urethral orifice
Body of clitoris, corpus cavernosum of clitoris
Frenulum of clitoris
Labium minus
Labium majus
External urethral orifice
Ureteric orifice

Sigmoid colon
● Median sacral artery
Recto-uterine fold**
Rectal ampulla; transverse rectal folds
Recto-uterine pouch***
Vaginal fornix; posterior part
Cervix of uterus; vaginal part
External os of uterus
Coccygeal body
Rectovaginal fascia [rectovaginal septum]
*

Fig. 1146   Pelvis in the female; median section; small and large intestines removed except for terminal parts of sigmoid colon and rectum; right lateral aspect.

*   Clinically: vesicovaginal septum.
**   Clinically: fold of DOUGLAS, sacro-uterine ligament.
*** Clinically: pouch of DOUGLAS.

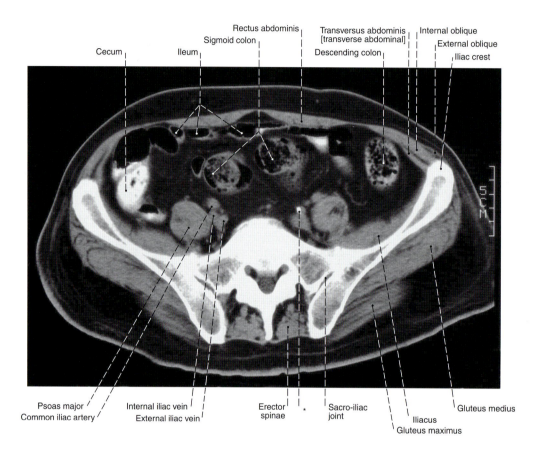

Cecum   Ileum   Rectus abdominis   Sigmoid colon   Transversus abdominis [transverse abdominal]   Descending colon   Internal oblique   External oblique   Iliac crest

Psoas major   Common iliac artery   Internal iliac vein   External iliac vein   Erector spinae   *   Sacro-iliac joint   Iliacus   Gluteus maximus   Gluteus medius

Fig. 1147   Pelvis; computer tomographic cross-section at level of 1st sacral segment after administration of contrast medium into the colon in supine position; caudal aspect.

* Calcification in the wall of the common iliac artery.

The contrast medium has become mixed with intestinal contents in the sigmoid and descending colon, while the cecum is almost entirely filled with contrast medium. The thickness of the subcutaneous fat in the gluteal region is well developed in this patient; this must be considered for intramuscular injections because many medications must only be injected into the musculature and not into the subcutaneous tissue.

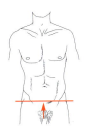

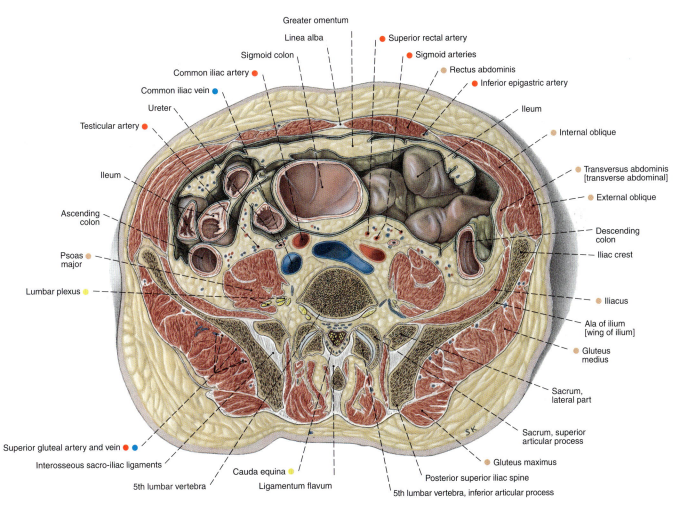

Greater omentum

Linea alba

Sigmoid colon

Common iliac artery ●

Common iliac vein ●

Ureter

Testicular artery ●

Ileum

Ascending colon

Psoas major ●

Lumbar plexus ●

Superior gluteal artery and vein ● ●

Interosseous sacro-iliac ligaments

5th lumbar vertebra

Superior rectal artery ●

Sigmoid arteries ●

Rectus abdominis ●

Inferior epigastric artery ●

Ileum

Internal oblique ●

Transversus abdominis [transverse abdominal] ●

External oblique ●

Descending colon

Iliac crest

Iliacus ●

Ala of ilium [wing of ilium]

Gluteus medius ●

Sacrum, lateral part

Sacrum, superior articular process

Gluteus maximus ●

Posterior superior iliac spine

5th lumbar vertebra, inferior articular process

Cauda equina ●

Ligamentum flavum

S K

Fig. 1148   Pelvis; transverse section at level of 5th lumbar vertebra; caudal aspect. This section is from another male than were the sections in Figs. 1140-1142. The sigmoid colon extends far cranially; thus, the top of the flexure is sectioned. The thickness of the subcutaneous fat in the gluteal region must be considered for intramuscular injections.

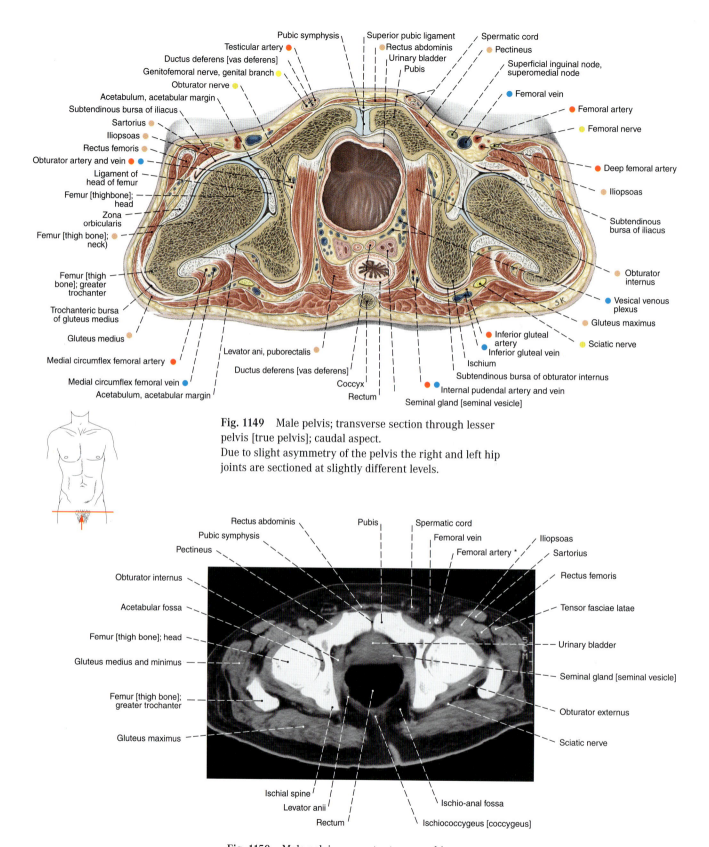

Pubic symphysis
Testicular artery ●
Ductus deferens [vas deferens]
Genitofemoral nerve, genital branch ●
Obturator nerve ●
Acetabulum, acetabular margin
Subtendinous bursa of iliacus
Sartorius ●
Iliopsoas
Rectus femoris ●
Obturator artery and vein ● ●
Ligament of head of femur
Femur [thighbone]; head
Zona orbicularis
Femur [thigh bone]; neck)
Femur [thigh bone]; greater trochanter
Trochanteric bursa of gluteus medius
Gluteus medius ●
Medial circumflex femoral artery ●
Medial circumflex femoral vein ●
Acetabulum, acetabular margin

Superior pubic ligament
Rectus abdominis ●
Urinary bladder
Pubis

Spermatic cord
Pectineus ●
Superficial inguinal node, superomedial node
Femoral vein ●
Femoral artery ●
Femoral nerve ●
Deep femoral artery ●
Iliopsoas ●
Subtendinous bursa of iliacus
Obturator internus ●
Vesical venous plexus ●
Gluteus maximus ●
Sciatic nerve ●

Levator ani, puborectalis ●
Ductus deferens [vas deferens]
Coccyx
Rectum

Inferior gluteal artery ●
Inferior gluteal vein ●
Ischium
Subtendinous bursa of obturator internus
Internal pudendal artery and vein ● ●
Seminal gland [seminal vesicle]

Fig. 1149 Male pelvis; transverse section through lesser pelvis [true pelvis]; caudal aspect.
Due to slight asymmetry of the pelvis the right and left hip joints are sectioned at slightly different levels.

Rectus abdominis
Pubic symphysis
Pectineus
Obturator internus
Acetabular fossa
Femur [thigh bone]; head
Gluteus medius and minimus
Femur [thigh bone]; greater trochanter
Gluteus maximus

Pubis
Femoral vein

Spermatic cord
Femoral artery *
Iliopsoas
Sartorius
Rectus femoris
Tensor fasciae latae
Urinary bladder
Seminal gland [seminal vesicle]
Obturator externus
Sciatic nerve

Ischial spine
Levator anii
Rectum
Ischio-anal fossa
Ischiococcygeus [coccygeus]

Fig. 1150 Male pelvis; computer tomographic cross-section through lesser pelvis [true pelvis] in supine position at approximately same level as in Fig. 1149; caudal aspect.

* Calcification in medial part of femoral artery.

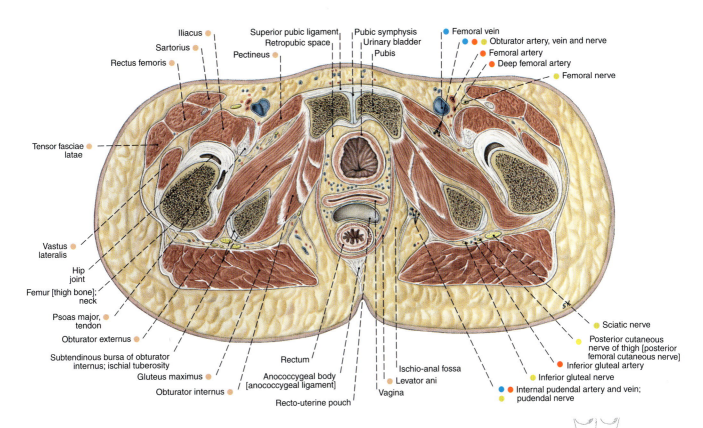

Fig. 1151 Female pelvis; transverse section through lesser pelvis [true pelvis] at level of pubic symphysis; caudal aspect.

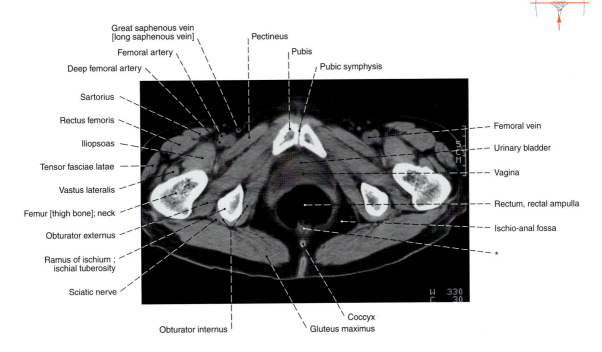

Fig. 1152 Female pelvis; computer tomographic cross-section through lesser pelvis [true pelvis] in supine position at approximately same level as in Fig. 1151; caudal aspect.

* Residua of contrast medium in intestinal contents.

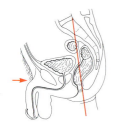

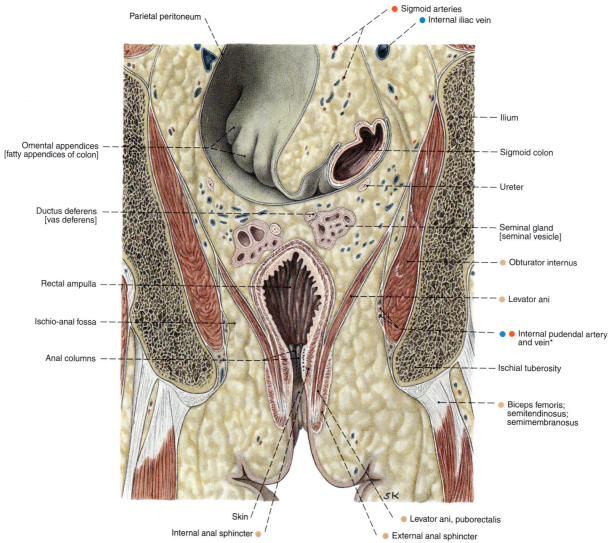

Parietal peritoneum

● Sigmoid arteries
● Internal iliac vein

Omental appendices
[fatty appendices of colon]

Ilium

Sigmoid colon

Ureter

Ductus deferens
[vas deferens]

Seminal gland
[seminal vesicle]

● Obturator internus

Rectal ampulla

● Levator ani

Ischio-anal fossa

● ● Internal pudendal artery
and vein*

Anal columns

Ischial tuberosity

● Biceps femoris;
semitendinosus;
semimembranosus

Skin

● Levator ani, puborectalis

Internal anal sphincter ●

● External anal sphincter

Fig. 1153 Male pelvis; frontal section
through lesser pelvis [true pelvis]; ventral
aspect.

* Clinically: ALCOCK's canal.

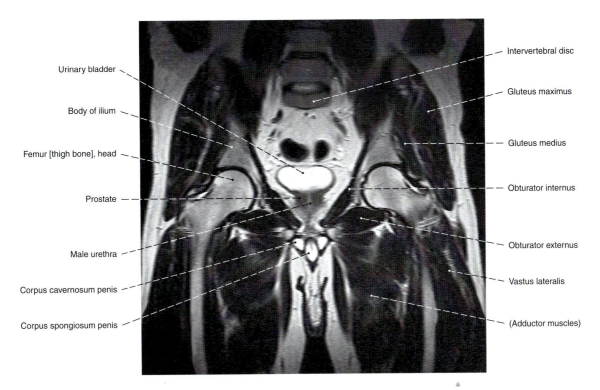

Urinary bladder

Body of ilium

Femur [thigh bone], head

Prostate

Male urethra

Corpus cavernosum penis

Corpus spongiosum penis

Intervertebral disc

Gluteus maximus

Gluteus medius

Obturator internus

Obturator externus

Vastus lateralis

(Adductor muscles)

Fig. 1154   Male pelvis; magnetic resonance image; frontal section at level of hip joints; ventral aspect.

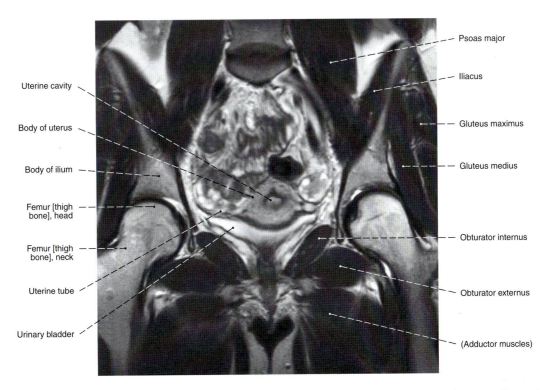

Uterine cavity

Body of uterus

Body of ilium

Femur [thigh bone], head

Femur [thigh bone], neck

Uterine tube

Urinary bladder

Psoas major

Iliacus

Gluteus maximus

Gluteus medius

Obturator internus

Obturator externus

(Adductor muscles)

Fig. 1155   Female pelvis; magnetic resonance image; frontal section at level of hip joints; ventral aspect.

When the urinary bladder is empty, the uterus lies on top of the urinary bladder due to its anteflexion.

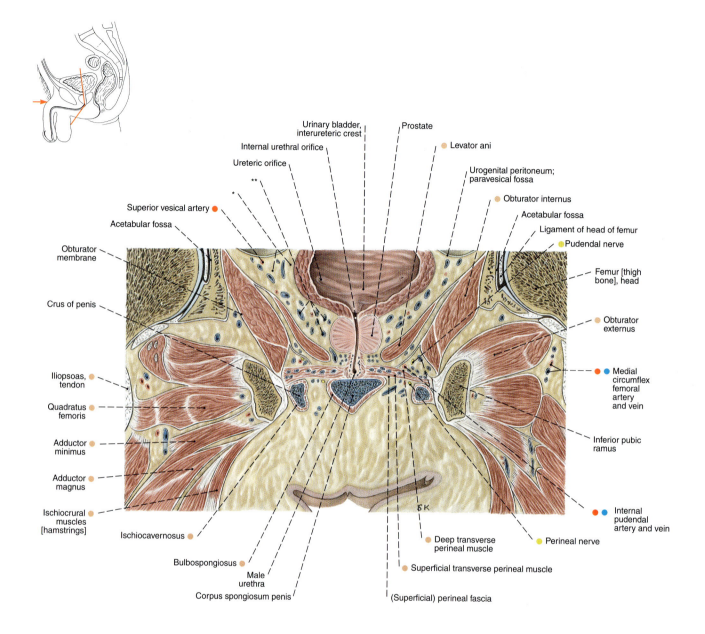

Urinary bladder, interureteric crest

Prostate

Levator ani

Internal urethral orifice

Urogenital peritoneum; paravesical fossa

Ureteric orifice

Obturator internus

**

Acetabular fossa

*

Ligament of head of femur

Superior vesical artery

Pudendal nerve

Acetabular fossa

Femur [thigh bone], head

Obturator membrane

Obturator externus

Crus of penis

Medial circumflex femoral artery and vein

Iliopsoas, tendon

Quadratus femoris

Inferior pubic ramus

Adductor minimus

Adductor magnus

Ischiocrural muscles [hamstrings]

Internal pudendal artery and vein

Ischiocavernosus

Perineal nerve

Bulbospongiosus

Deep transverse perineal muscle

Male urethra

Superficial transverse perineal muscle

Corpus spongiosum penis

(Superficial) perineal fascia

Fig. 1156   Male pelvis; oblique section through urinary bladder; ventral aspect.

 *   Clinically: paracystium.
** Clinically: prostatic venous plexus.

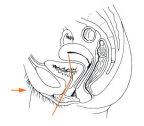

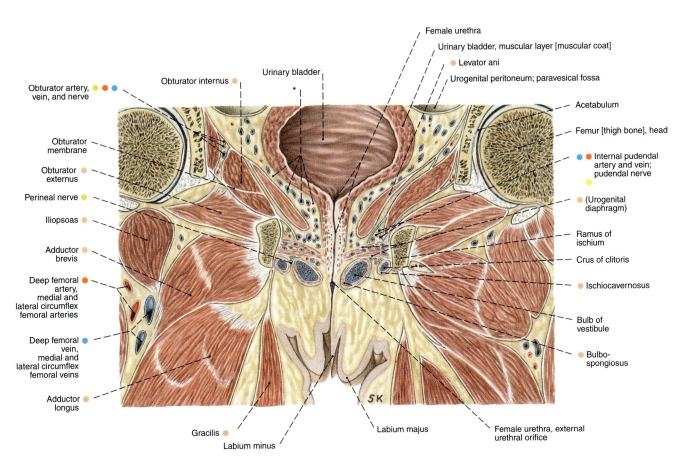

Female urethra

Urinary bladder, muscular layer [muscular coat]

Levator ani

Urogenital peritoneum; paravesical fossa

Obturator internus

Urinary bladder

*

Obturator artery,
vein, and nerve

Acetabulum

Femur [thigh bone], head

Obturator
membrane

Internal pudendal
artery and vein;
pudendal nerve

Obturator
externus

(Urogenital
diaphragm)

Perineal nerve

Iliopsoas

Ramus of
ischium

Adductor
brevis

Crus of clitoris

Deep femoral
artery,
medial and
lateral circumflex
femoral arteries

Ischiocavernosus

Deep femoral
vein,
medial and
lateral circumflex
femoral veins

Bulb of
vestibule

Bulbo-
spongiosus

Adductor
longus

SK

Gracilis

Labium majus

Female urethra, external
urethral orifice

Labium minus

Fig. 1157 Female pelvis; oblique section
through urinary bladder; ventral aspect.

* Clinically: paracystium with venous plexus.

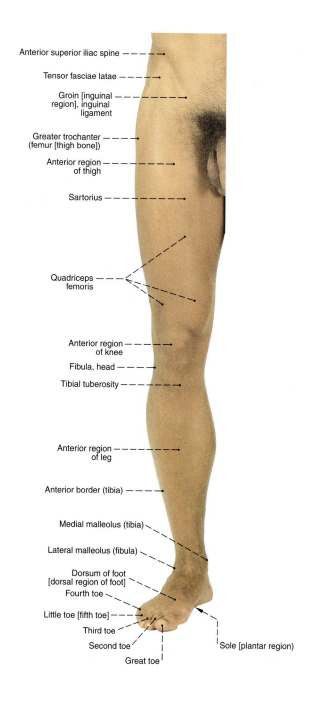

Anterior superior iliac spine

Tensor fasciae latae

Groin [inguinal region], inguinal ligament

Greater trochanter (femur [thigh bone])

Anterior region of thigh

Sartorius

Quadriceps femoris

Anterior region of knee

Fibula, head

Tibial tuberosity

Anterior region of leg

Anterior border (tibia)

Medial malleolus (tibia)

Lateral malleolus (fibula)

Dorsum of foot [dorsal region of foot]

Fourth toe

Little toe [fifth toe]

Third toe

Second toe

Great toe

Sole [plantar region]

Fig. 1158   Right lower limb; surface anatomy; anterior aspect.

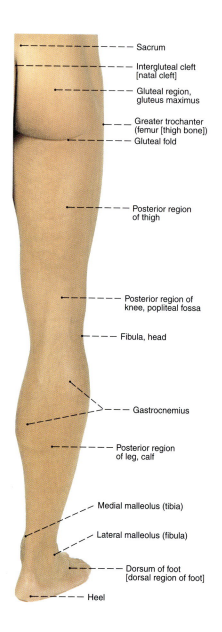

Sacrum

Intergluteal cleft [natal cleft]

Gluteal region, gluteus maximus

Greater trochanter (femur [thigh bone])

Gluteal fold

Posterior region of thigh

Posterior region of knee, popliteal fossa

Fibula, head

Gastrocnemius

Posterior region of leg, calf

Medial malleolus (tibia)

Lateral malleolus (fibula)

Dorsum of foot [dorsal region of foot]

Heel

Fig. 1159   Right lower limb; surface anatomy; posterior aspect.

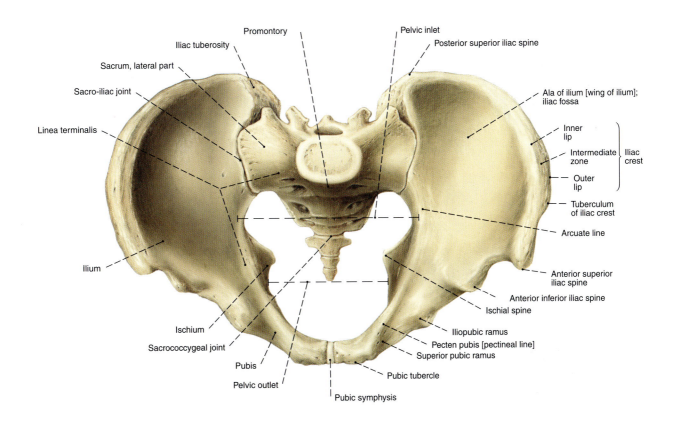

Fig. 1160 Sacrum and pelvic girdle; anterior
superior aspect (40%).
The area cranial of the linea terminalis is called the
greater pelvis [false pelvis]; the area caudal is called
the lesser pelvis [true pelvis].

Joints of pelvic girdle

Name	Type	Movements
Pubic symphysis	Synchondrosis with interpubic disc [interpubic fibrocartilage]	
Sacro-iliac joint	Amphiarthrosis	
Anterior sacro-iliac ligaments Posterior sacro-iliac ligaments Interosseous sacro-iliac ligaments Sacrotuberous ligament Sacrospinal ligament Superior pubic ligament Inferior pubic ligament	Fibrous joints	Minimal translation and rotation during pelvic deformation caused by different loads

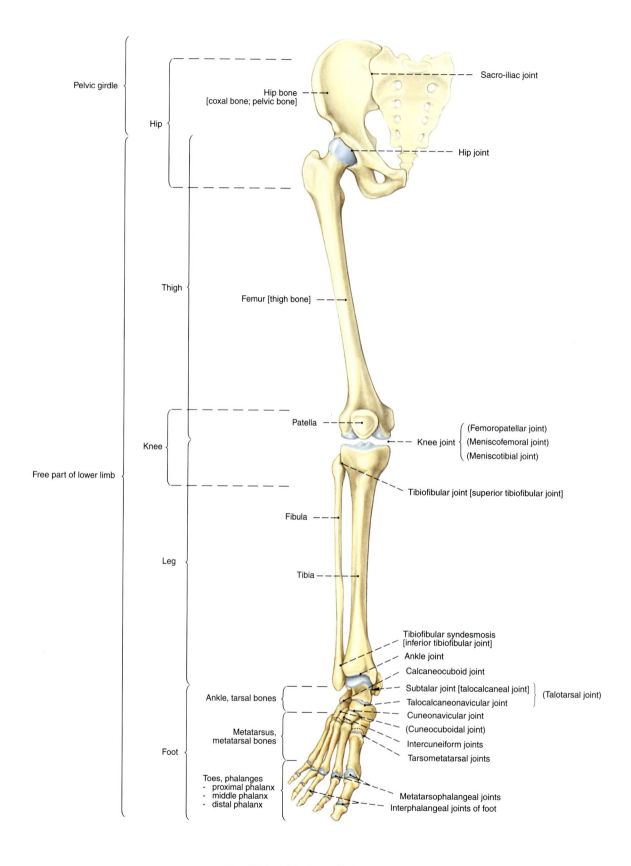

Pelvic girdle

Hip

Hip bone
[coxal bone; pelvic bone]

Sacro-iliac joint

Hip joint

Thigh

Femur [thigh bone]

Patella

Knee joint
(Femoropatellar joint)
(Meniscofemoral joint)
(Meniscotibial joint)

Knee

Free part of lower limb

Tibiofibular joint [superior tibiofibular joint]

Fibula

Leg

Tibia

Tibiofibular syndesmosis
[inferior tibiofibular joint]

Ankle joint

Calcaneocuboid joint

Ankle, tarsal bones

Subtalar joint [talocalcaneal joint]

Talocalcaneonavicular joint

(Talotarsal joint)

Cuneonavicular joint

Metatarsus,
metatarsal bones

(Cuneocuboidal joint)

Intercuneiform joints

Foot

Tarsometatarsal joints

Toes, phalanges
- proximal phalanx
- middle phalanx
- distal phalanx

Metatarsophalangeal joints

Interphalangeal joints of foot

Fig. 1161   Right lower limb; diagram of skeleton
and synovial joints; anterior aspect.

Joints of free lower limb (Fig. 1161)

Joint	Type	Movements
Hip joint	Ball-and-socket joint [spheroidal joint]	Flexion (anteversion), extension (retroversion), adduction, abduction. medial and lateral rotation
Knee joint	Pivot-hinge joint [trochoid joint and ginglymus]	Flexion, extension, medial and lateral rotation (only when knee is flexed)
Tibiofibular joint [superior tibiofibular joint]	Amphiarthrosis	Minimal translation in transverse and vertical directions, as well as minimal rotation
Tibiofibular syndesmosis [inferior tibiofibular joint]	Fibrous joint	Holds the malleoli together; in dorsiflexion of the ankle joint the malleoli drift somewhat apart
Ankle joint	Hinge joint [ginglymus]	Plantar flexion, dorsiflexion Supination (inversion), pronation (eversion)
Talotarsal joint a) Talocalcaneonavicular joint (anterior component) b) Subtalar joint [talocalcaneal joint] (posterior component)	Combined pivot-spherical joint	Little plantar and dorsiflexion and rotation; locks longitudinal arches of foot (key joint in talipes [flatfoot])
Transverse tarsal joint [CHOPART's joint] a) Talonavicular joint b) Calcaneocuboid joint	Amphiarthroses	Little movements causing deformation of foot during its adaptation to the floor (e.g. during walking)
Tarsal joints a) Cuneonavicular joint b) Intercuneiform joints c) Cuneocuboidal joint	Amphiarthroses	Little plantar and dorsiflexion and rotation of forefoot
Tarsometatarsal joints [LISFRANC's joint]	Amphiarthroses	Assist rotation of forefoot
Intermetatarsal joints	Amphiarthroses	
Metatarsophalangeal joints	Ball-and-socket joint [spheroidal joint], functionally limited	Flexion, extension of toes
Interphalangeal joints of foot	Hinge joints [ginglymi]	

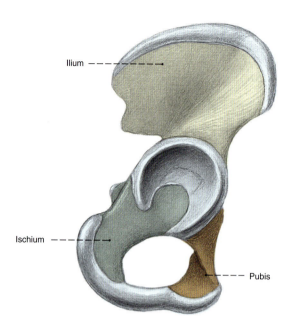

Ilium

Ischium

Pubis

Fig. 1162　Right hip bone [coxal bone; pelvic bone]; extension of its three bony components in the newborn; lateral aspect (110%).

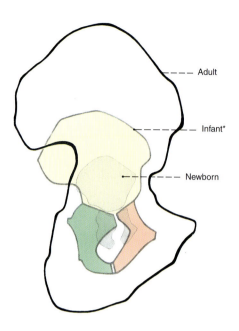

Adult

Infant*

Newborn

Fig. 1163　Right hip bone [coxal bone; pelvic bone]; extension of its three bony components at different ages; lateral aspect.

* Approximately 6 years of age.

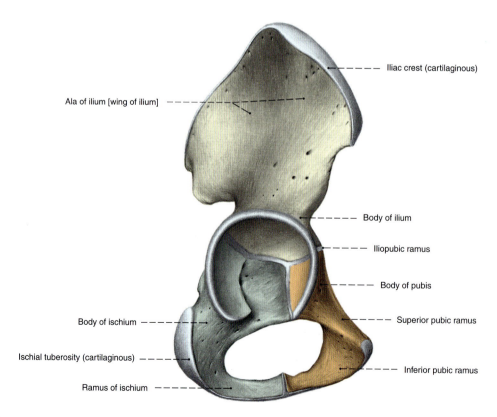

Iliac crest (cartilaginous)

Ala of ilium [wing of ilium]

Body of ilium

Iliopubic ramus

Body of pubis

Superior pubic ramus

Body of ischium

Ischial tuberosity (cartilaginous)

Inferior pubic ramus

Ramus of ischium

Fig. 1164　Right hip bone [coxal bone; pelvic bone]; developmental state at age of six; lateral aspect (90%). The three components of the hip bone [coxal bone; pelvic bone] are connected in the acetabulum by a Y-shaped cartilaginous joint, which ossifies at about 13–18 years of age.

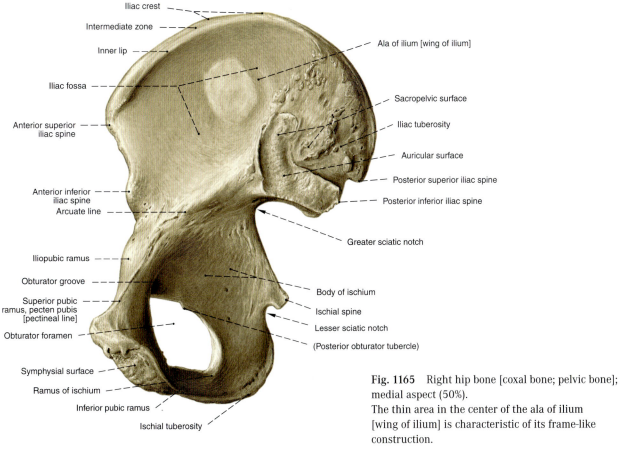

Iliac crest
Intermediate zone
Inner lip
Iliac fossa
Anterior superior iliac spine
Anterior inferior iliac spine
Arcuate line
Iliopubic ramus
Obturator groove
Superior pubic ramus, pecten pubis [pectineal line]
Obturator foramen
Symphysial surface
Ramus of ischium
Inferior pubic ramus
Ischial tuberosity

Ala of ilium [wing of ilium]
Sacropelvic surface
Iliac tuberosity
Auricular surface
Posterior superior iliac spine
Posterior inferior iliac spine
Greater sciatic notch
Body of ischium
Ischial spine
Lesser sciatic notch
(Posterior obturator tubercle)

Fig. 1165 Right hip bone [coxal bone; pelvic bone]; medial aspect (50%).
The thin area in the center of the ala of ilium [wing of ilium] is characteristic of its frame-like construction.

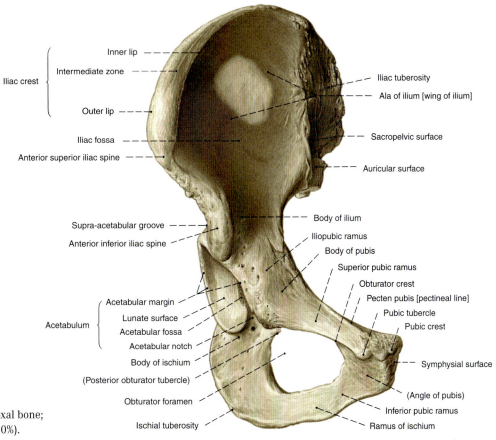

Iliac crest
Inner lip
Intermediate zone
Outer lip
Iliac fossa
Anterior superior iliac spine

Iliac tuberosity
Ala of ilium [wing of ilium]
Sacropelvic surface
Auricular surface
Body of ilium

Supra-acetabular groove
Anterior inferior iliac spine

Iliopubic ramus
Body of pubis
Superior pubic ramus
Obturator crest
Pecten pubis [pectineal line]
Pubic tubercle
Pubic crest

Acetabulum
Acetabular margin
Lunate surface
Acetabular fossa
Acetabular notch
Body of ischium
(Posterior obturator tubercle)
Obturator foramen
Ischial tuberosity

Symphysial surface
(Angle of pubis)
Inferior pubic ramus
Ramus of ischium

Fig. 1166 Right hip bone [coxal bone; pelvic bone]; ventral aspect (50%).

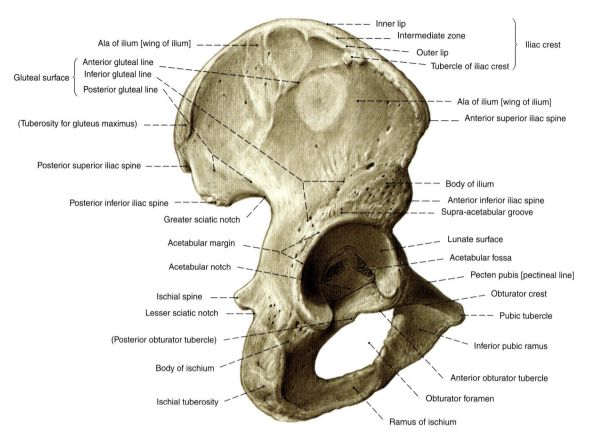

Fig. 1167 Right hip bone [coxal bone; pelvic bone];
lateral dorsal aspect (50%).

Labels (clockwise from top):
Inner lip — Intermediate zone — Outer lip — Tubercle of iliac crest — Iliac crest
Ala of ilium [wing of ilium]
Anterior superior iliac spine
Body of ilium
Anterior inferior iliac spine
Supra-acetabular groove
Lunate surface
Acetabular fossa
Pecten pubis [pectineal line]
Obturator crest
Pubic tubercle
Inferior pubic ramus
Anterior obturator tubercle
Obturator foramen
Ramus of ischium
Ischial tuberosity
Body of ischium
(Posterior obturator tubercle)
Lesser sciatic notch
Ischial spine
Acetabular notch
Acetabular margin
Greater sciatic notch
Posterior inferior iliac spine
Posterior superior iliac spine
(Tuberosity for gluteus maximus)
Gluteal surface — Anterior gluteal line / Inferior gluteal line / Posterior gluteal line
Ala of ilium [wing of ilium]

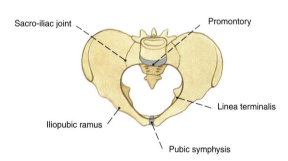

Fig. 1168 Pelvis; shape of pelvic inlet in the
male pelvis; superior aspect.

Labels: Sacro-iliac joint — Promontory — Linea terminalis — Pubic symphysis — Iliopubic ramus

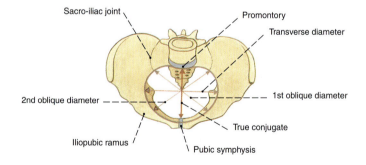

Fig. 1169 Pelvis; shape of pelvic inlet in the female pelvis;
superior aspect.

Labels: Sacro-iliac joint — Promontory — Transverse diameter — 1st oblique diameter — True conjugate — Pubic symphysis — Iliopubic ramus — 2nd oblique diameter

Gender differences in the pelvis

Compared to the male pelvis, in which the pelvic inlet is clearly narrowed by the promontory, the female pelvis has a more rounded and oval-shaped pelvic inlet. The two inferior pubic rami form a right angle (subpubic angle) in the male and an arch (pubic arch) in the female. The alae [wings] of ilia are wider apart in the female pelvis. The widest diameter of the obturator foramina is in the transverse plane in the female and in the vertical plane in the male.

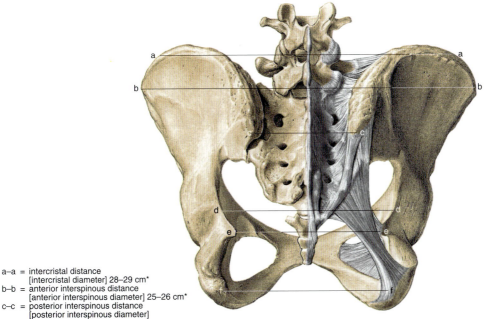

a–a = intercristal distance
[intercristal diameter] 28–29 cm*
b–b = anterior interspinous distance
[anterior interspinous diameter] 25–26 cm*
c–c = posterior interspinous distance
[posterior interspinous diameter]
(width of sacrum) 10 cm
* The intercristal distance [intercristal diameter]
seems to be smaller than the anterior
interspinous distance [anterior interspinous
diameter] due to the perspective.

Fig. 1170   Pelvis; diagram of dimension
of the female pelvis; dorsal aspect.

d–d = transverse diameter of
pelvic width
(interacetabular line)
12–12.5 cm
e–e = transverse diameter of
pelvic constriction
(interspinous line) 10.5 cm
f–f = transverse diameter of
pelvic outlet (tuberal
diameter) 11–12 cm

k–k = axis of pelvis
a–b = clinically: anatomical
conjugate
a–e = clinically: diagonal
conjugate
12.5–13 cm
a–c = clinically: true
conjugate
10.4–11 cm

h–d = clinically: sagittal
diameter of pelvic
width 12–12.5 cm
e–g = clinically: sagittal
diameter of pelvic
constriction
11–11.5 cm
e–f = clinically: sagittal
diameter of pelvic
outlet (pubococcygeal
distance) 9–10 cm

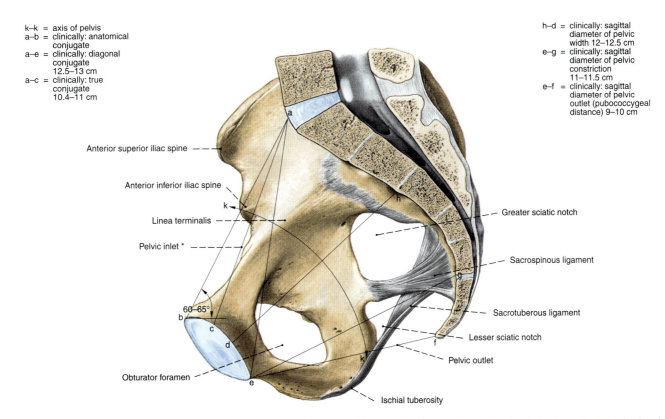

Anterior superior iliac spine
Anterior inferior iliac spine
Linea terminalis
Pelvic inlet *
60–65°
Obturator foramen

Greater sciatic notch
Sacrospinous ligament
Sacrotuberous ligament
Lesser sciatic notch
Pelvic outlet
Ischial tuberosity

Fig. 1171   Pelvis; diagram of dimension of the female pelvis;
median section; right medial aspect.

* The pelvic inlet is enclosed by the linea terminalis. Line a–c indicates the plan of
the pelvic inlet. The pelvic outlet is enclosed by the coccyx, the ischial tuberosity,
the ramus of ischium, and the inferior pelvic ramus on both sides.

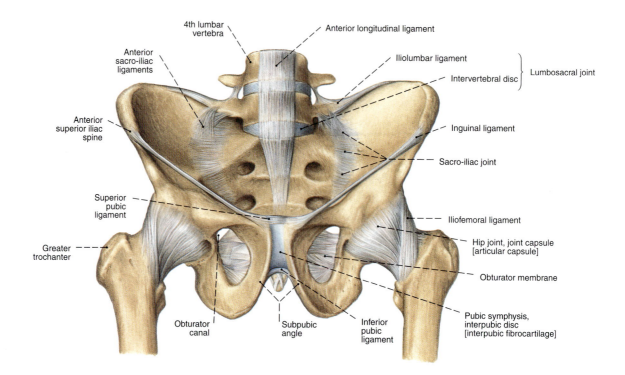

Fig. 1172   Joints of pelvic girdle and lumbosacral joint in the male; anterior inferior aspect (30%).

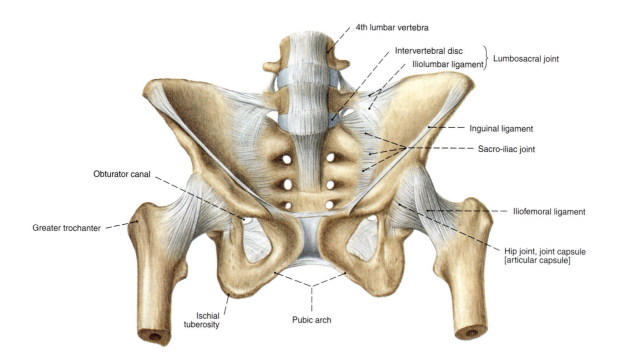

Fig. 1173   Joints of pelvic girdle and lumbosacral joint in the female; anterior inferior aspect (30%).

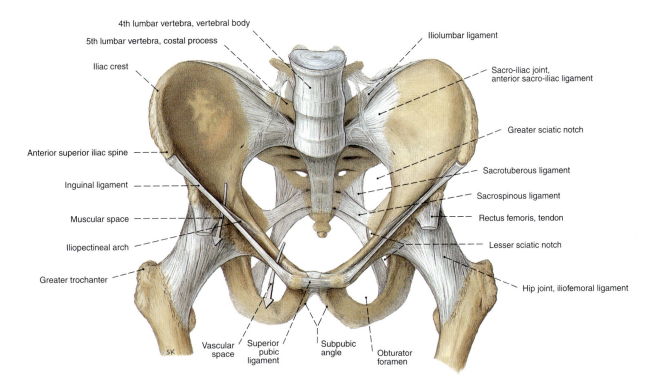

4th lumbar vertebra, vertebral body

5th lumbar vertebra, costal process

Iliac crest

Anterior superior iliac spine

Inguinal ligament

Muscular space

Iliopectineal arch

Greater trochanter

Vascular space

Superior pubic ligament

Subpubic angle

Obturator foramen

Iliolumbar ligament

Sacro-iliac joint, anterior sacro-iliac ligament

Greater sciatic notch

Sacrotuberous ligament

Sacrospinous ligament

Rectus femoris, tendon

Lesser sciatic notch

Hip joint, iliofemoral ligament

Fig. 1174 Joints of pelvic girdle and lumbosacral joint in the male; anterior superior aspect (30%).

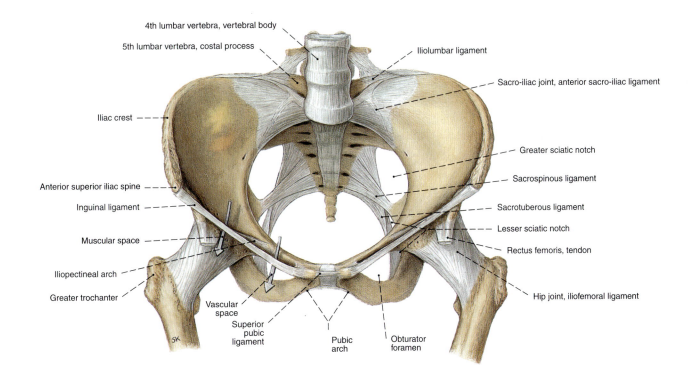

4th lumbar vertebra, vertebral body

5th lumbar vertebra, costal process

Iliac crest

Anterior superior iliac spine

Inguinal ligament

Muscular space

Iliopectineal arch

Greater trochanter

Vascular space

Superior pubic ligament

Pubic arch

Obturator foramen

Iliolumbar ligament

Sacro-iliac joint, anterior sacro-iliac ligament

Greater sciatic notch

Sacrospinous ligament

Sacrotuberous ligament

Lesser sciatic notch

Rectus femoris, tendon

Hip joint, iliofemoral ligament

Fig. 1175 Joints of pelvic girdle and lumbosacral joint in the female; anterior superior aspect (30%).

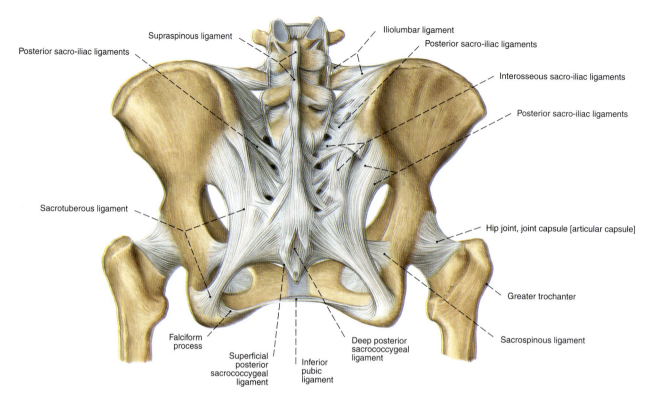

Fig. 1176   Joints of pelvic girdle and lumbosacral joint in the female; posterior aspect (30%).

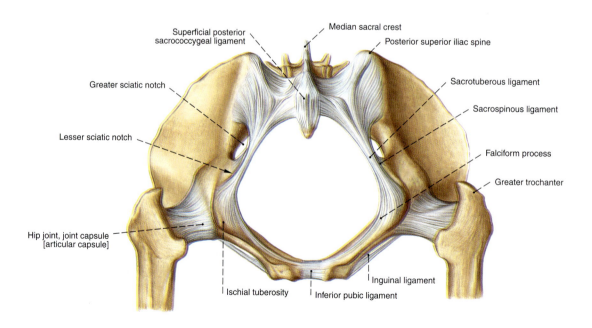

Fig. 1177   Joints of pelvic girdle in the female; inferior aspect (30%).

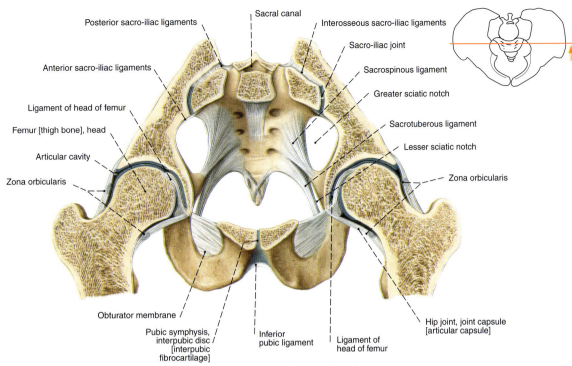

Posterior sacro-iliac ligaments

Anterior sacro-iliac ligaments

Ligament of head of femur

Femur [thigh bone], head

Articular cavity

Zona orbicularis

Sacral canal

Interosseous sacro-iliac ligaments

Sacro-iliac joint

Sacrospinous ligament

Greater sciatic notch

Sacrotuberous ligament

Lesser sciatic notch

Zona orbicularis

Obturator membrane

Pubic symphysis, interpubic disc [interpubic fibrocartilage]

Inferior pubic ligament

Ligament of head of femur

Hip joint, joint capsule [articular capsule]

Fig. 1178 Joints of pelvic girdle in the female; frontal section at level of middle of acetabulum; anterior aspect (30%).

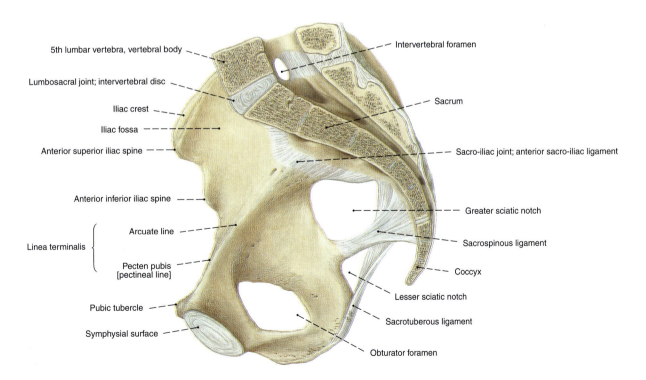

5th lumbar vertebra, vertebral body

Lumbosacral joint; intervertebral disc

Iliac crest

Iliac fossa

Anterior superior iliac spine

Anterior inferior iliac spine

Arcuate line

Linea terminalis

Pecten pubis [pectineal line]

Pubic tubercle

Symphysial surface

Intervertebral foramen

Sacrum

Sacro-iliac joint; anterior sacro-iliac ligament

Greater sciatic notch

Sacrospinous ligament

Coccyx

Lesser sciatic notch

Sacrotuberous ligament

Obturator foramen

Fig. 1179 Joints of pelvic girdle and lumbosacral joint in the female; median section; medial aspect (35%).
Normally, the anterior border of the lowest intervertebral disc forms the most ventral point of the posterior circumference of the pelvic inlet. In radiographs the most ventral point of the sacrum is called promontory.

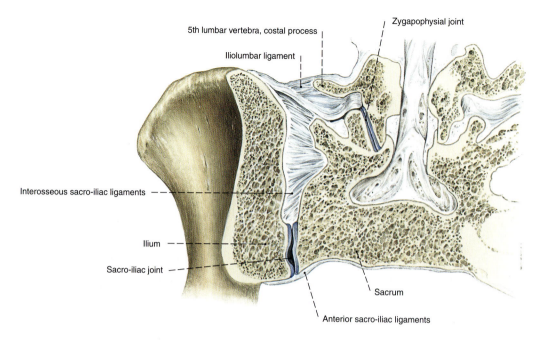

5th lumbar vertebra, costal process

Iliolumbar ligament

Zygapophysial joint

Interosseous sacro-iliac ligaments

Ilium

Sacro-iliac joint

Sacrum

Anterior sacro-iliac ligaments

Fig. 1180   Left sacro-iliac joint; frontal section; anterior aspect (45%).

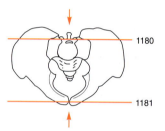

1180

1181

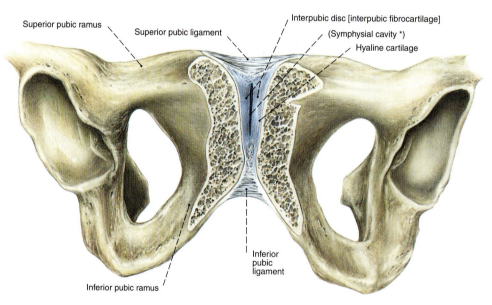

Superior pubic ramus

Superior pubic ligament

Interpubic disc [interpubic fibrocartilage]

(Symphysial cavity *)

Hyaline cartilage

Inferior pubic ligament

Inferior pubic ramus

Fig. 1181   Pubic symphysis; oblique section in the direction of the longitudinal axis of the pubic symphysis, slightly tilted toward the frontal plane; inferior anterior aspect (60%). The interpubic disc [interpubic fibrocartilage] is made of fibrocartilage; only the symphysial surfaces are covered with hyaline cartilage. Starting in the 1st decade a longitudinal cleft can be observed (*).

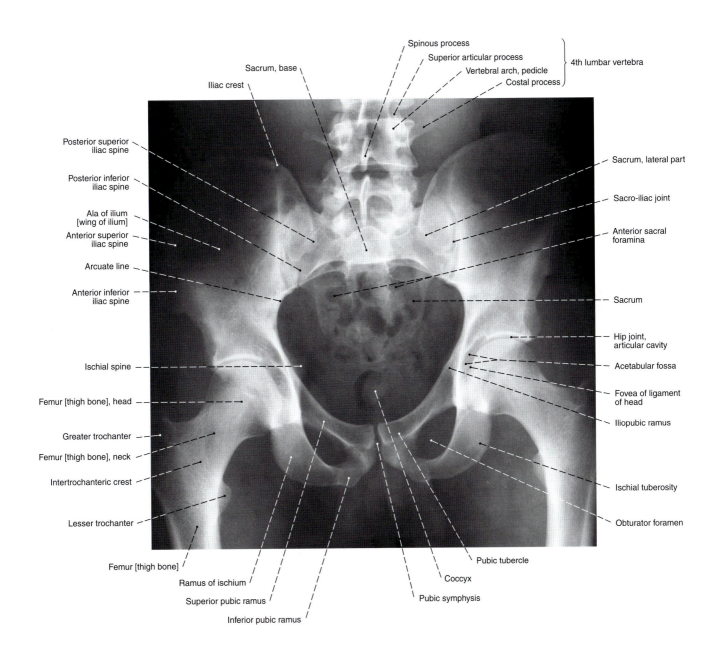

Spinous process

Superior articular process

Vertebral arch, pedicle

4th lumbar vertebra

Costal process

Sacrum, base

Iliac crest

Posterior superior
iliac spine

Posterior inferior
iliac spine

Ala of ilium
[wing of ilium]

Anterior superior
iliac spine

Arcuate line

Anterior inferior
iliac spine

Ischial spine

Femur [thigh bone], head

Greater trochanter

Femur [thigh bone], neck

Intertrochanteric crest

Lesser trochanter

Femur [thigh bone]

Ramus of ischium

Superior pubic ramus

Inferior pubic ramus

Sacrum, lateral part

Sacro-iliac joint

Anterior sacral
foramina

Sacrum

Hip joint,
articular cavity

Acetabular fossa

Fovea of ligament
of head

Iliopubic ramus

Ischial tuberosity

Obturator foramen

Pubic tubercle

Coccyx

Pubic symphysis

Fig. 1182 Male pelvis; AP radiograph in upright position;
central beam directed onto 3rd sacral segment.

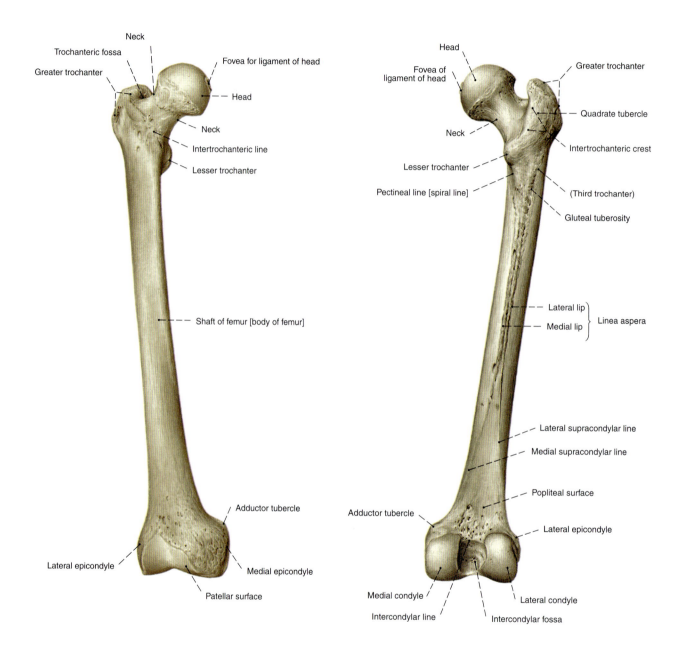

Neck

Trochanteric fossa

Greater trochanter

Fovea for ligament of head

Head

Neck

Intertrochanteric line

Lesser trochanter

Shaft of femur [body of femur]

Adductor tubercle

Lateral epicondyle

Medial epicondyle

Patellar surface

Head

Fovea of ligament of head

Greater trochanter

Quadrate tubercle

Neck

Intertrochanteric crest

Lesser trochanter

Pectineal line [spiral line]

(Third trochanter)

Gluteal tuberosity

Lateral lip

Medial lip

Linea aspera

Lateral supracondylar line

Medial supracondylar line

Popliteal surface

Adductor tubercle

Lateral epicondyle

Medial condyle

Lateral condyle

Intercondylar line

Intercondylar fossa

Fig. 1183   Right femur [thigh bone]; anterior aspect (30%).

Fig. 1184   Right femur [thigh bone]; posterior aspect (30%).

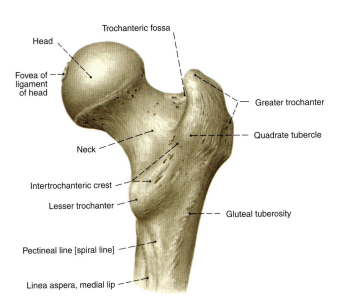

Head
Fovea of ligament of head
Neck
Intertrochanteric crest
Lesser trochanter
Pectineal line [spiral line]
Linea aspera, medial lip
Trochanteric fossa
Greater trochanter
Quadrate tubercle
Gluteal tuberosity

Fig. 1185   Right femur [thigh bone]; proximal extremity; posterior aspect (60%).

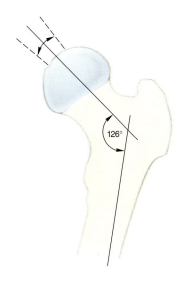

126°

Fig. 1186   Right femur [thigh bone]; variability of angle of the neck; posterior aspect.
The angle of the neck is also known as angle of inclination or angle of depression. It is 150° in the newborn and approximately 126° in the adult.

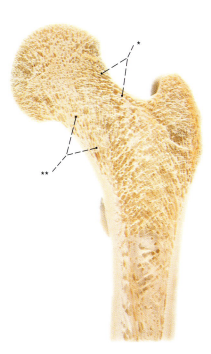

Fig. 1187   Femur [thigh bone]; structure of the spongy bone [trabecular bone] in large angle of inclination [angle of depression] (= coxa valga); section in the plane of the angle of anteversion [angle of declination] (60%). The lateral "tension bundle" (*) of the spongy bone [trabecular bone] is weakened; the medial "compression bundle" (**) is enlarged.

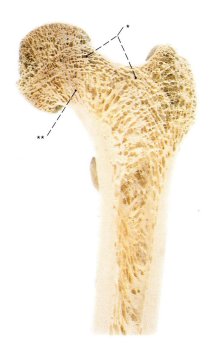

Fig. 1188   Femur [thigh bone]; structure of the spongy bone [trabecular bone] in small angle of inclination [angle of depression] (= coxa vara); section in the plane of the angle of anteversion [angle of declination] (60%). The lateral "tension bundle" (*) of the spongy bone [trabecular bone] is enlarged; the medial "compression bundle" (**) is weakened. Due to high-flexion stress the medial cortical bone of the neck is especially well developed.

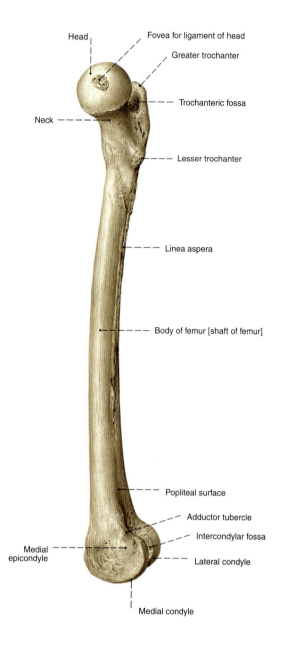

Head

Fovea for ligament of head

Greater trochanter

Trochanteric fossa

Neck

Lesser trochanter

Linea aspera

Body of femur [shaft of femur]

Popliteal surface

Adductor tubercle

Intercondylar fossa

Medial
epicondyle

Lateral condyle

Medial condyle

Fig. 1189   Right femur [thigh bone];
medial aspect (30%).

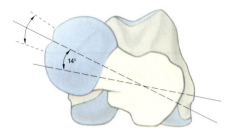

Fig. 1190   Right femur [thigh bone]; variability of angle
of declination [angle of anteversion]; proximal and distal
extremity projected over another; proximal aspect (70%).
**The angle of declination [angle of anteversion] is
approximately 30° in the infant and approximately
14° in the adult.**

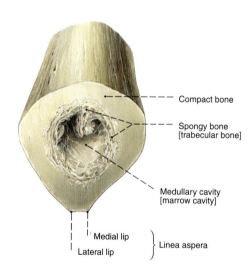

Compact bone

Spongy bone
[trabecular bone]

Medullary cavity
[marrow cavity]

Medial lip

Lateral lip

Linea aspera

Fig. 1191   Right femur [thigh bone]; cross-section
through middle of body of femur [shaft of femur];
distal aspect.

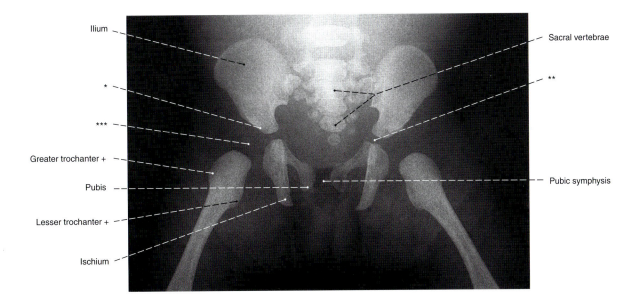

Ilium

Sacral vertebrae

*

**

***

Greater trochanter +

Pubis — Pubic symphysis

Lesser trochanter +

Ischium

Fig. 1192 Pelvis and femur [thigh bone]; AP radiograph of a premature born female (fetus in the 8th month of pregnancy).

* Bony roof of the acetabulum.
** Y-shaped epiphysial cartilage in acetabular fossa.
*** The ossification center in the head of femur does not appear before the 3rd to 5th month of life.
\+ Both trochanters are only bony projection of the diaphysis at this age.

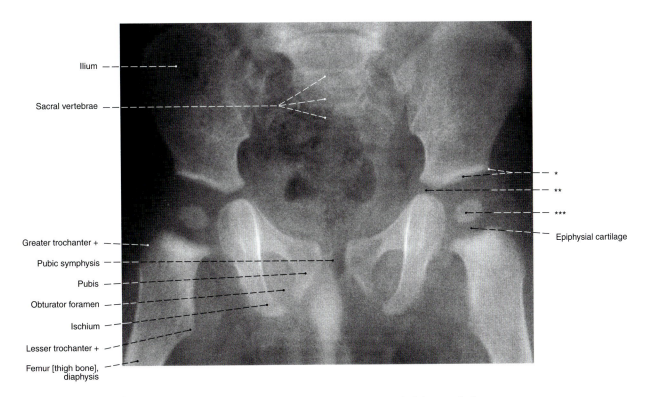

Ilium

Sacral vertebrae

*

**

***

Epiphysial cartilage

Greater trochanter +

Pubic symphysis

Pubis

Obturator foramen

Ischium

Lesser trochanter +

Femur [thigh bone], diaphysis

Fig. 1193 Pelvis and femur; AP radiograph of a 12-month-old boy.

* Bony roof of the acetabulum.
** Y-shaped epiphysial cartilage in acetabular fossa.
*** Ossification center in the head of femur.
\+ Both trochanters are only bony projection of the diaphysis at this age.

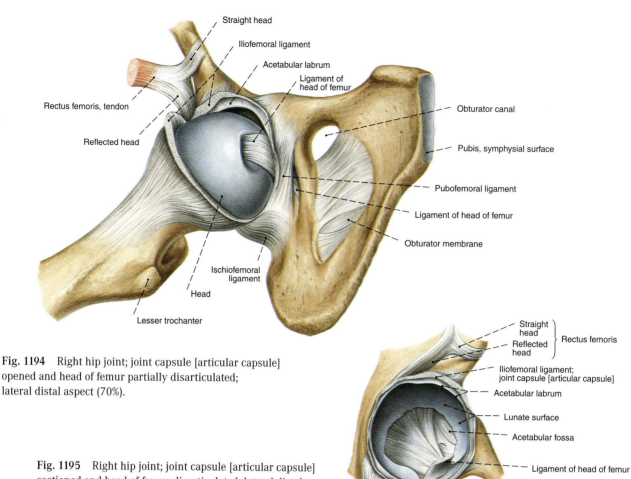

Straight head

Iliofemoral ligament

Acetabular labrum

Ligament of
head of femur

Rectus femoris, tendon

Obturator canal

Reflected head

Pubis, symphysial surface

Pubofemoral ligament

Ligament of head of femur

Obturator membrane

Ischiofemoral
ligament

Head

Lesser trochanter

Fig. 1194   Right hip joint; joint capsule [articular capsule]
opened and head of femur partially disarticulated;
lateral distal aspect (70%).

Straight
head
Reflected
head
} Rectus femoris

Iliofemoral ligament;
joint capsule [articular capsule]

Acetabular labrum

Lunate surface

Acetabular fossa

Fig. 1195   Right hip joint; joint capsule [articular capsule]
sectioned and head of femur disarticulated; lateral distal
aspect (50%).

Ligament of head of femur

Obturator canal

Transverse acetabular ligament

Ischiofemoral ligament;
joint capsule [articular capsule]

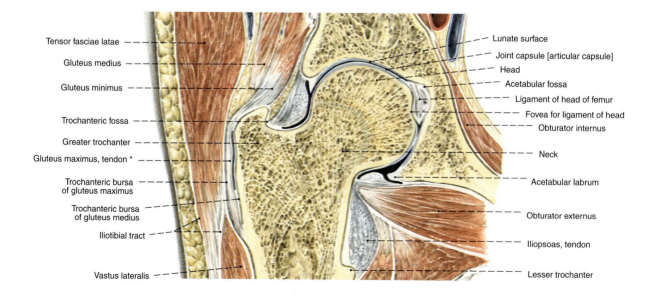

Tensor fasciae latae

Gluteus medius

Gluteus minimus

Trochanteric fossa

Greater trochanter

Gluteus maximus, tendon *

Trochanteric bursa
of gluteus maximus

Trochanteric bursa
of gluteus medius

Iliotibial tract

Vastus lateralis

Lunate surface

Joint capsule [articular capsule]

Head

Acetabular fossa

Ligament of head of femur

Fovea for ligament of head

Obturator internus

Neck

Acetabular labrum

Obturator externus

Iliopsoas, tendon

Lesser trochanter

Fig. 1196 Right hip joint; vertical section in plane of angle of
declination [angel of anteversion]; anterior aspect (65%).
* Merges into iliotibial tract.

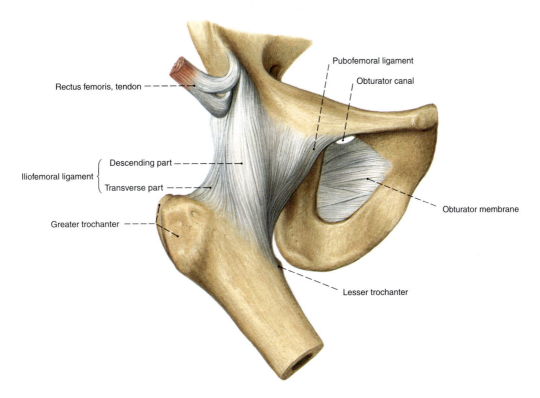

Rectus femoris, tendon

Iliofemoral ligament
  Descending part
  Transverse part

Greater trochanter

Pubofemoral ligament

Obturator canal

Obturator membrane

Lesser trochanter

Fig. 1197   Right hip joint; anterior distal aspect (50%).

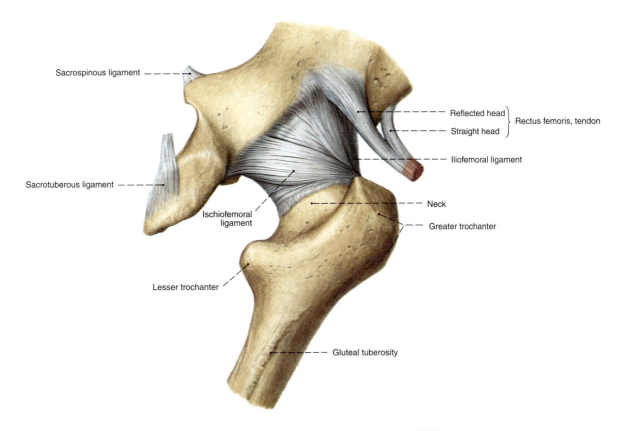

Sacrospinous ligament

Sacrotuberous ligament

Ischiofemoral
ligament

Lesser trochanter

Reflected head
Straight head   Rectus femoris, tendon

Iliofemoral ligament

Neck

Greater trochanter

Gluteal tuberosity

Fig. 1198   Right hip joint; posterior aspect (50%).

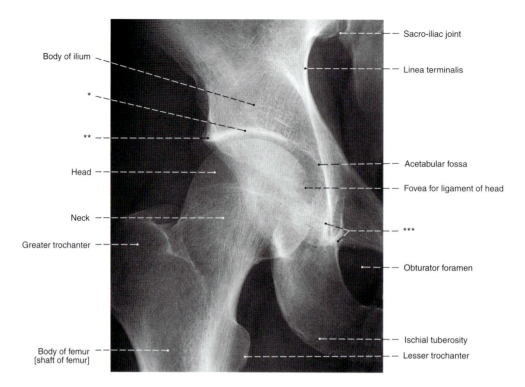

Body of ilium

*

**

Head

Neck

Greater trochanter

Body of femur
[shaft of femur]

Sacro-iliac joint

Linea terminalis

Acetabular fossa

Fovea for ligament of head

***

Obturator foramen

Ischial tuberosity

Lesser trochanter

Fig. 1199   Hip joint; AP radiograph in upright position, standing on both legs.

*   Clinically: roof of acetabulum = tangential projection of lunate surface.
**   Clinically: edge of roof of acetabulum = outermost part of acetabulum.
*** Clinically: KÖHLER'S teardrop = projection of acetabular fossa.

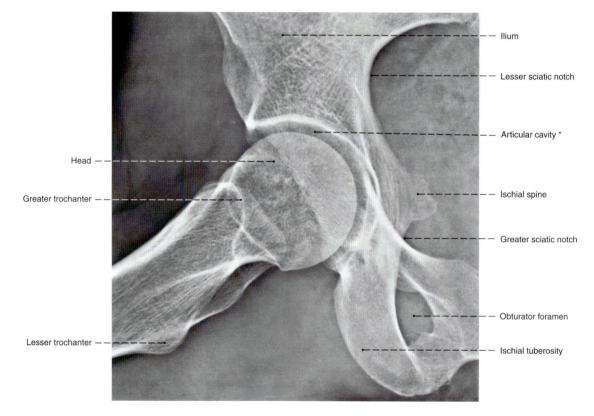

Head

Greater trochanter

Lesser trochanter

Ilium

Lesser sciatic notch

Articular cavity *

Ischial spine

Greater sciatic notch

Obturator foramen

Ischial tuberosity

Fig. 1200   Hip joint; AP radiograph in supine position and abduction and flexion of the thigh (so-called LAUENSTEIN projection).

* Due to little absorption of X-rays by cartilage, the articular cavity seems to be abnormally wide in radiographs.

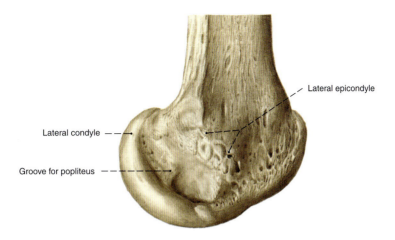

Fig. 1201   Right femur [thigh bone]; distal extremity; lateral aspect (80%).

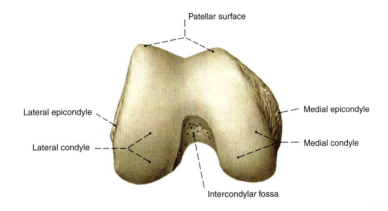

Fig. 1202   Right femur [thigh bone]; distal extremity; distal aspect (50%).

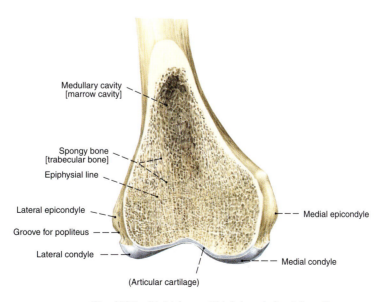

Fig. 1203   Right femur [thigh bone]; frontal section through distal extremity; anterior aspect (50%).

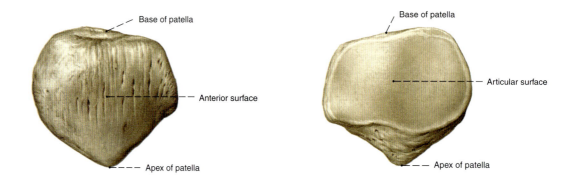

Fig. 1212 Right patella; anterior aspect (80%).

Fig. 1213 Right patella; posterior aspect (80%).

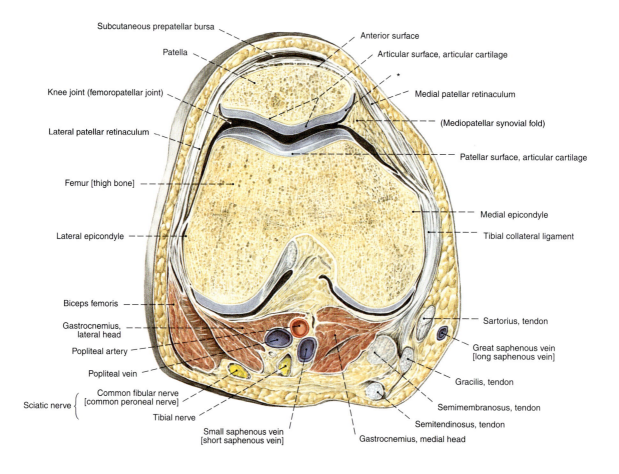

Fig. 1214 Right patella and femur [thigh bone]; cross-section through knee joint at level of middle of femoropatellar joint in extension; distal aspect (70%).

* Medial border facet.

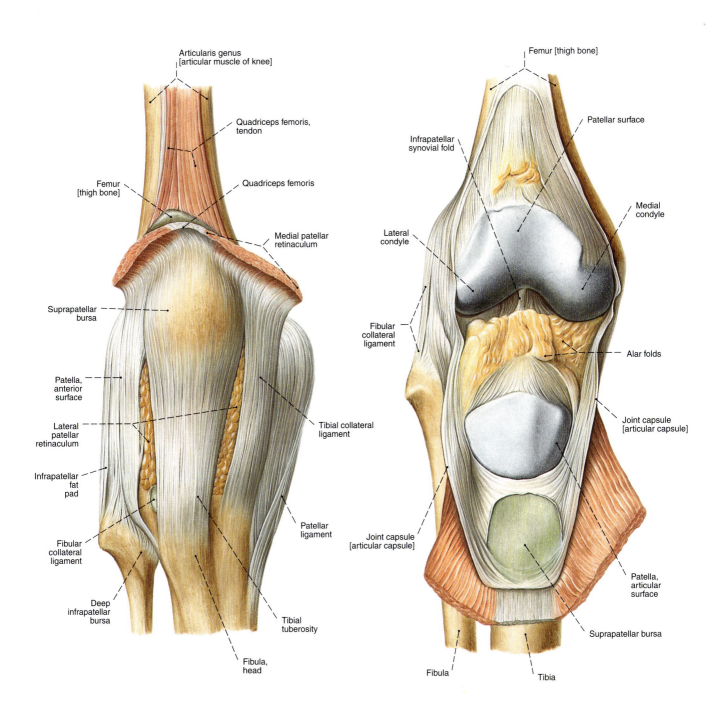

Articularis genus
[articular muscle of knee]

Quadriceps femoris,
tendon

Femur
[thigh bone]

Quadriceps femoris

Medial patellar
retinaculum

Suprapatellar
bursa

Patella,
anterior
surface

Lateral
patellar
retinaculum

Infrapatellar
fat
pad

Tibial collateral
ligament

Fibular
collateral
ligament

Patellar
ligament

Deep
infrapatellar
bursa

Tibial
tuberosity

Fibula,
head

Femur [thigh bone]

Infrapatellar
synovial fold

Patellar surface

Lateral
condyle

Medial
condyle

Fibular
collateral
ligament

Alar folds

Joint capsule
[articular capsule]

Joint capsule
[articular capsule]

Patella,
articular
surface

Suprapatellar bursa

Fibula

Tibia

Fig. 1215 Right knee joint with intact joint capsule [articular capsule]; anterior aspect [65%].

Fig. 1216 Right knee joint; quadriceps sectioned and anterior part of joint capsule [articular capsule] reflected distally; suprapatellar bursa opened; anterior aspect [65%].

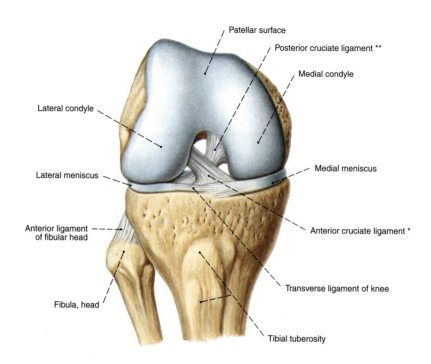

Patellar surface

Posterior cruciate ligament **

Medial condyle

Lateral condyle

Lateral meniscus

Medial meniscus

Anterior ligament
of fibular head

Anterior cruciate ligament *

Fibula, head

Transverse ligament of knee

Tibial tuberosity

Fig. 1217   Right knee joint in 90° flexion; joint capsule [articular capsule] and collateral ligaments removed; anterior aspect [65%].

*   Clinically: ACL.

**   Clinically: PCL.

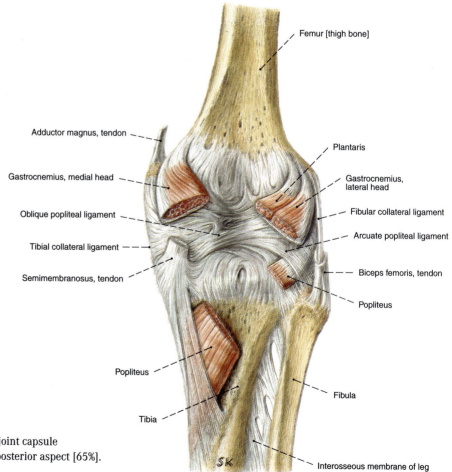

Femur [thigh bone]

Adductor magnus, tendon

Plantaris

Gastrocnemius, medial head

Gastrocnemius, lateral head

Oblique popliteal ligament

Fibular collateral ligament

Tibial collateral ligament

Arcuate popliteal ligament

Semimembranosus, tendon

Biceps femoris, tendon

Popliteus

Popliteus

Tibia

Fibula

Fig. 1218   Right knee joint with intact joint capsule [articular capsule] and muscle origins; posterior aspect [65%].

Interosseous membrane of leg

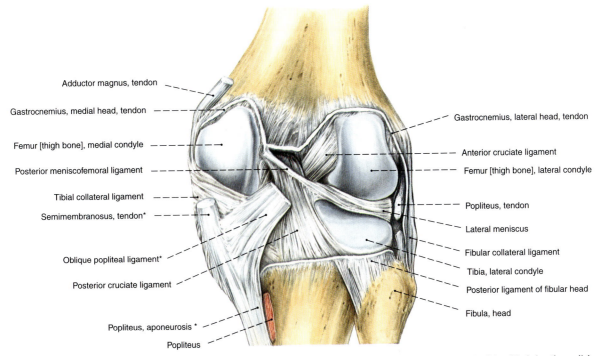

Adductor magnus, tendon

Gastrocnemius, medial head, tendon

Femur [thigh bone], medial condyle

Posterior meniscofemoral ligament

Tibial collateral ligament

Semimembranosus, tendon*

Oblique popliteal ligament*

Posterior cruciate ligament

Popliteus, aponeurosis *

Popliteus

Gastrocnemius, lateral head, tendon

Anterior cruciate ligament

Femur [thigh bone], lateral condyle

Popliteus, tendon

Lateral meniscus

Fibular collateral ligament

Tibia, lateral condyle

Posterior ligament of fibular head

Fibula, head

Fig. 1219 Right knee joint; cruciate ligaments and menisci exposed; posterior aspect (65%).

* Besides its bony insertion at the medial side of the tibia, below the medial condyle, the tendon of the semimembranosus also ends with the oblique popliteal ligament and an aponeurosis that covers the origin of the popliteus muscle.

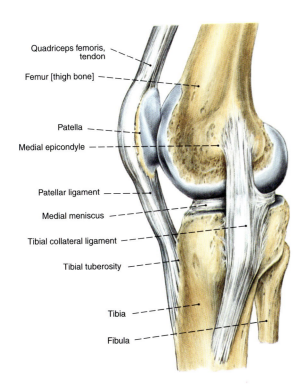

Quadriceps femoris, tendon

Femur [thigh bone]

Patella

Medial epicondyle

Patellar ligament

Medial meniscus

Tibial collateral ligament

Tibial tuberosity

Tibia

Fibula

Fig. 1220 Right knee joint; arrangement of fibers of tibial collateral ligament in extension; medial aspect (60%).
Only the posterior fibers of the tibial collateral ligament are attached to the medial meniscus.

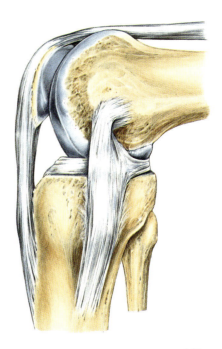

Fig. 1221 Right knee joint; arrangement of fibers of tibial collateral ligament in flexion; medial aspect (60%).
During flexion the posterior and proximal fibers of the tibial collateral ligament become twisted, which stabilizes the medial meniscus.

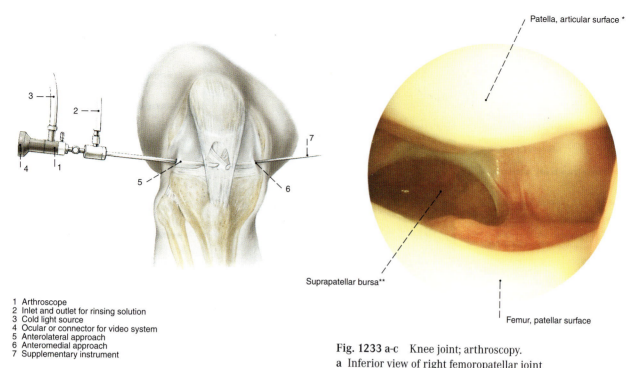

1 Arthroscope
2 Inlet and outlet for rinsing solution
3 Cold light source
4 Ocular or connector for video system
5 Anterolateral approach
6 Anteromedial approach
7 Supplementary instrument

Fig. 1232   Arthroscopic approaches.

Patella, articular surface *

Suprapatellar bursa**

Femur, patellar surface

Fig. 1233 a-c   Knee joint; arthroscopy.
a Inferior view of right femoropatellar joint

*   Patellar roof ridge: roof ridge between medial and lateral articular surface.
**   Clinically: suprapatellar recess.

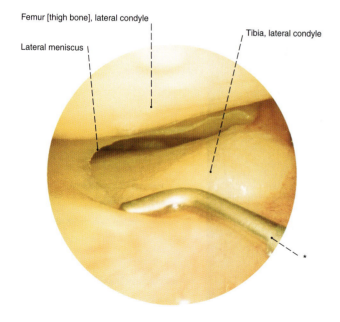

Femur [thigh bone], lateral condyle

Lateral meniscus

Tibia, lateral condyle

b   Medial view of free medial border of right lateral meniscus
The anterior part of the meniscus is depressed by a
probing hook (*).

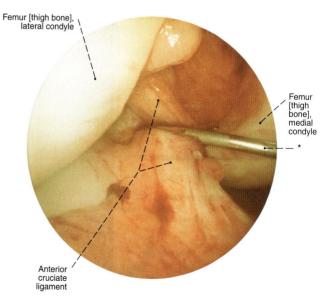

Femur [thigh bone],
lateral condyle

Femur [thigh bone], medial condyle

*

Anterior cruciate ligament

c   Anterolateral view of distal part of right anterior cruciate
ligament.
The ligament is covered with a rich-vascular synovial
membrane [synovial layer]; it is retracted medially by a
probing hook (*).

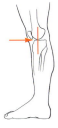

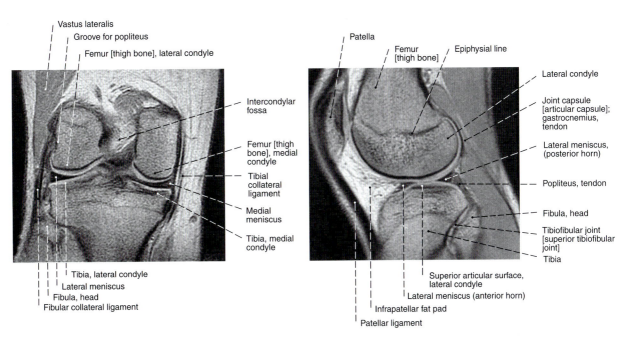

Vastus lateralis
Groove for popliteus
Femur [thigh bone], lateral condyle

Intercondylar fossa

Femur [thigh bone], medial condyle

Tibial collateral ligament

Medial meniscus

Tibia, medial condyle

Tibia, lateral condyle
Lateral meniscus
Fibula, head
Fibular collateral ligament

Patella
Femur [thigh bone]
Epiphysial line

Lateral condyle

Joint capsule [articular capsule]; gastrocnemius, tendon

Lateral meniscus, (posterior horn)

Popliteus, tendon

Fibula, head

Tibiofibular joint [superior tibiofibular joint]

Tibia

Superior articular surface, lateral condyle
Lateral meniscus (anterior horn)
Infrapatellar fat pad
Patellar ligament

Fig. 1234 Knee joint; magnetic resonance image; frontal section through middle of intercondylar eminence; knee in extension. Compact bone is visualized in black using this MRI technique.

Fig. 1235 Knee joint; magnetic resonance image; sagittal section through lateral part of joint; knee in extension.

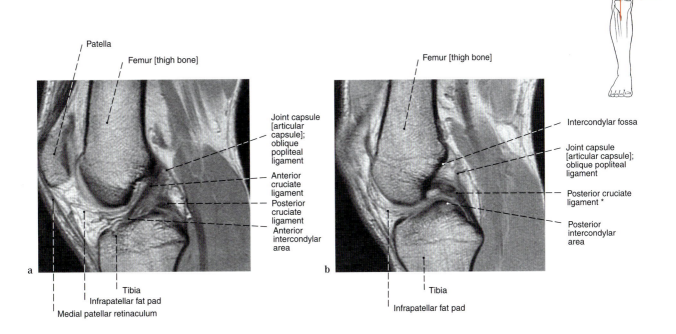

Patella
Femur [thigh bone]

Joint capsule [articular capsule]; oblique popliteal ligament

Anterior cruciate ligament

Posterior cruciate ligament

Anterior intercondylar area

Tibia
Infrapatellar fat pad
Medial patellar retinaculum

Femur [thigh bone]

Intercondylar fossa

Joint capsule [articular capsule]; oblique popliteal ligament

Posterior cruciate ligament *

Posterior intercondylar area

Tibia
Infrapatellar fat pad

Fig. 1236 a, b Knee joint; magnetic resonance image; sagittal sections; knee in extension.

a Anterior cruciate ligament
b Posterior cruciate ligament

* The inhomogeneity is caused by oblique sections of the fiber bundles.

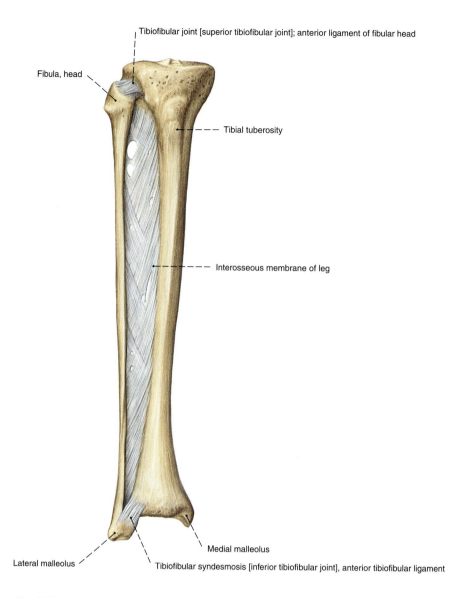

Tibiofibular joint [superior tibiofibular joint]; anterior ligament of fibular head

Fibula, head

Tibial tuberosity

Interosseous membrane of leg

Medial malleolus

Lateral malleolus

Tibiofibular syndesmosis [inferior tibiofibular joint], anterior tibiofibular ligament

Fig. 1237 Joints of right leg; anterior aspect (55%).

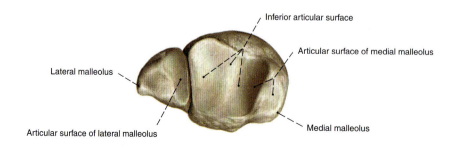

Inferior articular surface

Articular surface of medial malleolus

Lateral malleolus

Medial malleolus

Articular surface of lateral malleolus

Fig. 1238 Right tibia and fibula; distal aspect (55%).

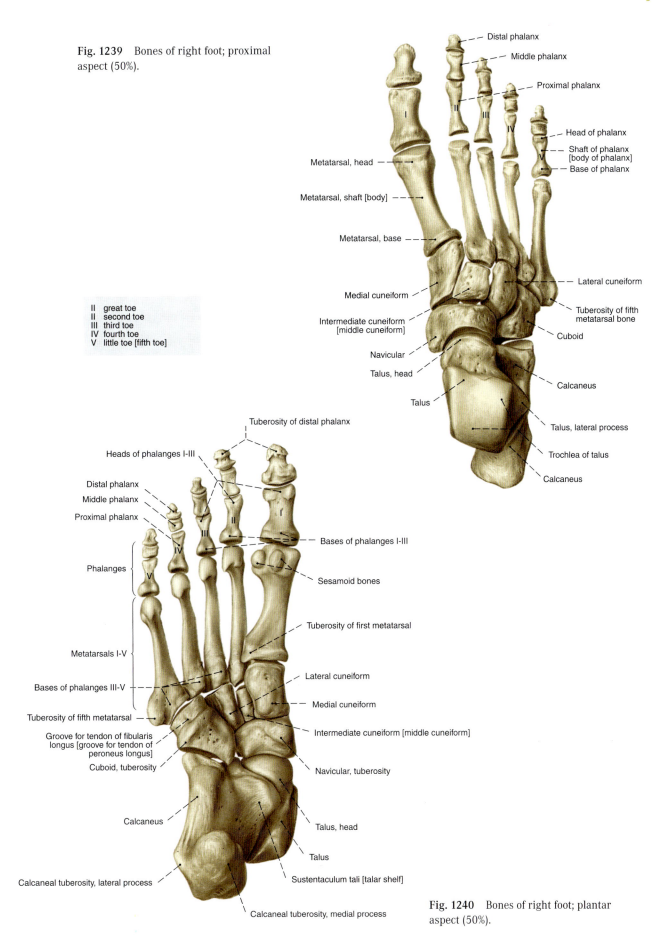

Fig. 1239 Bones of right foot; proximal aspect (50%).

Distal phalanx

Middle phalanx

Proximal phalanx

Head of phalanx

Shaft of phalanx [body of phalanx]

Base of phalanx

Metatarsal, head

Metatarsal, shaft [body]

Metatarsal, base

Lateral cuneiform

Medial cuneiform

Tuberosity of fifth metatarsal bone

Intermediate cuneiform [middle cuneiform]

Cuboid

Navicular

Talus, head

Calcaneus

Talus

Talus, lateral process

Trochlea of talus

Calcaneus

I great toe
II second toe
III third toe
IV fourth toe
V little toe [fifth toe]

Tuberosity of distal phalanx

Heads of phalanges I-III

Distal phalanx

Middle phalanx

Proximal phalanx

Bases of phalanges I-III

Phalanges

Sesamoid bones

Tuberosity of first metatarsal

Metatarsals I-V

Lateral cuneiform

Bases of phalanges III-V

Medial cuneiform

Tuberosity of fifth metatarsal

Intermediate cuneiform [middle cuneiform]

Groove for tendon of fibularis longus [groove for tendon of peroneus longus]

Navicular, tuberosity

Cuboid, tuberosity

Calcaneus

Talus, head

Calcaneal tuberosity, lateral process

Talus

Sustentaculum tali [talar shelf]

Calcaneal tuberosity, medial process

Fig. 1240 Bones of right foot; plantar aspect (50%).

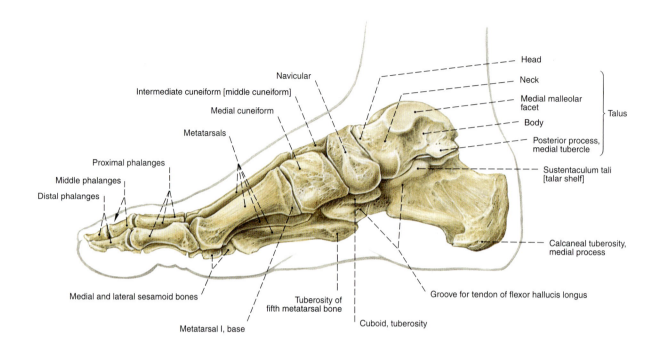

Fig. 1241   Bones of right foot; medial aspect (45%).

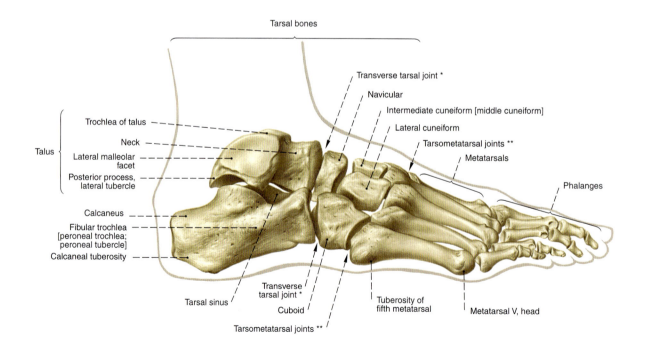

Fig. 1242   Bones of right foot; lateral aspect (45%).

*   Also: CHOPART's joint.
**   Also: LISFRANC's joint.

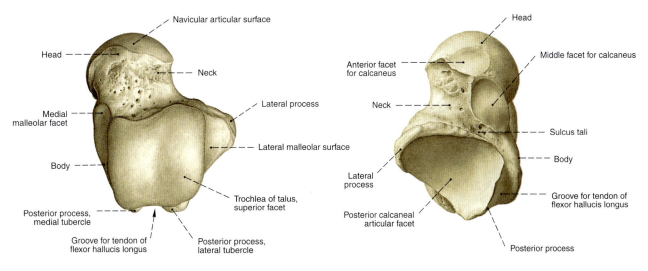

Navicular articular surface

Head

Neck

Medial malleolar facet

Lateral process

Lateral malleolar surface

Body

Trochlea of talus, superior facet

Posterior process, medial tubercle

Groove for tendon of flexor hallucis longus

Posterior process, lateral tubercle

Fig. 1243   Right talus; proximal aspect (85%).

Head

Anterior facet for calcaneus

Middle facet for calcaneus

Neck

Sulcus tali

Body

Lateral process

Groove for tendon of flexor hallucis longus

Posterior calcaneal articular facet

Posterior process

Fig. 1244   Right talus; plantar aspect (85%).

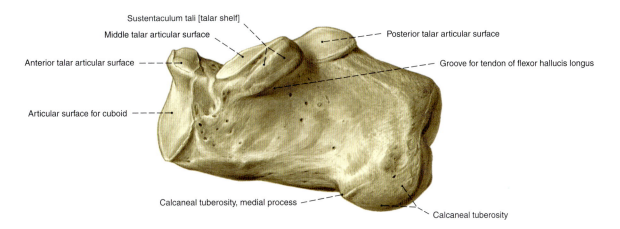

Sustentaculum tali [talar shelf]

Middle talar articular surface

Posterior talar articular surface

Anterior talar articular surface

Groove for tendon of flexor hallucis longus

Articular surface for cuboid

Calcaneal tuberosity, medial process

Calcaneal tuberosity

Fig. 1245   Right calcaneus; medial aspect (90%).

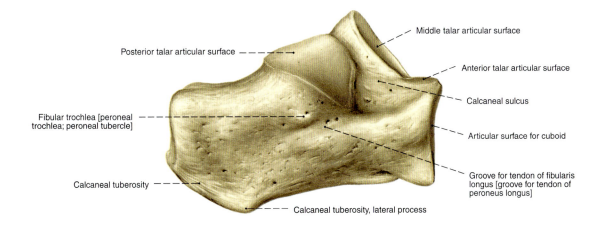

Posterior talar articular surface

Middle talar articular surface

Anterior talar articular surface

Calcaneal sulcus

Fibular trochlea [peroneal trochlea; peroneal tubercle]

Articular surface for cuboid

Groove for tendon of fibularis longus [groove for tendon of peroneus longus]

Calcaneal tuberosity

Calcaneal tuberosity, lateral process

Fig. 1246   Right calcaneus; lateral aspect (90%).

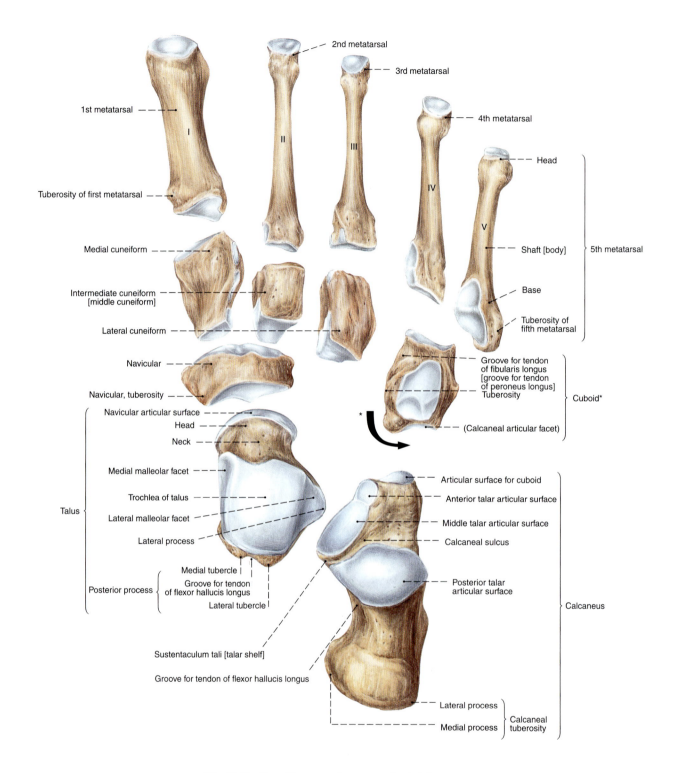

2nd metatarsal

3rd metatarsal

1st metatarsal — I

II

III

4th metatarsal

Head

Tuberosity of first metatarsal

IV

V

Shaft [body]

5th metatarsal

Medial cuneiform

Base

Intermediate cuneiform
[middle cuneiform]

Tuberosity of
fifth metatarsal

Lateral cuneiform

Navicular

Groove for tendon
of fibularis longus
[groove for tendon
of peroneus longus]
Tuberosity

Cuboid*

Navicular, tuberosity

Navicular articular surface

(Calcaneal articular facet)

Head

*

Neck

Medial malleolar facet

Articular surface for cuboid

Trochlea of talus

Anterior talar articular surface

Lateral malleolar facet

Middle talar articular surface

Lateral process

Calcaneal sulcus

Talus

Medial tubercle

Posterior talar
articular surface

Groove for tendon
of flexor hallucis longus

Posterior process

Calcaneus

Lateral tubercle

Sustentaculum tali [talar shelf]

Groove for tendon of flexor hallucis longus

Lateral process

Calcaneal
tuberosity

Medial process

Fig. 1247   Tarsal bones and metatarsals of right
foot; distances between bones increased for
didactic reasons; proximal aspect (80%).
* The cuboid is shown from the medial aspect.

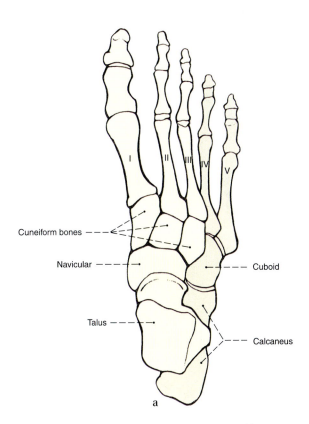
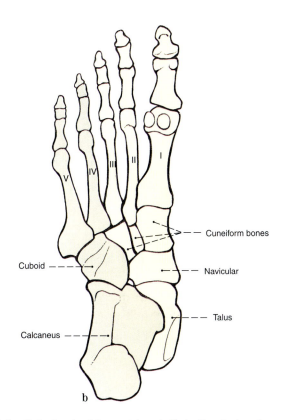

Fig. 1248 a, b Bones of right foot; arrangement of bones.
a Proximal aspect
b Plantar aspect

While all the heads of the metatarsals lie in the plantar plane, the cuneiform bones, the navicular, and the talus lie more and more dorsally above the lateral skeletal parts, so that the talus lies over the calcaneus. Thus, the longitudinal arch is formed on the medial side.

The wedge-shaped cross-section of the cuneiform bones and the bases of the metatarsals create the formation of the transverse arch.

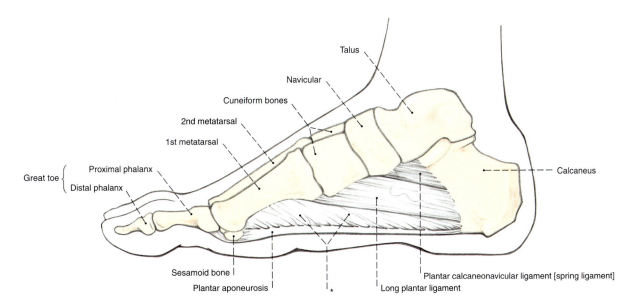

Fig. 1249 Bracing of the medial longitudinal arch of the right foot; medial aspect.

*Medial intermuscular septum.

The shown longitudinal ligamentous structures brace the longitudinal arch passively. These ligaments are supported by the short muscles of the foot.

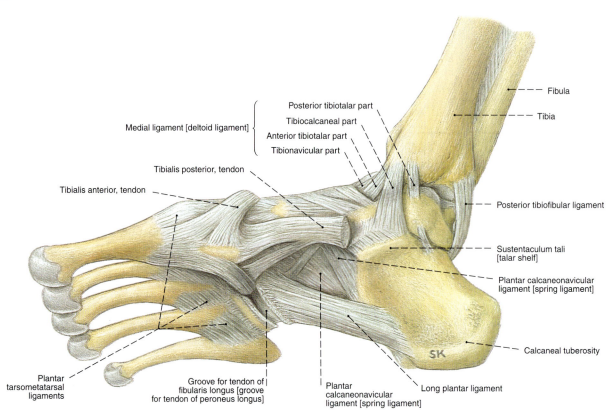

Fibula

Tibia

Medial ligament [deltoid ligament] {
Posterior tibiotalar part
Tibiocalcaneal part
Anterior tibiotalar part
Tibionavicular part

Tibialis posterior, tendon

Tibialis anterior, tendon

Posterior tibiofibular ligament

Sustentaculum tali [talar shelf]

Plantar calcaneonavicular ligament [spring ligament]

Calcaneal tuberosity

SK

Plantar tarsometatarsal ligaments

Groove for tendon of fibularis longus [groove for tendon of peroneus longus]

Plantar calcaneonavicular ligament [spring ligament]

Long plantar ligament

Fig. 1250   Joints of right foot; ligaments and tendons of tarsus and ankle joint; medial aspect (70%).

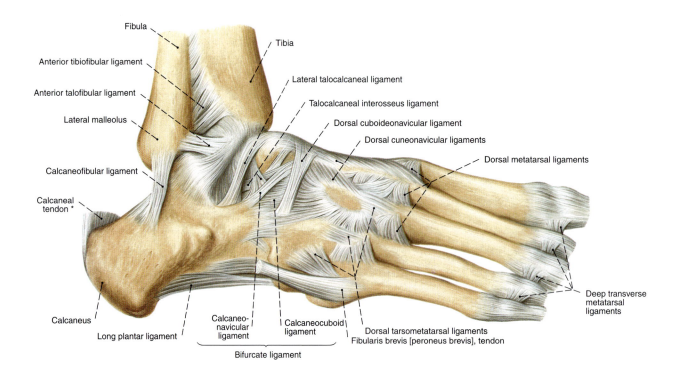

Fibula

Tibia

Anterior tibiofibular ligament

Lateral talocalcaneal ligament

Anterior talofibular ligament

Talocalcaneal interosseus ligament

Lateral malleolus

Dorsal cuboideonavicular ligament

Dorsal cuneonavicular ligaments

Calcaneofibular ligament

Dorsal metatarsal ligaments

Calcaneal tendon *

Calcaneus

Long plantar ligament

Calcaneo-navicular ligament

Calcaneocuboid ligament

Dorsal tarsometatarsal ligaments

Fibularis brevis [peroneus brevis], tendon

Deep transverse metatarsal ligaments

Bifurcate ligament

Fig. 1251   Joints of right foot; ligaments and tendons of tarsus and metatarsus; lateral aspect (70%).

*Also ACHILLES tendon.

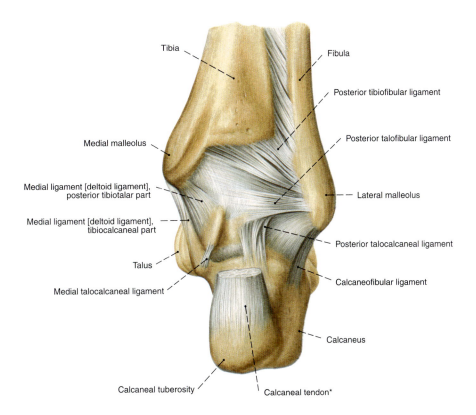

Tibia

Fibula

Posterior tibiofibular ligament

Posterior talofibular ligament

Medial malleolus

Medial ligament [deltoid ligament], posterior tibiotalar part

Lateral malleolus

Medial ligament [deltoid ligament], tibiocalcaneal part

Posterior talocalcaneal ligament

Talus

Calcaneofibular ligament

Medial talocalcaneal ligament

Calcaneus

Calcaneal tuberosity

Calcaneal tendon*

Fig. 1252   Joints of right foot; ligaments and tendons of tarsus; posterior aspect (70%).
*Also ACHILLES tendon.

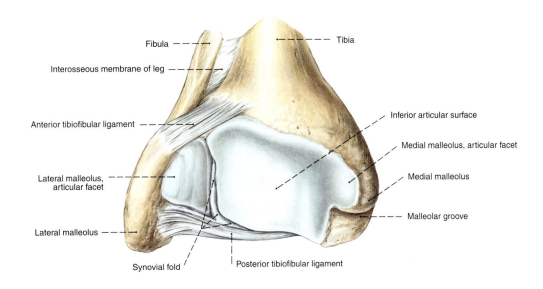

Fibula

Tibia

Interosseous membrane of leg

Anterior tibiofibular ligament

Inferior articular surface

Medial malleolus, articular facet

Lateral malleolus, articular facet

Medial malleolus

Lateral malleolus

Malleolar groove

Synovial fold

Posterior tibiofibular ligament

Fig. 1253   Right ankle joint; proximal articular surfaces; distal aspect (120%).

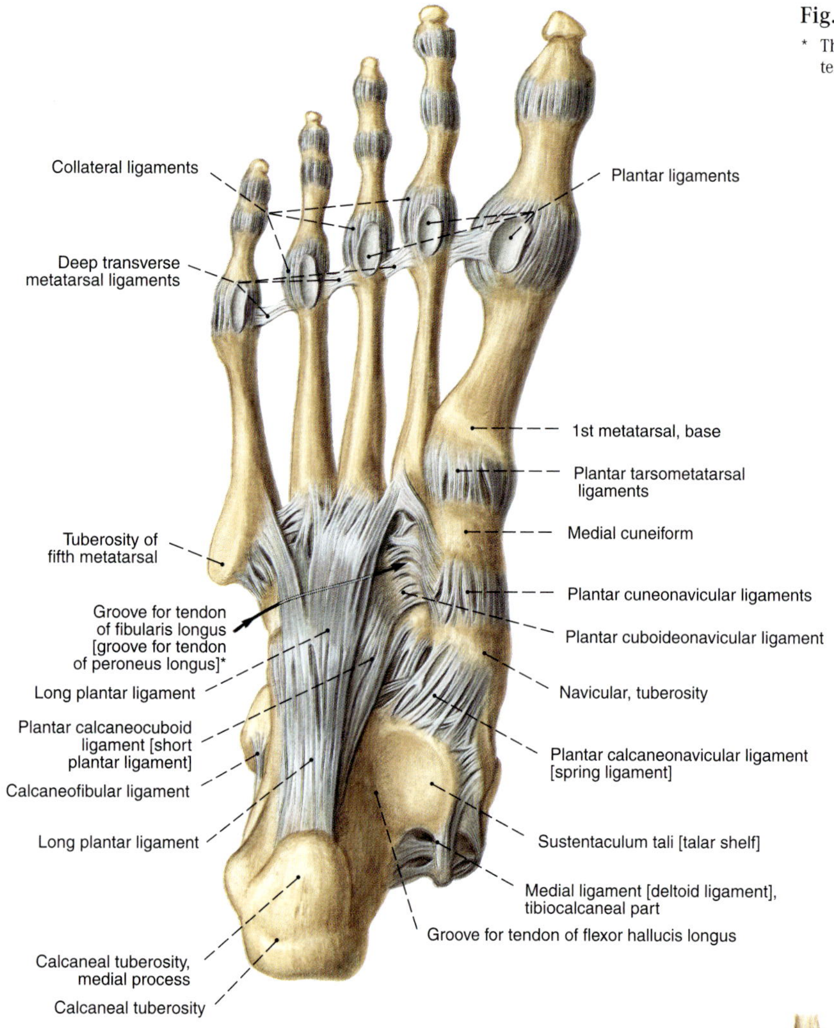

Collateral ligaments

Deep transverse metatarsal ligaments

Plantar ligaments

Fig. 1254   Joints of right foot; plantar aspect (55%).
* The long plantar ligament closes the groove, creating a canal for tendon of fibularis [peroneus] longus.

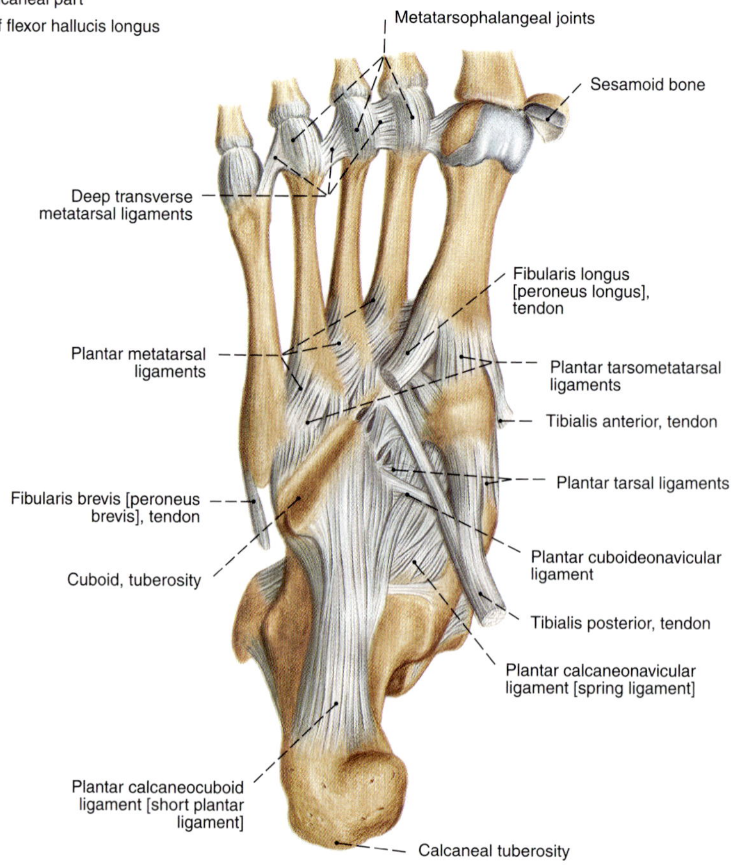

1st metatarsal, base

Plantar tarsometatarsal ligaments

Medial cuneiform

Tuberosity of fifth metatarsal

Plantar cuneonavicular ligaments

Plantar cuboideonavicular ligament

Groove for tendon of fibularis longus [groove for tendon of peroneus longus]*

Navicular, tuberosity

Long plantar ligament

Plantar calcaneocuboid ligament [short plantar ligament]

Plantar calcaneonavicular ligament [spring ligament]

Calcaneofibular ligament

Long plantar ligament

Sustentaculum tali [talar shelf]

Medial ligament [deltoid ligament], tibiocalcaneal part

Calcaneal tuberosity, medial process

Groove for tendon of flexor hallucis longus

Calcaneal tuberosity

Metatarsophalangeal joints

Sesamoid bone

Deep transverse metatarsal ligaments

Fibularis longus [peroneus longus], tendon

Plantar metatarsal ligaments

Plantar tarsometatarsal ligaments

Tibialis anterior, tendon

Plantar tarsal ligaments

Fibularis brevis [peroneus brevis], tendon

Plantar cuboideonavicular ligament

Cuboid, tuberosity

Tibialis posterior, tendon

Plantar calcaneonavicular ligament [spring ligament]

Plantar calcaneocuboid ligament [short plantar ligament]

Calcaneal tuberosity

Fig. 1255   Joints of right foot; ligaments and tendons of tarsus and metatarsus; plantar aspect (55%).

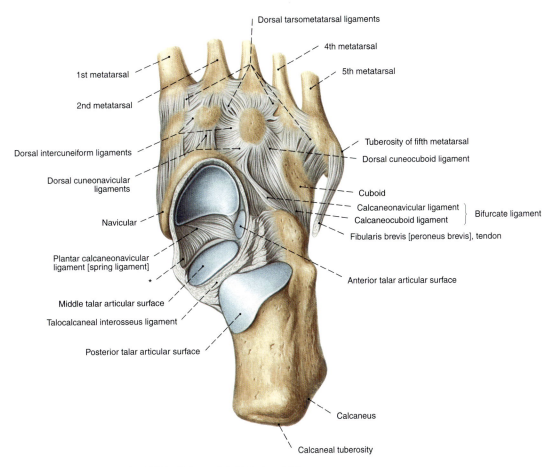

Dorsal tarsometatarsal ligaments

4th metatarsal

5th metatarsal

1st metatarsal

2nd metatarsal

Tuberosity of fifth metatarsal

Dorsal intercuneiform ligaments

Dorsal cuneocuboid ligament

Dorsal cuneonavicular ligaments

Cuboid

Calcaneonavicular ligament

Calcaneocuboid ligament } Bifurcate ligament

Navicular

Fibularis brevis [peroneus brevis], tendon

Plantar calcaneonavicular ligament [spring ligament]

Anterior talar articular surface

*

Middle talar articular surface

Talocalcaneal interosseus ligament

Posterior talar articular surface

Calcaneus

Calcaneal tuberosity

Fig. 1256 Joints of right foot; subtalar [talocalcaneal] and talocalcaneonavicular joints disarticulated; proximal aspect (70%).
* See Fig. 1257.

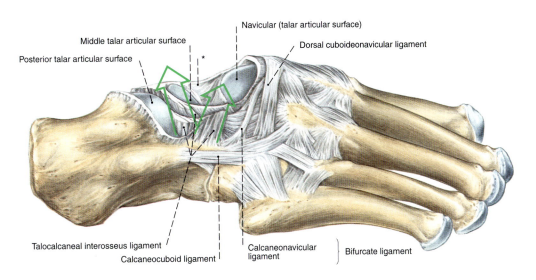

Middle talar articular surface

Posterior talar articular surface

Navicular (talar articular surface)

Dorsal cuboideonavicular ligament

*

Talocalcaneal interosseus ligament

Calcaneocuboid ligament

Calcaneonavicular ligament } Bifurcate ligament

Fig. 1257 Subtalar [talocalcaneal] and talocalcaneonavicular joints of right foot; talus and lateral ligaments removed; lateral aspect (70%).
The two arrows indicate the torsion of the talocalcaneal interosseus ligament.

* Sheet of dense connective tissue between the plantar calcaneonavicular ligament [spring ligament] and the tibionavicular part of the medial ligament [deltoid ligament] that opposes the medially directed shearing force of the head of talus.
Weakening of this sheet causes flattening of the medial longitudinal arch (flatfoot; splayfoot; talipes planus).

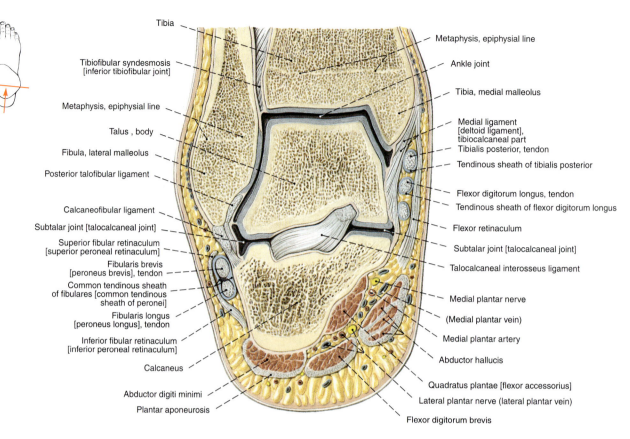

Tibia

Tibiofibular syndesmosis
[inferior tibiofibular joint]

Metaphysis, epiphysial line

Talus , body

Fibula, lateral malleolus

Posterior talofibular ligament

Calcaneofibular ligament

Subtalar joint [talocalcaneal joint]

Superior fibular retinaculum
[superior peroneal retinaculum]

Fibularis brevis
[peroneus brevis], tendon

Common tendinous sheath
of fibulares [common tendinous
sheath of peronei]

Fibularis longus
[peroneus longus], tendon

Inferior fibular retinaculum
[inferior peroneal retinaculum]

Calcaneus

Abductor digiti minimi

Plantar aponeurosis

Metaphysis, epiphysial line

Ankle joint

Tibia, medial malleolus

Medial ligament
[deltoid ligament],
tibiocalcaneal part

Tibialis posterior, tendon

Tendinous sheath of tibialis posterior

Flexor digitorum longus, tendon

Tendinous sheath of flexor digitorum longus

Flexor retinaculum

Subtalar joint [talocalcaneal joint]

Talocalcaneal interosseus ligament

Medial plantar nerve

(Medial plantar vein)

Medial plantar artery

Abductor hallucis

Quadratus plantae [flexor accessorius]

Lateral plantar nerve (lateral plantar vein)

Flexor digitorum brevis

Fig. 1258 Subtalar [talocalcaneal] and talocalcaneonavicular joints of right foot; frontal section through malleoli distal aspect (90%).
* See Fig. 1257.

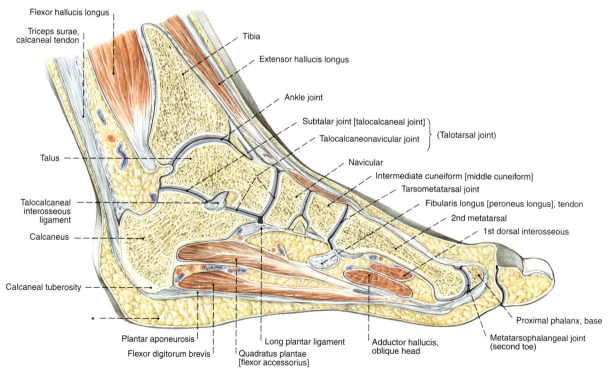

Flexor hallucis longus

Triceps surae,
calcaneal tendon

Talus

Talocalcaneal
interosseous
ligament

Calcaneus

Calcaneal tuberosity

*

Plantar aponeurosis

Flexor digitorum brevis

Tibia

Extensor hallucis longus

Ankle joint

Subtalar joint [talocalcaneal joint]

Talocalcaneonavicular joint } (Talotarsal joint)

Navicular

Intermediate cuneiform [middle cuneiform]

Tarsometatarsal joint

Fibularis longus [peroneus longus], tendon

2nd metatarsal

1st dorsal interosseous

Proximal phalanx, base

Metatarsophalangeal joint
(second toe)

Adductor hallucis,
oblique head

Quadratus plantae
[flexor accessorius]

Long plantar ligament

Fig. 1259 Subtalar [talocalcaneal] and talocalcaneonavicular joints of right foot; sagittal section through middle of trochlea of talus; lateral aspect (50%).

* Calcaneal fat pad.

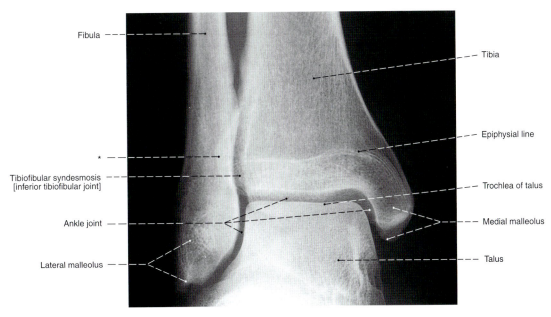

Fibula

Tibia

Epiphysial line

*

Tibiofibular syndesmosis [inferior tibiofibular joint]

Trochlea of talus

Ankle joint

Medial malleolus

Lateral malleolus

Talus

Fig. 1260 Ankle and talocalcaneonavicular joints; AP radiograph in supine position; central beam directed tangential to the trochlea of talus.

* Clinically the posterior border of the fibular notch is also called third malleolus.

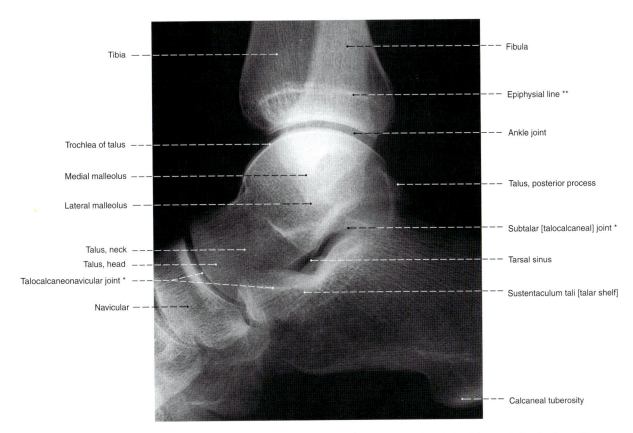

Tibia

Fibula

Epiphysial line **

Ankle joint

Trochlea of talus

Medial malleolus

Talus, posterior process

Lateral malleolus

Subtalar [talocalcaneal] joint *

Talus, neck

Tarsal sinus

Talus, head

Talocalcaneonavicular joint *

Sustentaculum tali [talar shelf]

Navicular

Calcaneal tuberosity

Fig. 1261 Subtalar [talocalcaneal] and talocalcaneonavicular joints; lateral radiograph in supine position; central beam directed onto the top of the trochlea of talus.

* Due to their torsion the articular clefts are not viewed orthogonally.
** Superposition of epiphysial lines of tibia and fibula.

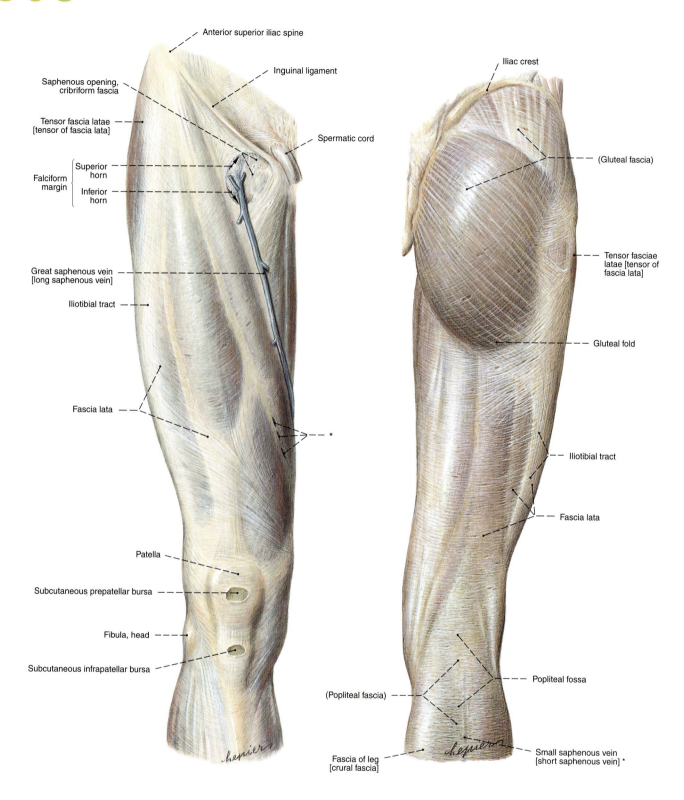

Fig. 1262   Fascia lata of right thigh; anterior aspect.
The transition zone between the aponeurosis of the external oblique and the fascia lata is called inguinal ligament. This ligament is attached laterally to the anterior superior iliac spine and medially to the pubic tubercle.

* Openings for perforating veins (DODD's veins).

Fig. 1263   Fascia lata of right thigh; posterior aspect.

* Sub- or intrafascial course of small saphenous vein [short saphenous vein].

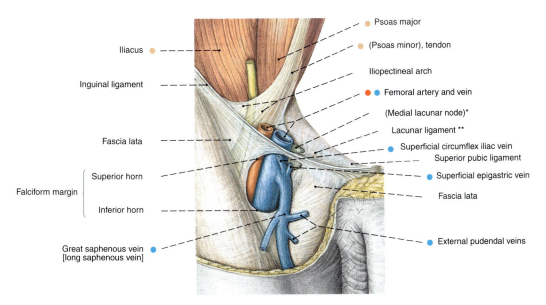

Iliacus

Inguinal ligament

Fascia lata

Falciform margin
- Superior horn
- Inferior horn

Great saphenous vein
[long saphenous vein]

Psoas major

(Psoas minor), tendon

Iliopectineal arch

Femoral artery and vein

(Medial lacunar node)*

Lacunar ligament **

Superficial circumflex iliac vein

Superior pubic ligament

Superficial epigastric vein

Fascia lata

External pudendal veins

Fig. 1264 Right saphenous opening and vascular space; anterior abdominal wall, contents of abdomen, iliac fascia, and femoral septum (CLOQUET's septum) removed; anterior aspect.

* Also: ROSNEMUELLER'S gland [node].
** Also: GIMBERNAT's ligament.

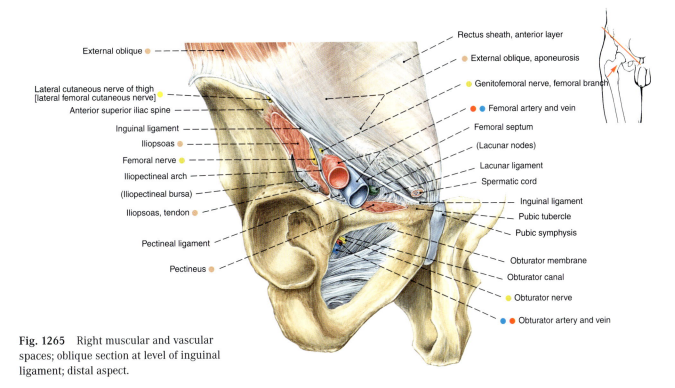

External oblique

Lateral cutaneous nerve of thigh [lateral femoral cutaneous nerve]

Anterior superior iliac spine

Inguinal ligament

Iliopsoas

Femoral nerve

Iliopectineal arch

(Iliopectineal bursa)

Iliopsoas, tendon

Pectineal ligament

Pectineus

Rectus sheath, anterior layer

External oblique, aponeurosis

Genitofemoral nerve, femoral branch

Femoral artery and vein

Femoral septum

(Lacunar nodes)

Lacunar ligament

Spermatic cord

Inguinal ligament

Pubic tubercle

Pubic symphysis

Obturator membrane

Obturator canal

Obturator nerve

Obturator artery and vein

Fig. 1265 Right muscular and vascular spaces; oblique section at level of inguinal ligament; distal aspect.

Muscular and vascular spaces of the groin [inguinal region]

The space beneath the inguinal ligament is divided into two passage spaces by the iliopectineal arch. Lateral to this arch lies the muscular space, medial the vascular space. Through the muscular space pass the iliopsoas, the lateral cutaneous nerve of thigh [lateral femoral cutaneous nerve], and the femoral nerve to reach the thigh. In the vascular space are the femoral artery and vein, the femoral branch of genitofemoral nerve, and the lacunar nodes (lateral, medial, and intermediate), as well as lymphatic vessels. The space between the femoral vein (lateral), the sharp-edged lacunar ligament (medial), the inguinal ligament (ventral), and the pectineal ligament (dorsal) is filled with loose connective tissue, the femoral septum (CLOQUETS' s septum) and is also called femoral ring or femoral canal.

Here a femoral hernia may develop; the femoral ring then becomes the inner and the saphenous opening the outer opening of the hernia.

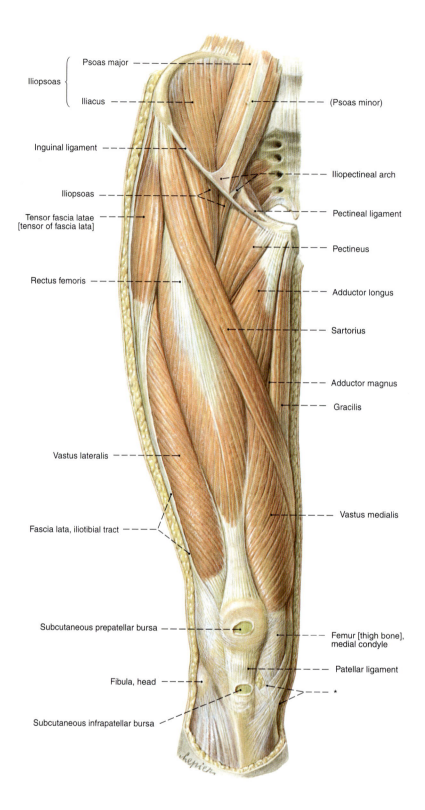

Iliopsoas {
  Psoas major
  Iliacus

Inguinal ligament

Iliopsoas

Tensor fascia latae
[tensor of fascia lata]

Rectus femoris

Vastus lateralis

Fascia lata, iliotibial tract

Subcutaneous prepatellar bursa

Fibula, head

Subcutaneous infrapatellar bursa

(Psoas minor)

Iliopectineal arch

Pectineal ligament

Pectineus

Adductor longus

Sartorius

Adductor magnus

Gracilis

Vastus medialis

Femur [thigh bone],
medial condyle

Patellar ligament

*

Fig. 1266   Muscles of right thigh and hip; fascia lata except
iliotibial tract removed; anterior aspect.

*   Common insertion of sartorius, gracilis, and semitendinosus beneath the
     medial condyle of tibia (formerly superficial pes anserinus).

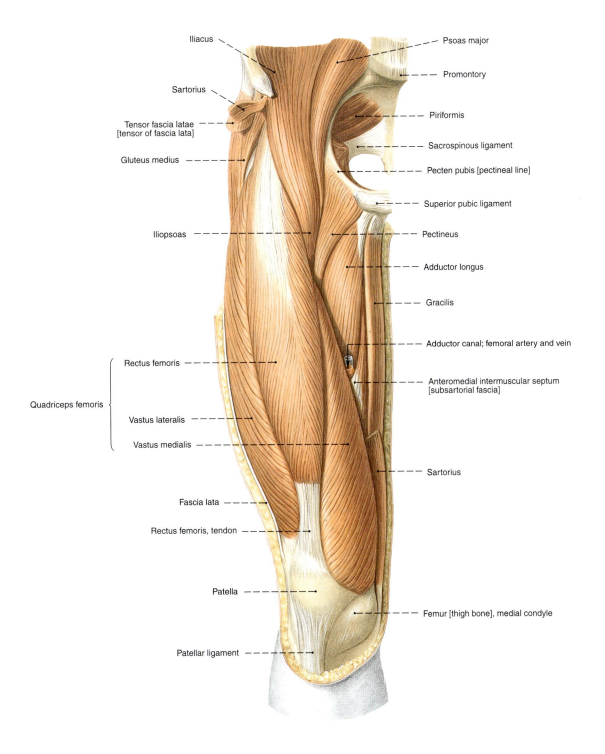

Iliacus

Sartorius

Tensor fascia latae
[tensor of fascia lata]

Gluteus medius

Iliopsoas

Rectus femoris

Quadriceps femoris

Vastus lateralis

Vastus medialis

Fascia lata

Rectus femoris, tendon

Patella

Patellar ligament

Psoas major

Promontory

Piriformis

Sacrospinous ligament

Pecten pubis [pectineal line]

Superior pubic ligament

Pectineus

Adductor longus

Gracilis

Adductor canal; femoral artery and vein

Anteromedial intermuscular septum
[subsartorial fascia]

Sartorius

Femur [thigh bone], medial condyle

Fig. 1267 Muscles of right thigh and hip; fascia lata,
tensor fasciae latae [tensor of fascia lata], and sartorius
removed; anterior aspect.

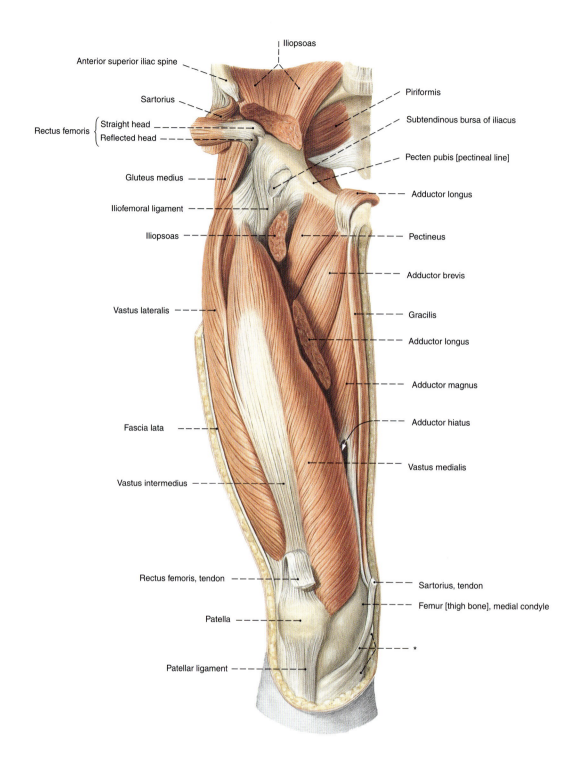

Anterior superior iliac spine

Sartorius

Rectus femoris { Straight head

Reflected head }

Gluteus medius

Iliofemoral ligament

Iliopsoas

Vastus lateralis

Fascia lata

Vastus intermedius

Rectus femoris, tendon

Patella

Patellar ligament

Iliopsoas

Piriformis

Subtendinous bursa of iliacus

Pecten pubis [pectineal line]

Adductor longus

Pectineus

Adductor brevis

Gracilis

Adductor longus

Adductor magnus

Adductor hiatus

Vastus medialis

Sartorius, tendon

Femur [thigh bone], medial condyle

*

Fig. 1268   Muscles of right thigh and hip; deep layer after removal of sartorius, rectus femoris, and adductor longus as well as partial removal of iliopsoas in the region of the joint; anterior and lateral wall of adductor canal and anteromedial intermuscular septum [subsartorial fascia] removed to expose adductor hiatus; anterior aspect.

*   Common insertion of sartorius, gracilis, and semitendinosus beneath the medial condyle of tibia.
**   Origin of rectus femoris reflected laterally.

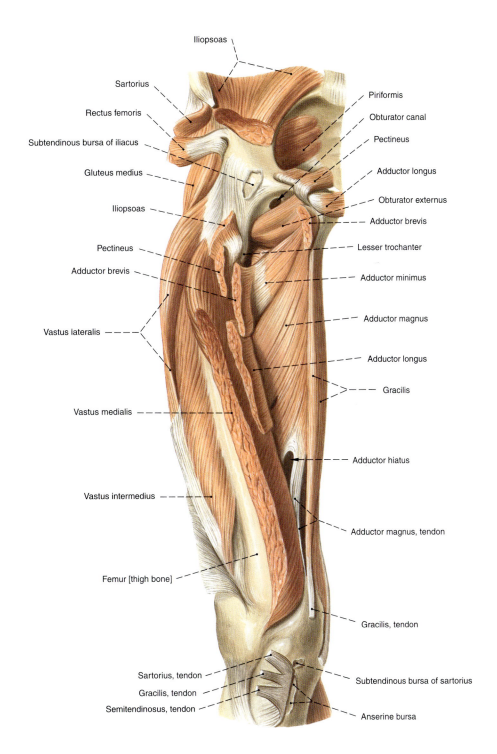

Iliopsoas

Sartorius

Rectus femoris

Subtendinous bursa of iliacus

Gluteus medius

Iliopsoas

Pectineus

Adductor brevis

Vastus lateralis

Vastus medialis

Vastus intermedius

Femur [thigh bone]

Sartorius, tendon

Gracilis, tendon

Semitendinosus, tendon

Piriformis

Obturator canal

Pectineus

Adductor longus

Obturator externus

Adductor brevis

Lesser trochanter

Adductor minimus

Adductor magnus

Adductor longus

Gracilis

Adductor hiatus

Adductor magnus, tendon

Gracilis, tendon

Subtendinous bursa of sartorius

Anserine bursa

Fig. 1269   Muscles of right thigh and hip;
superficial muscles extensively and also several
deep muscle removed; anterior and lateral wall
of adductor canal removed; anterior aspect.

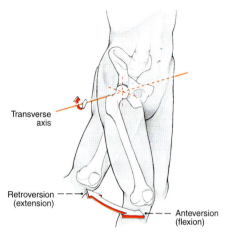

Fig. 1270   Hip joint; movement in the sagittal plane.

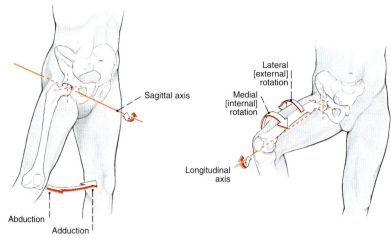

Fig. 1271   Hip joint; movement in the frontal plane.

Fig. 1272   Hip joint; movement in the transverse plane.

Ventral muscles of hip (Figs. 1266-1268, 1285)

This group comprises only the iliacus and psoas major, which assemble the iliopsoas. The iliopsoas is the only muscle passing only the hip joint anteriorly. The other muscles ventral to the hip joint also pass the knee joint and, thus, are explained with the muscles of the thigh.

Muscle *Innervation*	Origin	Insertion	Function
1. Iliacus *Muscular branches (lumbar plexus)*	Iliac fossa and anterior inferior iliac spine, anterior part of joint capsule of hip joint	Lesser trochanter and adjacent area of medial lip of linea aspera	
2. Psoas major *Muscular branches (lumbar plexus)*	**Superficial part:** vertebral bodies of 12th thoracic–4th lumbar vertebrae (lateral surfaces), intervertebral discs	Lesser trochanter	**Lumbar vertebral column:** Lateral flexion, extension (increases lumbar lordosis)
3. Psoas minor *Muscular branches (lumbar plexus)* (inconstant muscle)	**Deep part:** costal processes of 1st–4th lumbar vertebrae Vertebral bodies of 12th thoracic and 1st lumbar vertebrae (lateral surfaces)	Fascia of iliopsoas, iliopectineal arch (frequently via along flat tendon)	**Hip joint :** Flexion, medial rotation (lateral rotation when gluteal muscles contract simultaneously)

Ventral muscles of thigh (Figs. 1266, 1267, 1285)

Sartorius spirals from proximal lateral across the thigh toward its distal medial insertion. The short muscle belly of tensor fascia latae lies most lateral, embedded in the fascia lata, that blends with the iliotibial tract. The majority of the ventral muscles of thigh is made by the quadriceps femoris.

Muscle *Innervation*	Origin	Insertion	Function
1. Quadriceps femoris *Femoral nerve (lumbar plexus)* Rectus femoris acts on two joints Vastus medialis, lateralis, and intermedius acts on one joint	**Rectus femoris, straight head:** anterior inferior iliac spine **Rectus femoris, reflected head:** superior border of acetabulum **Vastus medialis:** medial lip of linea aspera (lower 2/3)	Patella (proximal and lateral borders), tibial tuberosity (via patellar ligament), proximal extremity of tibia (regions lateral and medial to tibial tuberosity, via patellar retinacula)	**Hip joint** (rectus femoris only): flexion **Knee joint:** extension

Muscle *Innervation*	Origin	Insertion	Function
	Vastus lateralis: greater trochanter (distal circumference), lateral lip of linea aspera		
	Vastus intermedius : anterior surface of femur (upper 2/3)		
	Articularis genus [articular muscle of knee]: anterior surface of femur (distal 1/3)		
2. **Sartorius** *Femoral nerve (lumbar plexus)*	Anterior superior iliac spine	Tibial tuberosity (medial facet)	**Hip joint:** Flexion, lateral rotation, abduction **Knee joint:** Flexion, medial rotation
3. **Tensor fasciae latae [tensor of fascia lata]** *Superior gluteal nerve (sacral plexus)*	Anterior superior iliac spine	Lateral surface of tibia (via iliotibial tract beneath lateral condyle)	**Hip joint:** Flexion, abduction, medial rotation **Knee joint:** Stabilization in extended position

Medial muscles of thigh (Figs. 1266, 1268, 1269, 1285, 1286)

The medial group of muscles of thigh are also known as the adductor compartment due to their main function. They form the triangular medial compartment of thigh. Most medial lies gracilis. From proximal to distal pectineus is followed by adductor brevis, adductor longus, and adductor magnus. Obturator externus lies deep to pectineus and close to the inferior circumference of the femoral neck.

Muscle *Innervation*	Origin	Insertion	Function
1. **Gracilis** *Obturator nerve (lumbar plexus)*	Inferior pubic ramus (medial border, near symphysis)	Proximal extremity of tibia (medial to tibial tuberosity)	**Hip joint:** Adduction, flexion, lateral rotation **Knee joint:** Flexion, medial rotation
2. **Pectineus** *Femoral and obturator nerves (lumbar plexus)*	Pecten pubis [pectineal line]	Pectineal line [spiral line] of femur [thigh bone]	**Hip joint:** Adduction, flexion, lateral rotation
3. **Adductor brevis** *Obturator nerve (lumbar plexus)*	Inferior pubic ramus (closer to obturator foramen compared to adductor longus)	Medial lip of linea aspera (proximal 1/3)	**Hip joint:** Adduction, flexion, lateral rotation
4. **Adductor longus** *Obturator nerve (lumbar plexus)*	Pubis (beneath pubic crest up to symphysis)	Medial lip of linea aspera (middle 1/3)	**Hip joint:** Adduction, flexion, lateral rotation (most anterior fibers rotate medially)
5. **Adductor magnus** *Obturator nerve (lumbar plexus) and sciatic nerve (tibial part-sacral plexus) The adductor minimus is a proximal part of adductor magnus*	Inferior pubic ramus and ramus of ischium (medial border)	Medial lip of linea aspera (proximal 2/3), gluteal tuberosity, adductor tubercle (adductor hiatus between both insertions)	**Hip joint:** Adduction, lateral rotation, flexion (anterior part), extension (posterior part)
6. **Obturator externus** *Obturator nerve (lumbar plexus)*	Circumference of obturator foramen (lateral surface), obturator membrane	Trochanteric fossa	**Hip joint:** Lateral rotation, adduction, flexion

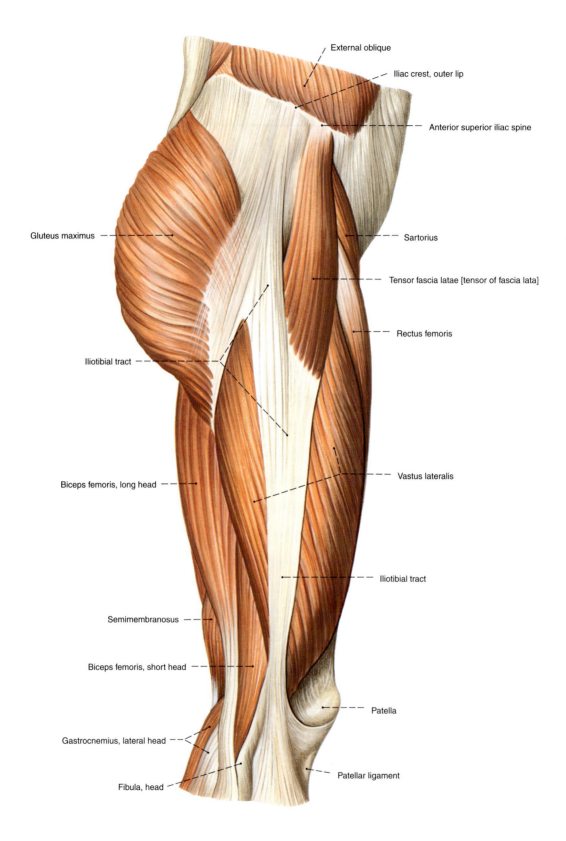

Fig. 1273   Muscles of right thigh and hip; fascia lata
removed except for iliotibial tract; lateral aspect.

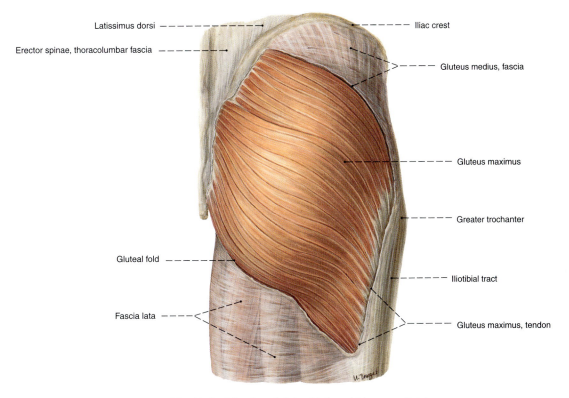

Latissimus dorsi — Iliac crest

Erector spinae, thoracolumbar fascia — Gluteus medius, fascia

Gluteus maximus

Greater trochanter

Iliotibial tract

Gluteal fold — Gluteus maximus, tendon

Fascia lata —

Fig. 1274 Muscles of right thigh and hip; superficial muscles after removal of fascia of gluteus maximus; dorsal aspect.

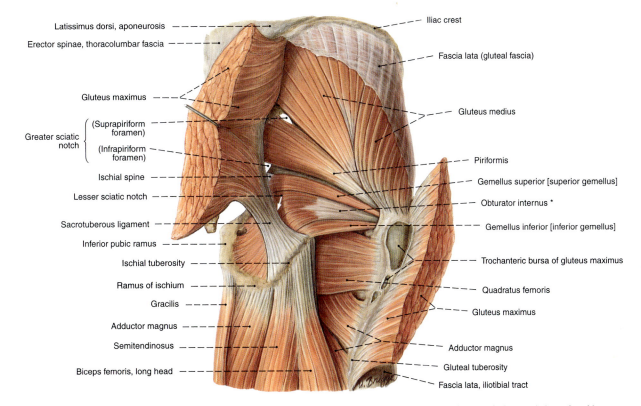

Latissimus dorsi, aponeurosis — Iliac crest

Erector spinae, thoracolumbar fascia — Fascia lata (gluteal fascia)

Gluteus maximus — Gluteus medius

Greater sciatic notch { (Suprapiriform foramen) — Piriformis

(Infrapiriform foramen) — Gemellus superior [superior gemellus]

Ischial spine — Obturator internus *

Lesser sciatic notch — Gemellus inferior [inferior gemellus]

Sacrotuberous ligament — Trochanteric bursa of gluteus maximus

Inferior pubic ramus — Quadratus femoris

Ischial tuberosity — Gluteus maximus

Ramus of ischium — Adductor magnus

Gracilis — Gluteal tuberosity

Adductor magnus — Fascia lata, iliotibial tract

Semitendinosus —

Biceps femoris, long head —

Fig. 1275 Muscles of right thigh and hip; deep muscles after sectioning of gluteus maximus; dorsal aspect.

* The part of obturator internus between the lesser sciatic notch and its insertion is frequently made only of tendinous bands.

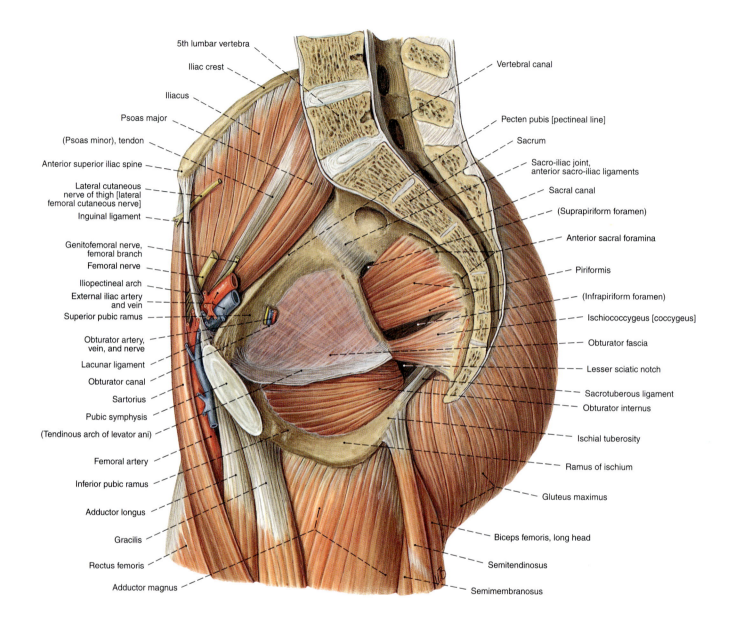

5th lumbar vertebra

Iliac crest

Iliacus

Psoas major

(Psoas minor), tendon

Anterior superior iliac spine

Lateral cutaneous nerve of thigh [lateral femoral cutaneous nerve]

Inguinal ligament

Genitofemoral nerve, femoral branch

Femoral nerve

Iliopectineal arch

External iliac artery and vein

Superior pubic ramus

Obturator artery, vein, and nerve

Lacunar ligament

Obturator canal

Sartorius

Pubic symphysis

(Tendinous arch of levator ani)

Femoral artery

Inferior pubic ramus

Adductor longus

Gracilis

Rectus femoris

Adductor magnus

Vertebral canal

Pecten pubis [pectineal line]

Sacrum

Sacro-iliac joint, anterior sacro-iliac ligaments

Sacral canal

(Suprapiriform foramen)

Anterior sacral foramina

Piriformis

(Infrapiriform foramen)

Ischiococcygeus [coccygeus]

Obturator fascia

Lesser sciatic notch

Sacrotuberous ligament

Obturator internus

Ischial tuberosity

Ramus of ischium

Gluteus maximus

Biceps femoris, long head

Semitendinosus

Semimembranosus

Fig. 1276   Muscles of right thigh and hip; pelvis and lumbar vertebral column sectioned in the median plane; medial aspect.

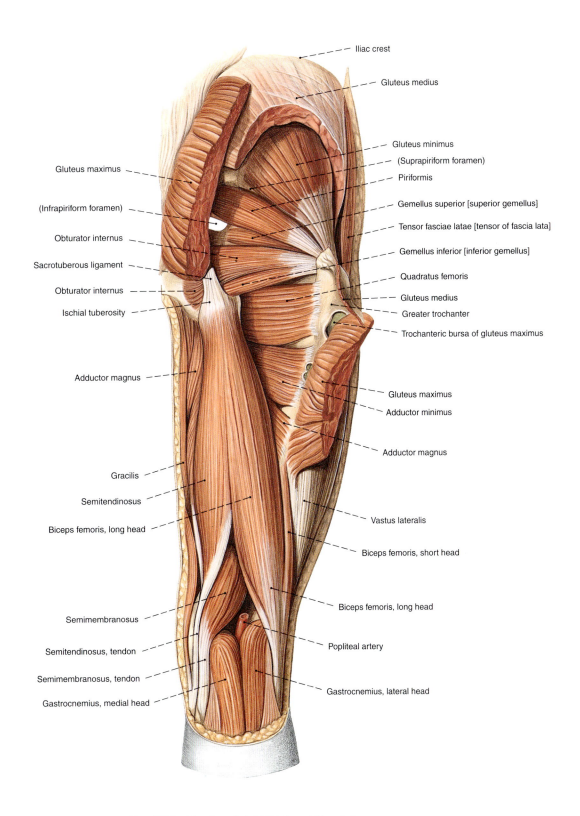

Iliac crest

Gluteus medius

Gluteus minimus

(Suprapiriform foramen)

Piriformis

Gluteus maximus

Gemellus superior [superior gemellus]

(Infrapiriform foramen)

Tensor fasciae latae [tensor of fascia lata]

Obturator internus

Gemellus inferior [inferior gemellus]

Sacrotuberous ligament

Quadratus femoris

Obturator internus

Gluteus medius

Ischial tuberosity

Greater trochanter

Trochanteric bursa of gluteus maximus

Adductor magnus

Gluteus maximus

Adductor minimus

Adductor magnus

Gracilis

Semitendinosus

Vastus lateralis

Biceps femoris, long head

Biceps femoris, short head

Biceps femoris, long head

Semimembranosus

Semitendinosus, tendon

Popliteal artery

Semimembranosus, tendon

Gastrocnemius, medial head

Gastrocnemius, lateral head

Fig. 1277   Muscles of right thigh and hip; gluteus maximus and medius partially removed; posterior aspect.

Posterior muscles of thigh (Figs. 1277, 1286)

The posterior muscles of thigh comprise the biceps femoris, semitendinosus, and semimembranosus from lateral to medial.

Muscle *Innervation*	Origin	Insertion	Function
1. **Biceps femoris** Long head: *Sciatic nerve, tibial part [sacral plexus]* Short head: *Sciatic nerve, fibular part [sacral plexus]* Long head acts at two joints; short head acts at one joint	**Long head:** ischial tuberosity (common head with semitendinosus) **Short head:** lateral lip of linea aspera (middle 1/3)	Head of fibula (embraces fibular collateral ligament) Blends with crural fascia [fascia of leg]	**Hip joint:** Extension, adduction, lateral rotation **Knee joint:** Flexion, lateral rotation
2. **Semitendinosus** *Sciatic nerve, tibial part [sacral plexus]*	Ischial tuberosity (common head with long head of biceps femoris)	Tibial tuberosity (medial surface)	**Hip joint:** Extension, adduction, lateral rotation **Knee joint:** Flexion, medial rotation
3. **Semimembranosus** *Sciatic nerve, tibial part [sacral plexus]*	Ischial tuberosity	Proximal extremity of fibula (beneath medial condyle)	**Hip joint:** Extension, adduction, lateral rotation **Knee joint:** Flexion, medial rotation

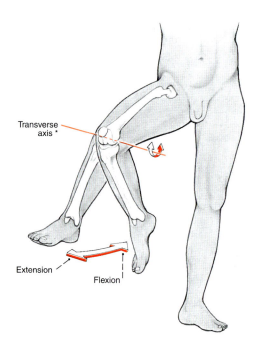

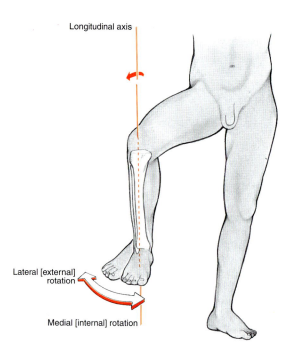

Fig. 1279   Knee joint; movement in the sagittal plane.

* Due to the inhomogeneous curvature of the condyles of femur [thigh bone] the position of this axis changes during movement (instantaneous axis).

Fig. 1280   Knee joint; movement in the transverse plane.

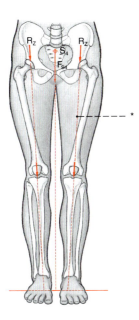

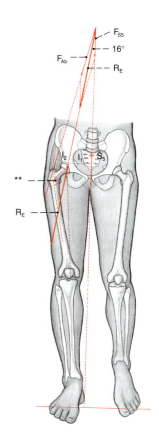

S₄   center of gravity of 4/6 parts of body weight
F_{S4}   load of parts of body weight effective in the hip joints
R_Z   resulting force in each hip joint in two-legged standing
S₆   center of gravity of 5/6 parts of body weight
F_{S5}   load of parts of body weight effective in the hip joints
R_E   resulting force in each hip joint in one-legged standing
F_{Ab}   force of abductors
I₁   lever arm of F_{S5}
I₂   lever arm of F_{Ab}
*   Centroidal axis.
**   Angle of inclination [depression] of neck (approx. 125°).

Fig. 1281   Load on hip joints in two-legged standing.

Fig. 1282   Unilateral load on hip joint in the stance phase.

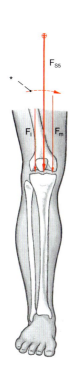

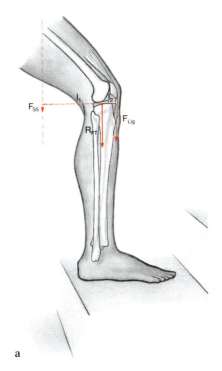

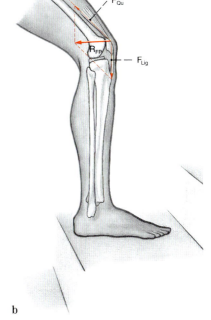

a

b

F_l   partial force effective in lateral compartment
F_m   partial force effective in medial compartment
F_{S5}   load of approx. 5/6 parts of body weight effective in the knee joints

F_{Qu}   force of quadriceps femoris
F_{Lig}   force of patellar ligament
R_{FP}   resulting force in femoropatellar joint
R_{FT}   resulting force in femorotibial joint

I₁   lever arm of 5/6 parts of body weight effective in this position
I₂   lever arm of patellar ligament
*   Torque of body

Fig. 1283   Load on knee joint in the frontal plane.

Fig. 1284 a, b   Load on knee joint in the sagittal plane.
a   Femorotibial joint
b   Femoropatellar joint

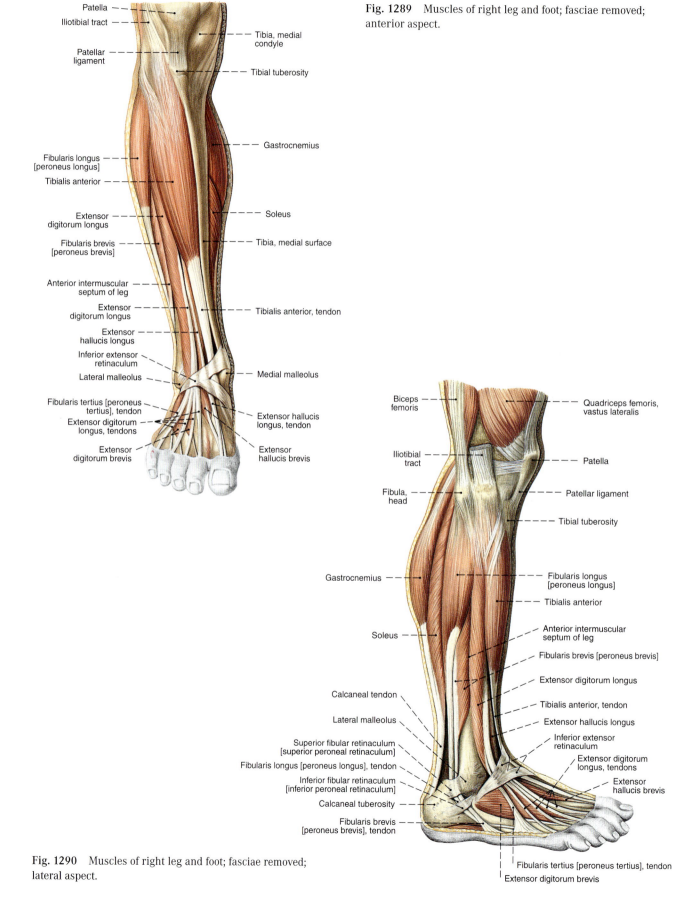

Patella
Iliotibial tract
Patellar ligament
Tibia, medial condyle
Tibial tuberosity
Gastrocnemius
Fibularis longus [peroneus longus]
Tibialis anterior
Soleus
Extensor digitorum longus
Fibularis brevis [peroneus brevis]
Tibia, medial surface
Anterior intermuscular septum of leg
Extensor digitorum longus
Tibialis anterior, tendon
Extensor hallucis longus
Inferior extensor retinaculum
Lateral malleolus
Medial malleolus
Fibularis tertius [peroneus tertius], tendon
Extensor digitorum longus, tendons
Extensor hallucis longus, tendon
Extensor digitorum brevis
Extensor hallucis brevis

Fig. 1289 Muscles of right leg and foot; fasciae removed; anterior aspect.

Biceps femoris
Quadriceps femoris, vastus lateralis
Iliotibial tract
Patella
Fibula, head
Patellar ligament
Tibial tuberosity
Gastrocnemius
Fibularis longus [peroneus longus]
Tibialis anterior
Soleus
Anterior intermuscular septum of leg
Fibularis brevis [peroneus brevis]
Extensor digitorum longus
Calcaneal tendon
Tibialis anterior, tendon
Lateral malleolus
Extensor hallucis longus
Inferior extensor retinaculum
Superior fibular retinaculum [superior peroneal retinaculum]
Fibularis longus [peroneus longus], tendon
Extensor digitorum longus, tendons
Inferior fibular retinaculum [inferior peroneal retinaculum]
Extensor hallucis brevis
Calcaneal tuberosity
Fibularis brevis [peroneus brevis], tendon
Fibularis tertius [peroneus tertius], tendon
Extensor digitorum brevis

Fig. 1290 Muscles of right leg and foot; fasciae removed; lateral aspect.

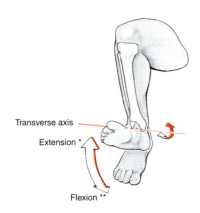

Fig. 1291   Ankle joint; movement in the sagittal plane.

Flexion and extension are the main movements of the ankle joint.

To avoid misunderstanding, flexion** is also known as plantar flexion and extension* is also known as dorsiflexion.

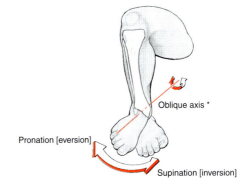

Fig. 1292   Ankle joint; rotation movements.
Starting from maximal plantar flexion, pronation is also known as lateral abduction and supination is also known as medial abduction.

* This axis courses from the medial side of the neck of talus posteriorly beneath the lateral process of the calcaneal tuberosity. It is slightly more exaggerated than shown in this figure for didactic reasons (see Fig. 1310).

Ventral muscles of leg (Figs. 1289, 1300, 1308, 1310)

Most superficially and medially, tibialis anterior bulges the fascia of leg. Medially follows extensor digitorum longus, which laterally frequently ends in fibularis [peroneus] tertius. The deepest muscle is the extensor hallucis longus.

Muscle *Innervation*	Origin	Insertion	Function
1. Tibialis anterior *Deep fibular [peroneal] nerve (sciatic nerve)*	Proximal extremity of tibia (beneath lateral condyle), lateral surface of tibia [upper 2/3], interosseous membrane of leg, fascia of leg	Base of 1st metatarsal (medial border), medial cuneiform (plantar surface)	**Ankle joint:** Dorsiflexion **Talotarsal joint:** Supination
2. Extensor hallucis longus *Deep fibular [peroneal] nerve (sciatic nerve)*	Medial surface of fibula (distal 2/3), interosseous membrane of leg, fascia of leg	Base of distal phalanx of great toe, proximal phalanx	**Ankle joint:** Dorsiflexion **Talotarsal joint:** Supination **Joints of great toe:** Extension
3. Extensor digitorum longus *Deep fibular [peroneal] nerve (sciatic nerve)*	Proximal extremity of tibia (beneath lateral condyle), anterior border of fibula, interosseous membrane of leg, anterior intermuscular septum of leg, fascia of leg	Extensor expansion of 2nd–5th toes	**Ankle joint:** Dorsiflexion **Talotarsal joint:** Pronation **Joints of toes:** Extension
4. Fibularis [peroneus] longus *Deep fibular [peroneal] nerve (sciatic nerve) (variable)*	Limb of extensor digitorum longus	Base of 5th metatarsal	

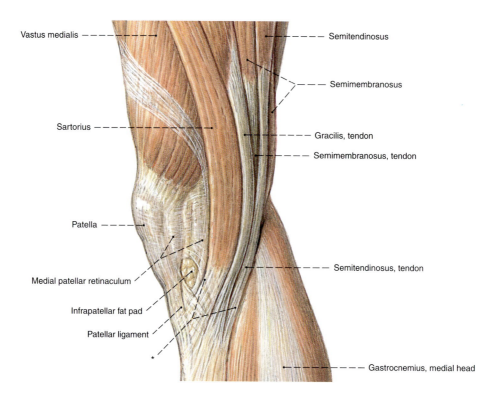

Fig. 1293   Muscles in the region of the right knee joint; fasciae removed; medial aspect.

*   Common insertion of sartorius, gracilis, and semitendinosus beneath the medial condyle of tibia (formerly superficial pes anserinus).

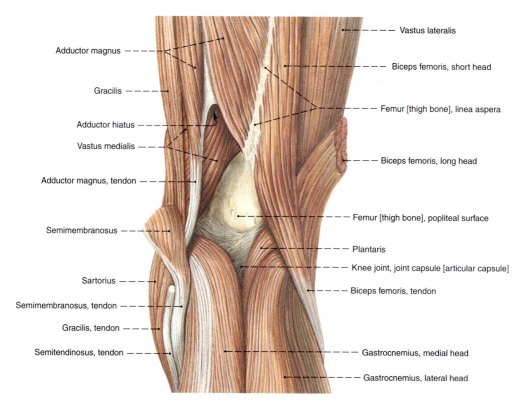

Fig. 1294   Muscles in the region of the right knee joint; fasciae and ischiocrural muscles [hamstrings] extensively removed; posterior aspect.

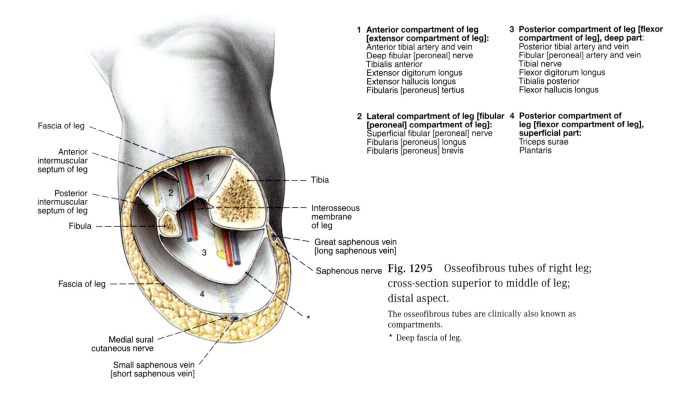

1 **Anterior compartment of leg [extensor compartment of leg]:**
Anterior tibial artery and vein
Deep fibular [peroneal] nerve
Tibialis anterior
Extensor digitorum longus
Extensor hallucis longus
Fibularis [peroneus] tertius

2 **Lateral compartment of leg [fibular [peroneal] compartment of leg]:**
Superficial fibular [peroneal] nerve
Fibularis [peroneus] longus
Fibularis [peroneus] brevis

3 **Posterior compartment of leg [flexor compartment of leg], deep part:**
Posterior tibial artery and vein
Fibular [peroneal] artery and vein
Tibial nerve
Flexor digitorum longus
Tibialis posterior
Flexor hallucis longus

4 **Posterior compartment of leg [flexor compartment of leg], superficial part:**
Triceps surae
Plantaris

Labels on figure: Fascia of leg · Anterior intermuscular septum of leg · Posterior intermuscular septum of leg · Fibula · Fascia of leg · Medial sural cutaneous nerve · Small saphenous vein [short saphenous vein] · Tibia · Interosseous membrane of leg · Great saphenous vein [long saphenous vein] · Saphenous nerve

Fig. 1295 Osseofibrous tubes of right leg; cross-section superior to middle of leg; distal aspect.

The osseofibrous tubes are clinically also known as compartments.

* Deep fascia of leg.

The strong fascia of leg and the equally strong intermuscular septa of leg together with the interosseous membrane and the bones of leg form osseofibrous tubes that are also known as compartments. Anterior, lateral, superficial posterior, and deep posterior compartments can be differentiated. In addition to a girding function to decrease flexion forces on the bones of leg,

they increase pressure during muscle action. When the venous valves are intact they essentially support venous drainage. When physiologic pressure equilibrium is disturbed, e.g. due to effusion of blood, compression of nerves and blood vessels within the osseofibrous tube may cause the so-called compartment syndrome.

Lateral muscles of leg (Fig.1290)

Lateral superficial lies the fibularis [peroneus] longus, beneath it the fibularis [peroneus] brevis.

Muscle *Innervation*	Origin	Insertion	Function*
1. **Fibularis [peroneus] longus** *Superficial fibular [peroneal] nerve (sciatic nerve)*	Head of fibula, lateral surface and posterior border of fibula (proximal 2/3), anterior and posterior intermuscular septa of leg, fascia of leg	Tuberosity of 1st metatarsal, intermediate [middle] cuneiform (plantar surface)	**Ankle joint:** Plantar flexion **Talotarsal joint:** Pronation
2. **Fibularis [peroneus] brevis** *Superficial fibular [peroneal] nerve (sciatic nerve)*	Lateral surface and anterior border of fibula (distal 1/2), anterior and posterior intermuscular septa of leg	Tuberosity of 5th metatarsal, tendinous slip to little toe	**Ankle joint:** Plantar flexion **Talotarsal joint:** Pronation

*Plantar flexion is also known as flexion, dorsiflexion is also known as extension.

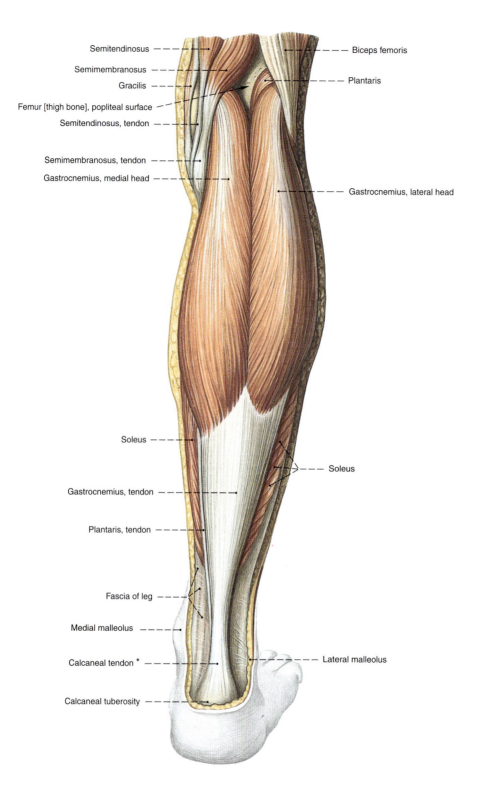

Semitendinosus

Semimembranosus

Gracilis

Femur [thigh bone], popliteal surface

Semitendinosus, tendon

Semimembranosus, tendon

Gastrocnemius, medial head

Biceps femoris

Plantaris

Gastrocnemius, lateral head

Soleus

Gastrocnemius, tendon

Plantaris, tendon

Soleus

Fascia of leg

Medial malleolus

Calcaneal tendon *

Calcaneal tuberosity

Lateral malleolus

Fig. 1296   Muscles of right leg;
fascia of leg removed;
posterior aspect.

* Also: ACHILLES tendon.

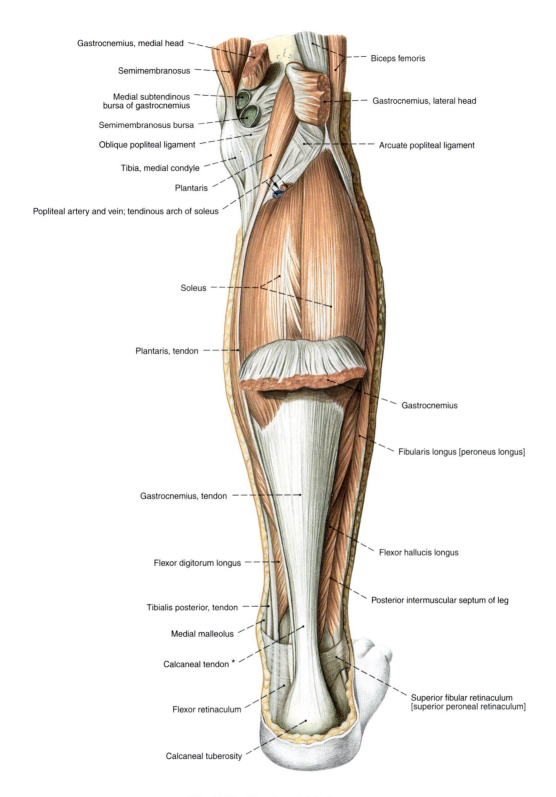

Gastrocnemius, medial head

Semimembranosus

Medial subtendinous bursa of gastrocnemius

Semimembranosus bursa

Oblique popliteal ligament

Tibia, medial condyle

Plantaris

Popliteal artery and vein; tendinous arch of soleus

Soleus

Plantaris, tendon

Gastrocnemius, tendon

Flexor digitorum longus

Tibialis posterior, tendon

Medial malleolus

Calcaneal tendon *

Flexor retinaculum

Calcaneal tuberosity

Biceps femoris

Gastrocnemius, lateral head

Arcuate popliteal ligament

Gastrocnemius

Fibularis longus [peroneus longus]

Flexor hallucis longus

Posterior intermuscular septum of leg

Superior fibular retinaculum [superior peroneal retinaculum]

Fig. 1297   Muscles of right leg; gastrocnemius partially removed; posterior aspect.

* Also: ACHILLES tendon.

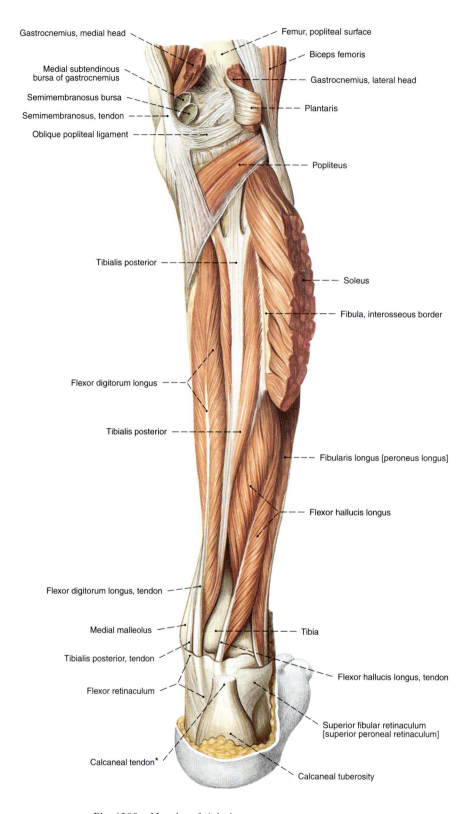

Gastrocnemius, medial head

Medial subtendinous bursa of gastrocnemius

Semimembranosus bursa

Semimembranosus, tendon

Oblique popliteal ligament

Tibialis posterior

Flexor digitorum longus

Tibialis posterior

Flexor digitorum longus, tendon

Medial malleolus

Tibialis posterior, tendon

Flexor retinaculum

Calcaneal tendon*

Femur, popliteal surface

Biceps femoris

Gastrocnemius, lateral head

Plantaris

Popliteus

Soleus

Fibula, interosseous border

Fibularis longus [peroneus longus]

Flexor hallucis longus

Tibia

Flexor hallucis longus, tendon

Superior fibular retinaculum [superior peroneal retinaculum]

Calcaneal tuberosity

Fig. 1298   Muscles of right leg; superficial muscles extensively removed; posterior aspect.

* Also: ACHILLES tendon.

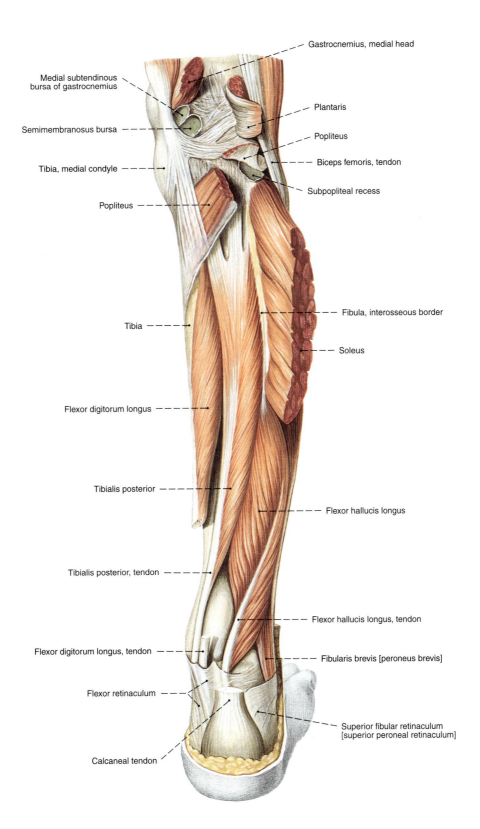

Gastrocnemius, medial head

Medial subtendinous bursa of gastrocnemius

Plantaris

Semimembranosus bursa

Popliteus

Tibia, medial condyle

Biceps femoris, tendon

Subpopliteal recess

Popliteus

Fibula, interosseous border

Tibia

Soleus

Flexor digitorum longus

Tibialis posterior

Flexor hallucis longus

Tibialis posterior, tendon

Flexor hallucis longus, tendon

Flexor digitorum longus, tendon

Fibularis brevis [peroneus brevis]

Flexor retinaculum

Superior fibular retinaculum [superior peroneal retinaculum]

Calcaneal tendon

Fig. 1299   Muscles of right leg; superficial muscles extensively removed; popliteus sectioned and tendon of flexor digitorum longus removed at crossing with tendon of tibialis posterior (crural chiasm); posterior aspect.

Superficial dorsal muscles of leg (Figs. 1296, 1297, 1301)

The surface relief of the calf is formed by the two heads of gastrocnemius. It overlies the soleus and together with the soleus forms the triceps surae. The tiny plantaris may be considered a fourth head of this muscle

Muscle *Innervation*	Origin	Insertion	Function
1. **Triceps surae** *Tibial nerve (sciatic nerve)*	**Gastrocnemius, medial head:** popliteal surface of femur (proximal of medial condyle) **Gastrocnemius, lateral head:** popliteal surface of femur (proximal of lateral condyle) **Soleus:** head of fibula, posterior surface and posterior border of fibula (proximal 1/3), posterior surface of tibia (from and beneath soleal line), tendinous arch of soleus **Plantaris:** popliteal surface of femur (proximal of lateral condyle)	Calcaneal tuberosity via calcaneal tenodn [ACHILLES tendon]	**Knee joint** (gastrocnemius and plantaris only): Flexion **Ankle joint:** Plantar flexion **Talotarsal joint:** Supination

* Plantar flexion is also known as flexion; dorsiflexion is also known as extension.

Deep dorsal muscles of leg (Figs. 1298, 1301, 1313, 1314, 1318)

Most proximal the popliteus courses obliquely to the lateral region of the knee joint. Of the muscles in the foot the tibialis posterior is the most superficial. Beneath it are medial the flexor digitorum longus and lateral the flexor hallucis longus.

Muscle *Innervation*	Origin	Insertion	Function
1. **Popliteus** *Tibial nerve (sciatic nerve)*	Lateral epicondyle of femur	Posterior surface of tibia above soleal line	**Knee joint:** Medial rotation, flexion
2. **Tibialis posterior** *Tibial nerve (sciatic nerve)*	Interosseous membrane of leg, posterior surfaces of tibia and fibula (proximal 1/2 adjacent to interosseous membrane)	Tuberosity of navicular, lateral, intermediate [middle], and medial cuneiform (plantar surfaces), bases of 2nd–4th metatarsals	**Ankle joint:** Plantar flexion **Talotarsal joint:** Supination
3. **Flexor digitorum longus** *Tibial nerve (sciatic nerve)*	Posterior surface of tibia (beneath soleal line), tendinous arch between tibia and fibula (above crural chiasm)	Distal phalanges 2nd–5th metatarsals	**Ankle joint:** Plantar flexion **Talotarsal joint:** Supination **Joints of toes:** Flexion
4. **Flexor hallucis longus** *Tibial nerve (sciatic nerve)*	Posterior surface of fibula (distal 2/3), interosseous membrane of leg, posterior intermuscular septum of leg	Distal phalanx of great toe	**Ankle joint:** Plantar flexion **Talotarsal joint:** Supination **Joints of great toe:** Flexion

*Plantar flexion is also known as flexion; dorsiflexion is also known as extension.

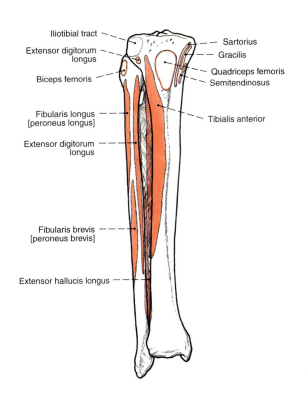

Iliotibial tract
Extensor digitorum longus
Biceps femoris
Fibularis longus [peroneus longus]
Extensor digitorum longus
Fibularis brevis [peroneus brevis]
Extensor hallucis longus

Sartorius
Gracilis
Quadriceps femoris
Semitendinosus
Tibialis anterior

Fig. 1300   Muscle origins and insertions on the bones of right leg; anterior aspect.

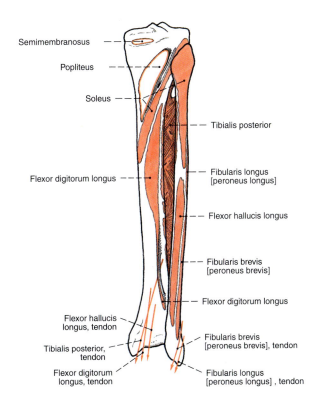

Semimembranosus
Popliteus
Soleus
Flexor digitorum longus

Flexor hallucis longus, tendon
Tibialis posterior, tendon
Flexor digitorum longus, tendon

Tibialis posterior
Fibularis longus [peroneus longus]
Flexor hallucis longus
Fibularis brevis [peroneus brevis]
Flexor digitorum longus
Fibularis brevis [peroneus brevis], tendon
Fibularis longus [peroneus longus] , tendon

Fig. 1301   Muscle origins and insertions on the bones of right leg; posterior aspect.

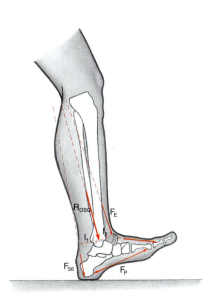

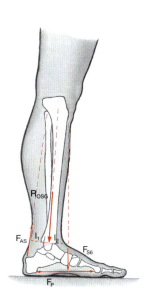

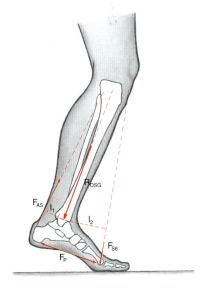

F_{S6} force of body weight (6/6)
R_{OSG} resulting force in ankle joint
[REMARK: OSG *may* be changed to AJ for ankle joint both in figures and legend]

F_{AS} tractive force of Achilles tendon
[REMARK: AS *may* be changed to AT for Achilles tendon both in figures and legend]
F_E tractive force of extensor muscles

F_P tractive force effective on plantar aponeurosis
l_1 lever arm
l_2 lever arm

Fig. 1302   Forces in the foot during heel-strikeposition (standing on calcaneal tuberosity).

Fig. 1303   Forces in the foot during support phase (static load on sole).

Fig. 1304   Forces in the foot during toe-off position (standing on balls of toes).

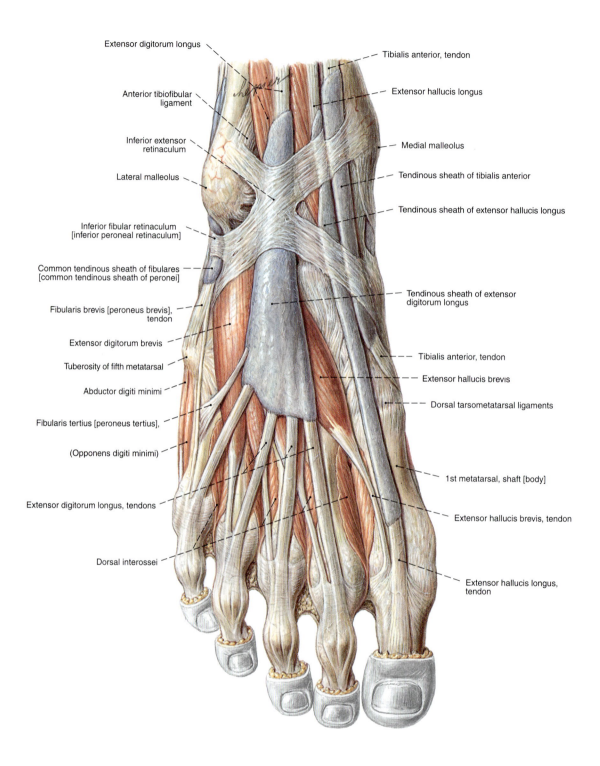

Extensor digitorum longus

Anterior tibiofibular ligament

Inferior extensor retinaculum

Lateral malleolus

Inferior fibular retinaculum [inferior peroneal retinaculum]

Common tendinous sheath of fibulares [common tendinous sheath of peronei]

Fibularis brevis [peroneus brevis], tendon

Extensor digitorum brevis

Tuberosity of fifth metatarsal

Abductor digiti minimi

Fibularis tertius [peroneus tertius]

(Opponens digiti minimi)

Extensor digitorum longus, tendons

Dorsal interossei

Tibialis anterior, tendon

Extensor hallucis longus

Medial malleolus

Tendinous sheath of tibialis anterior

Tendinous sheath of extensor hallucis longus

Tendinous sheath of extensor digitorum longus

Tibialis anterior, tendon

Extensor hallucis brevis

Dorsal tarsometatarsal ligaments

1st metatarsal, shaft [body]

Extensor hallucis brevis, tendon

Extensor hallucis longus, tendon

Fig. 1305   Tendinous sheaths of right foot; anterior aspect.

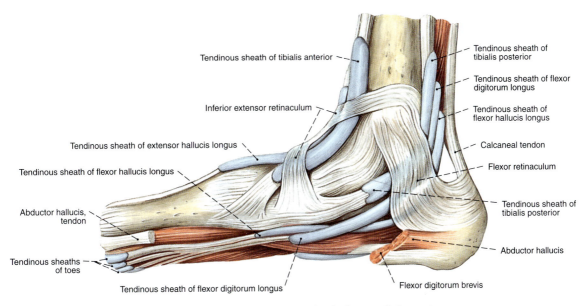

Tendinous sheath of tibialis anterior

Inferior extensor retinaculum

Tendinous sheath of extensor hallucis longus

Tendinous sheath of flexor hallucis longus

Abductor hallucis, tendon

Tendinous sheaths of toes

Tendinous sheath of flexor digitorum longus

Tendinous sheath of tibialis posterior

Tendinous sheath of flexor digitorum longus

Tendinous sheath of flexor hallucis longus

Calcaneal tendon

Flexor retinaculum

Tendinous sheath of tibialis posterior

Abductor hallucis

Flexor digitorum brevis

Fig. 1306   Tendinous sheaths of right foot; medial aspect.

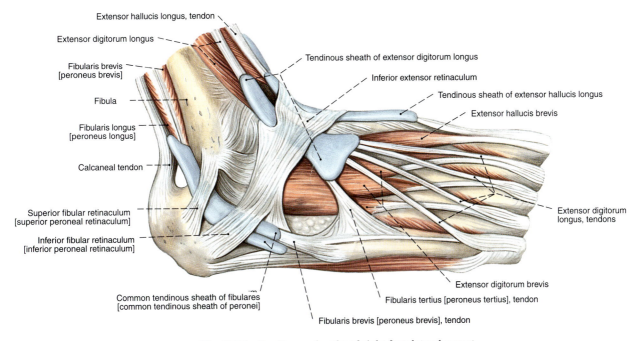

Extensor hallucis longus, tendon

Extensor digitorum longus

Fibularis brevis [peroneus brevis]

Fibula

Fibularis longus [peroneus longus]

Calcaneal tendon

Superior fibular retinaculum [superior peroneal retinaculum]

Inferior fibular retinaculum [inferior peroneal retinaculum]

Common tendinous sheath of fibulares [common tendinous sheath of peronei]

Fibularis brevis [peroneus brevis], tendon

Fibularis tertius [peroneus tertius], tendon

Extensor digitorum brevis

Tendinous sheath of extensor digitorum longus

Inferior extensor retinaculum

Tendinous sheath of extensor hallucis longus

Extensor hallucis brevis

Extensor digitorum longus, tendons

Fig. 1307   Tendinous sheaths of right foot; lateral aspect.

Tendinous sheaths of foot

Anterior tarsal tendinous sheaths: On the dorsum of foot beneath the superior and inferior extensor retinacula for tendons of tibialis anterior, extensor hallucis longus, and extensor digitorum longus.

Tibial tarsal tendinous sheaths: Behind the medial malleolus beneath the flexor retinaculum for tendons of tibialis posterior, flexor digitorum longus, and flexor hallucis longus.

Fibular tarsal tendinous sheaths: Behind the lateral malleolus beneath the superior and inferior fibular [peroneal] retinacula usually a common tendinous sheath for tendons of fibulares [peronei] longus and brevis. The tendinous sheath of fibularis [peroneus] longus extends further distally under the long plantar ligament to the insertion at the plantar surface of the base of the 1st metatarsal and the medial cuneiform.

Tendinous sheaths of toes: On the plantar side of toes for flexor digitorum longus and flexor digitorum brevis.

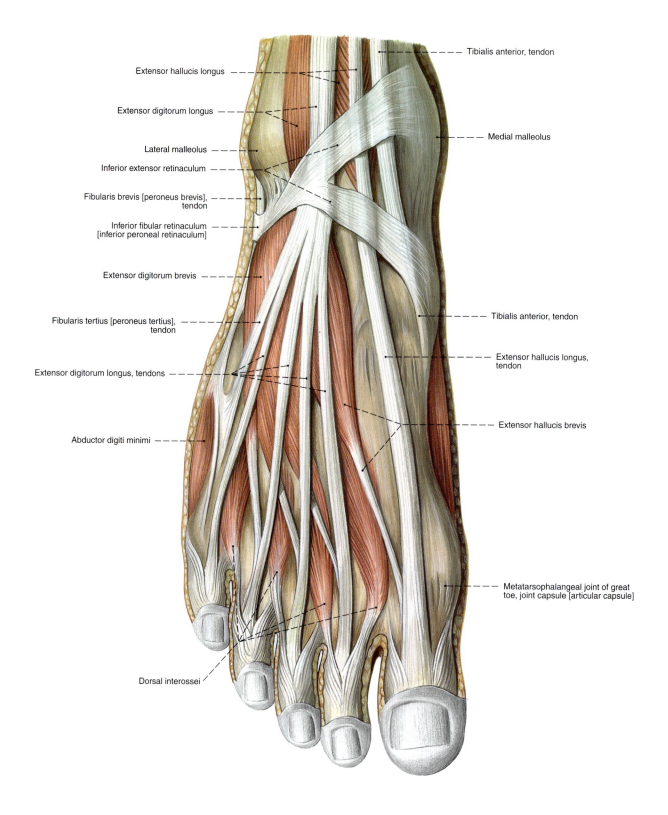

Extensor hallucis longus

Extensor digitorum longus

Lateral malleolus

Inferior extensor retinaculum

Fibularis brevis [peroneus brevis], tendon

Inferior fibular retinaculum [inferior peroneal retinaculum]

Extensor digitorum brevis

Fibularis tertius [peroneus tertius], tendon

Extensor digitorum longus, tendons

Abductor digiti minimi

Dorsal interossei

Tibialis anterior, tendon

Medial malleolus

Tibialis anterior, tendon

Extensor hallucis longus, tendon

Extensor hallucis brevis

Metatarsophalangeal joint of great toe, joint capsule [articular capsule]

Fig. 1308 Muscles of right foot; tendinous sheath removed; anterior aspect.

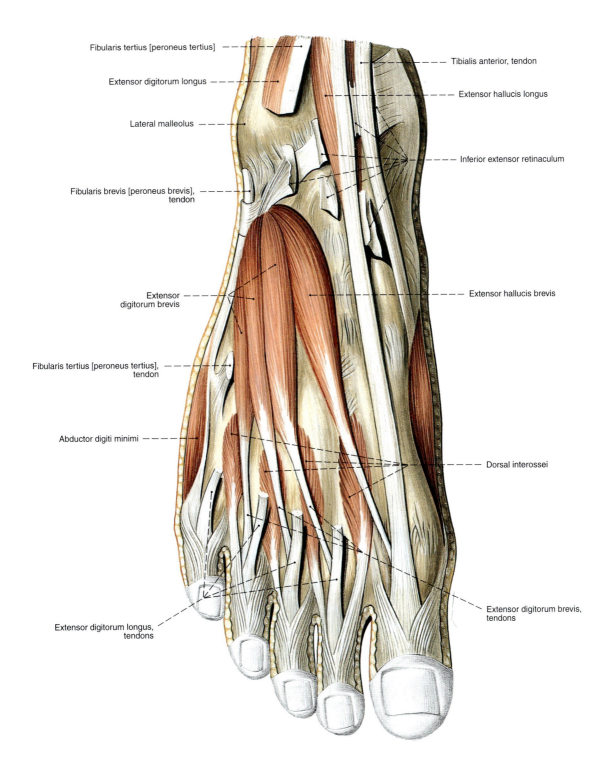

Fibularis tertius [peroneus tertius]

Extensor digitorum longus

Lateral malleolus

Fibularis brevis [peroneus brevis], tendon

Extensor digitorum brevis

Fibularis tertius [peroneus tertius], tendon

Abductor digiti minimi

Extensor digitorum longus, tendons

Tibialis anterior, tendon

Extensor hallucis longus

Inferior extensor retinaculum

Extensor hallucis brevis

Dorsal interossei

Extensor digitorum brevis, tendons

Fig. 1309   Muscles of right foot; inferior extensor retinaculum split and extensor digitorum longus extensively removed; anterior aspect.

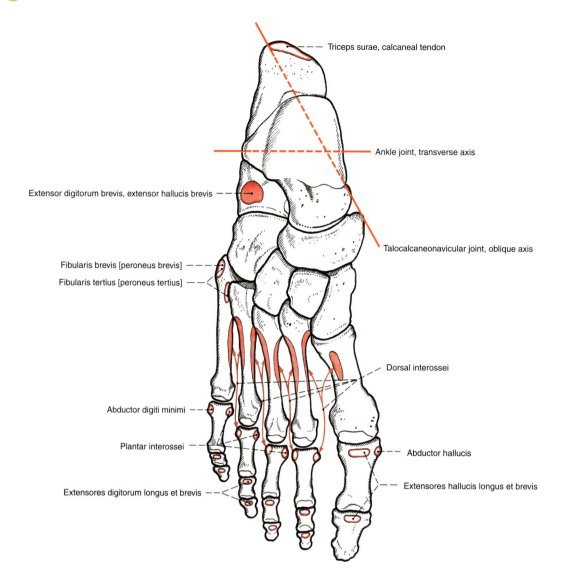

Triceps surae, calcaneal tendon

Ankle joint, transverse axis

Extensor digitorum brevis, extensor hallucis brevis

Talocalcaneonavicular joint, oblique axis

Fibularis brevis [peroneus brevis]

Fibularis tertius [peroneus tertius]

Dorsal interossei

Abductor digiti minimi

Plantar interossei

Abductor hallucis

Extensores digitorum longus et brevis

Extensores hallucis longus et brevis

Fig. 1310　Muscle origins and insertions on bones of right foot; dorsal aspect.
The axes of the ankle joint and the talotarsal joints are indicated.

Muscles of dorsum of foot (Fig. 1308)

Both muscles of the dorsum of foot protrude only little through the skin. From a small area of origin the extensor hallucis brevis courses to the great toe and the extensor digitorum brevis to the other toes.

Muscle *Innervation*	Origin	Insertion	Function
1. **Extensor digitorum brevis** *Deep fibular [peroneal] nerve (Common fibular [peroneal] nerve)*	Calcaneus (dorsal and lateral surface)	Extensor expansion of 2nd–4th toes	**Joints of toes:** Extension
2. **Extensor hallucis brevis** *Deep fibular [peroneal nerve (Common fibular [peroneal] nerve)*	Calcaneus (dorsal and lateral surface)	Proximal phalanx of great toe	**Joints of great toe:** Extension

* Plantar flexion is also known as flexion, dorsiflexion is also known as extension.

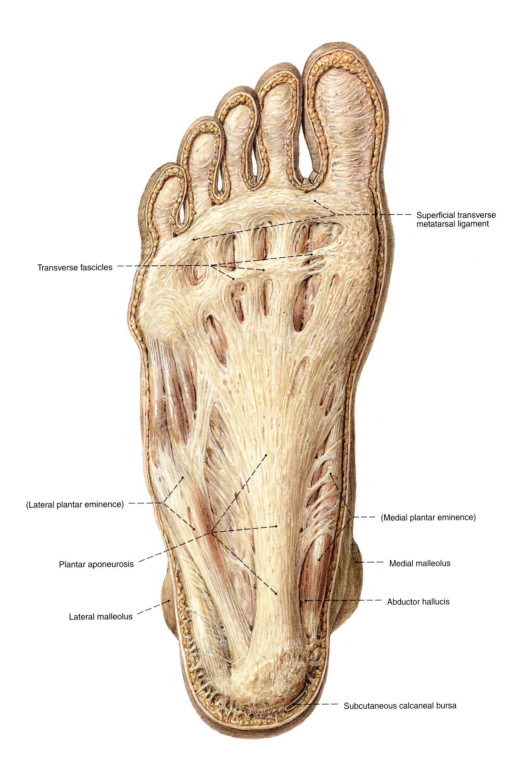

Superficial transverse metatarsal ligament

Transverse fascicles

(Lateral plantar eminence)

Plantar aponeurosis

Lateral malleolus

(Medial plantar eminence)

Medial malleolus

Abductor hallucis

Subcutaneous calcaneal bursa

Fig. 1311 Muscles of right foot; demonstration of plantar aponeurosis; plantar aspect.

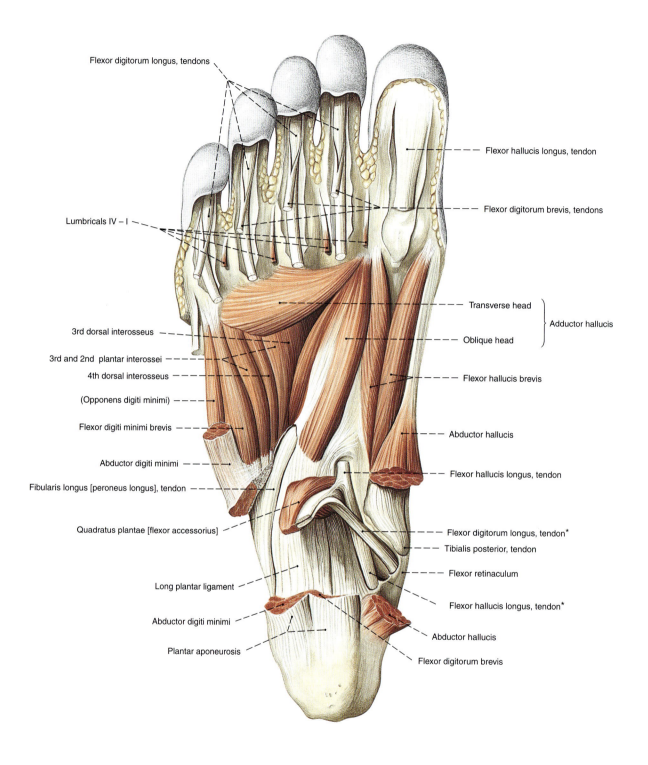

Flexor digitorum longus, tendons

Flexor hallucis longus, tendon

Flexor digitorum brevis, tendons

Lumbricals IV – I

Transverse head

Oblique head

Adductor hallucis

3rd dorsal interosseus

3rd and 2nd plantar interossei

4th dorsal interosseus

Flexor hallucis brevis

(Opponens digiti minimi)

Flexor digiti minimi brevis

Abductor hallucis

Abductor digiti minimi

Flexor hallucis longus, tendon

Fibularis longus [peroneus longus], tendon

Quadratus plantae [flexor accessorius]

Flexor digitorum longus, tendon*

Tibialis posterior, tendon

Flexor retinaculum

Long plantar ligament

Flexor hallucis longus, tendon*

Abductor digiti minimi

Abductor hallucis

Plantar aponeurosis

Flexor digitorum brevis

Fig. 1314   Muscles of right foot; deep layer; superficial muscles, flexor digitorum and hallucis longus extensively removed; plantar aspect.

* The crossing over of the tendons of flexor digitorum longus and flexor hallucis longus is also known as plantar chiasm.

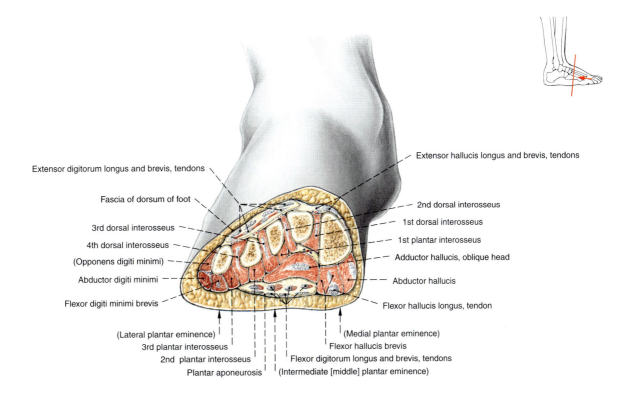

Extensor digitorum longus and brevis, tendons
Fascia of dorsum of foot
3rd dorsal interosseus
4th dorsal interosseus
(Opponens digiti minimi)
Abductor digiti minimi
Flexor digiti minimi brevis

Extensor hallucis longus and brevis, tendons
2nd dorsal interosseus
1st dorsal interosseus
1st plantar interosseus
Adductor hallucis, oblique head
Abductor hallucis
Flexor hallucis longus, tendon

(Lateral plantar eminence)
3rd plantar interosseus
2nd plantar interosseus
Plantar aponeurosis
(Medial plantar eminence)
Flexor hallucis brevis
Flexor digitorum longus and brevis, tendons
(Intermediate [middle] plantar eminence)

Fig. 1315 Osseofibrous tubes of right foot; frontal section through metatarsus; distal aspect.

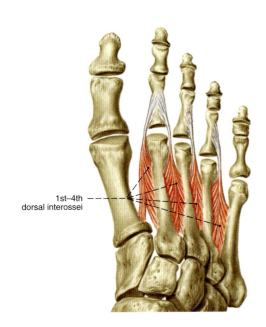

1st–4th
dorsal interossei

Fig. 1316 Muscles of right foot; dorsal interossei; dorsal aspect.

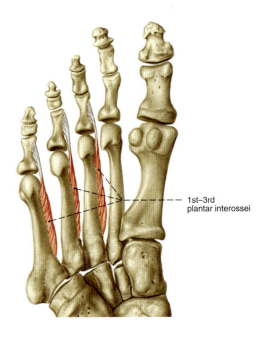

1st–3rd
plantar interossei

Fig. 1317 Muscles of right foot; plantar interossei; plantar aspect.

Medial plantar muscles (Figs. 1312, 1318)

The medial border of the foot, the medial plantar eminence, is formed mainly by the abductor hallucis. Neighboring are the flexor hallucis brevis and the adductor hallucis laterally.

Muscle *Innervation*	Origin	Insertion	Function*
1. Abductor hallucis *Medial plantar nerve (tibial nerve)*	Medial process of calcaneal tuberosity, plantar aponeurosis, flexor retinaculum	Medial sesamoid bone of capsule of metatarsophalangeal joint of great toe, base of proximal phalanx of great toe (medial edge)	**Metatarsophalangeal joint of great toe :** Abduction, flexion
2. Flexor hallucis brevis *Medial part: medial plantar nerve (tibial nerve)* *Lateral part: lateral plantar nerve (tibial nerve)*	Cuneiform bones (plantar surface), plantar calcaneocuboid ligament [short plantar ligament], tendon of tibialis posterior	**Medial part:** medial sesamoid bone of capsule of metatarsophalangeal joint of great toe, base of proximal phalanx of great toe **Lateral part:** lateral sesamoid bone of capsule of metatarsophalangeal joint of great toe, base of proximal phalanx of great toe	**Metatarsophalangeal joint of great toe :** Flexion
3. Adductor hallucis *Medial plantar nerve (tibial nerve)*	**Oblique head:** cuboid, lateral cuneiform, long plantar ligament, plantar calcaneocuboid ligament [short plantar ligament] **Transverse head:** joint capsules of metatarsophalangeal joints of 3rd–5th toes; deep transverse metatarsal ligament	Lateral sesamoid bone of capsule of metatarsophalangeal joint of great toe, base of proximal phalanx of great toe	**Metatarsophalangeal joint of great toe :** Adduction toward 2nd toe, flexion

* Explanation see page 347.

Middle plantar muscles (Figs. 1312, 1318)

Small muscles are located in the depth of the longitudinal arch of foot. The flexor digitorum brevis is attached to the plantar aponeurosis proximally. Beneath this muscle the quadratus plantae [flexor accessorius] blends with the main tendon of the flexor digitorum longus. The four lumbricals originate from its four tendons. The three plantar and the four dorsal interossei fill the space between the metatarsals.

Muscle/*Innervation*	Origin	Insertion	Function*
1. Flexor digitorum brevis *Medial plantar nerve (tibial nerve)*	Calcaneal tuberosity (plantar surface), plantar aponeurosis	Middle phalanges of 2nd–4th toes (penetrated by tendons of flexor digitorum longus)	**Metatarsophalangeal joints of toes:** Flexion **Interphalangeal joints of toes:** Flexion
2. Quadratus plantae [flexor accessorius] *Lateral plantar nerve (tibial nerve)*	Calcaneal tuberosity (plantar surface), long plantar ligament	Tendon of flexor digitorum longus (lateral border before its division)	Changes direction of flexor digitorum longus
3. 1st–4th lumbricals *Medial(1st) and lateral (2nd–4th) plantar nerve (tibial nerve)*	**1st lumbrical:** tendon of flexor digitorum longus of 2nd toe (medial side) **2nd–4th lumbricals:** tendons of flexor digitorum longus of 3rd–5th toes (adjacent sides)	Proximal phalanges of 2nd–5th toes (medial side), occasionally into the extensor expansion [extensor hood]	**Metatarsophalangeal joints of toes:** Flexion
4. 1st–3rd plantar interossei *Lateral plantar nerve (tibial nerve)*	3rd–5th metatarsals (plantar surface), long plantar ligament	Bases of proximal phalanges of 3rd–5th toes (medial sides)	**Metatarsophalangeal joints of toes:**
5. 1st–4th plantar interossei *Lateral plantar nerve (tibial nerve)*	Adjacent sides of 1st–5th metatarsal (by two heads), long plantar ligament	**1st dorsal interosseus:** Base of proximal phalanx of 2nd toe (medial side) **2nd–4th dorsal interossei:** Bases of proximal phalanges of 3rd and 4th toes (lateral side), blend with the extensor expansions [extensor hoods]	**Metatarsophalangeal joints of toes:** Flexion, lateral abduction (3rd and 4th toes), medial abduction (2nd toe) **Interphalangeal joints of toes:** Extension

* Explanation see page 347.

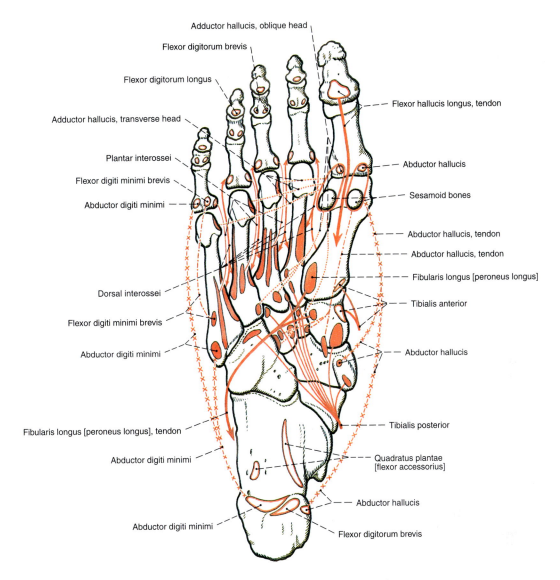

Fig. 1318 Muscle origins and insertions on the bones of right foot; plantar aspect.

Lateral plantar muscles (Fig. 1312)

The lateral border of the foot, the lateral plantar eminence, is formed mainly by the abductor digiti minimi. Beneath are the flexor digiti minimi brevis and opponens digiti minimi.

Muscle/*Innervation*	Origin	Insertion	Function
1. Abductor digiti minimi *Lateral plantar nerve* *(tibial nerve)*	Lateral and medial process (deep head) of calcaneal tuberosity, plantar aponeurosis	Base of proximal phalanx of 5th toe, tuberosity of 5th metatarsal	**Metatarsophalangeal joint of 5th toe :** Abduction, flexion, opposition
2. Flexor digiti minimi brevis *Lateral plantar nerve* *(tibial nerve)*	Base of 5th metatarsal, long plantar ligament, plantar tendinous sheath of fibularis [peroneus] longus	Proximal phalanx of 5th toe	**Metatarsophalangeal joint of 5th toe :** Abduction, flexion, opposition
3. Opponens digiti minimi *Lateral plantar nerve* *(tibial nerve)* *(variable)*	Base of 5th metatarsal, long plantar ligament, plantar tendinous sheath of fibularis [peroneus] longus	5th metatarsal (lateral border)	**Metatarsophalangeal joint of 5th toe :** Abduction, flexion, opposition

* Plantar flexion is also known as flexion; dorsiflexion is also known as extension.

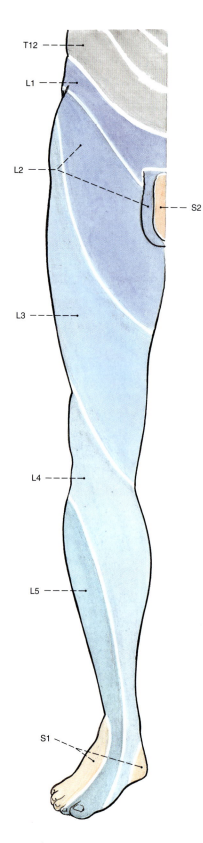

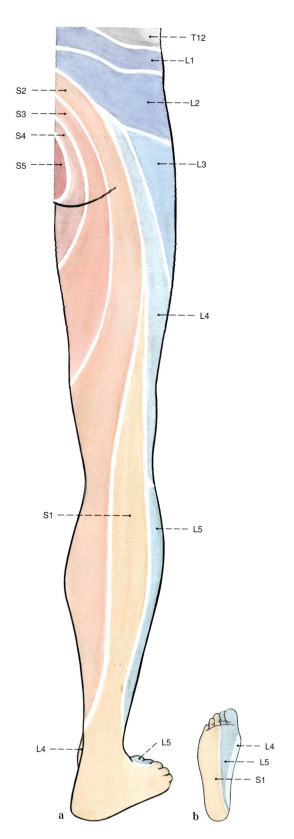

Fig. 1319   Segmental cutaneous innervation (dermatomes) of right lower limb; anterior aspect.

Fig. 1320 a, b   Segmental cutaneous innervation (dermatomes) of right lower limb.
a   Posterior aspect
b   Plantar aspect

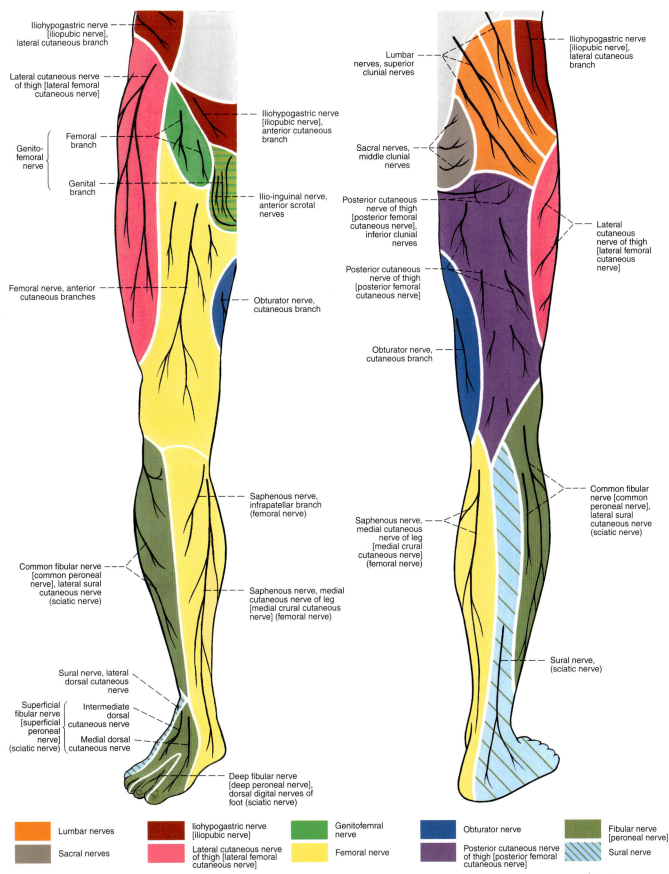

Iliohypogastric nerve [iliopubic nerve], lateral cutaneous branch

Lateral cutaneous nerve of thigh [lateral femoral cutaneous nerve]

Genito-femoral nerve — Femoral branch

Genital branch

Femoral nerve, anterior cutaneous branches

Iliohypogastric nerve [iliopubic nerve], anterior cutaneous branch

Ilio-inguinal nerve, anterior scrotal nerves

Obturator nerve, cutaneous branch

Saphenous nerve, infrapatellar branch (femoral nerve)

Common fibular nerve [common peroneal nerve], lateral sural cutaneous nerve (sciatic nerve)

Saphenous nerve, medial cutaneous nerve of leg [medial crural cutaneous nerve] (femoral nerve)

Sural nerve, lateral dorsal cutaneous nerve

Superficial fibular nerve [superficial peroneal nerve] (sciatic nerve) — Intermediate dorsal cutaneous nerve

Medial dorsal cutaneous nerve

Deep fibular nerve [deep peroneal nerve], dorsal digital nerves of foot (sciatic nerve)

Lumbar nerves, superior clunial nerves

Sacral nerves, middle clunial nerves

Posterior cutaneous nerve of thigh [posterior femoral cutaneous nerve], inferior clunial nerves

Posterior cutaneous nerve of thigh [posterior femoral cutaneous nerve]

Obturator nerve, cutaneous branch

Saphenous nerve, medial cutaneous nerve of leg [medial crural cutaneous nerve] (femoral nerve)

Iliohypogastric nerve [iliopubic nerve], lateral cutaneous branch

Lateral cutaneous nerve of thigh [lateral femoral cutaneous nerve]

Common fibular nerve [common peroneal nerve], lateral sural cutaneous nerve (sciatic nerve)

Sural nerve, (sciatic nerve)

Legend:
- Lumbar nerves
- Sacral nerves
- Iliohypogastric nerve [iliopubic nerve]
- Lateral cutaneous nerve of thigh [lateral femoral cutaneous nerve]
- Genitofemral nerve
- Femoral nerve
- Obturator nerve
- Posterior cutaneous nerve of thigh [posterior femoral cutaneous nerve]
- Fibular nerve [peroneal nerve]
- Sural nerve

Fig. 1321 Cutaneous nerves of right lower limb; anterior aspect.

Fig. 1322 Cutaneous nerves of right lower limb; posterior aspect.

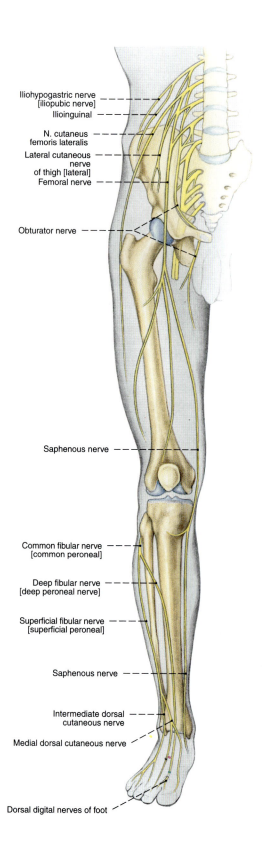

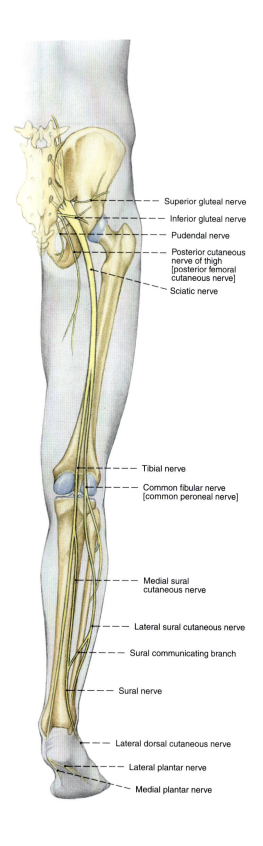

Iliohypogastric nerve [iliopubic nerve]

Ilioinguinal

N. cutaneus femoris lateralis

Lateral cutaneous nerve of thigh [lateral]

Femoral nerve

Obturator nerve

Saphenous nerve

Common fibular nerve [common peroneal]

Deep fibular nerve [deep peroneal nerve]

Superficial fibular nerve [superficial peroneal]

Saphenous nerve

Intermediate dorsal cutaneous nerve

Medial dorsal cutaneous nerve

Dorsal digital nerves of foot

Superior gluteal nerve

Inferior gluteal nerve

Pudendal nerve

Posterior cutaneous nerve of thigh [posterior femoral cutaneous nerve]

Sciatic nerve

Tibial nerve

Common fibular nerve [common peroneal nerve]

Medial sural cutaneous nerve

Lateral sural cutaneous nerve

Sural communicating branch

Sural nerve

Lateral dorsal cutaneous nerve

Lateral plantar nerve

Medial plantar nerve

Fig. 1323   Nerves of right lower limb; general survey; anterior aspect.

Fig. 1324   Nerves of right lower limb; general survey; posterior aspect.

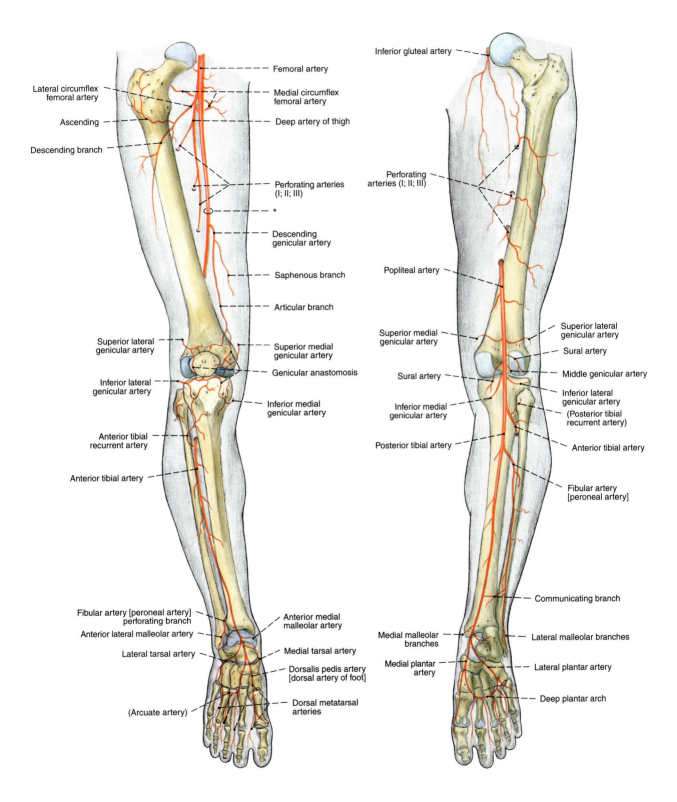

Femoral artery

Lateral circumflex femoral artery

Medial circumflex femoral artery

Ascending

Deep artery of thigh

Descending branch

Perforating arteries (I; II; III)

*

Descending genicular artery

Saphenous branch

Articular branch

Superior lateral genicular artery

Superior medial genicular artery

Genicular anastomosis

Inferior lateral genicular artery

Inferior medial genicular artery

Anterior tibial recurrent artery

Anterior tibial artery

Fibular artery [peroneal artery] perforating branch

Anterior medial malleolar artery

Anterior lateral malleolar artery

Lateral tarsal artery

Medial tarsal artery

Dorsalis pedis artery [dorsal artery of foot]

(Arcuate artery)

Dorsal metatarsal arteries

Inferior gluteal artery

Perforating arteries (I; II; III)

Popliteal artery

Superior medial genicular artery

Superior lateral genicular artery

Sural artery

Sural artery

Middle genicular artery

Inferior medial genicular artery

Inferior lateral genicular artery

(Posterior tibial recurrent artery)

Posterior tibial artery

Anterior tibial artery

Fibular artery [peroneal artery]

Communicating branch

Medial malleolar branches

Lateral malleolar branches

Medial plantar artery

Lateral plantar artery

Deep plantar arch

Fig. 1325 Arteries of right lower limb; general survey; anterior aspect.
The segment of the femoral artery between the origin of the deep artery of thigh and its entrance into the adductor canal (*) is clinically also known as superficial femoral artery.

Fig. 1326 Arteries of right lower limb; general survey; posterior aspect.

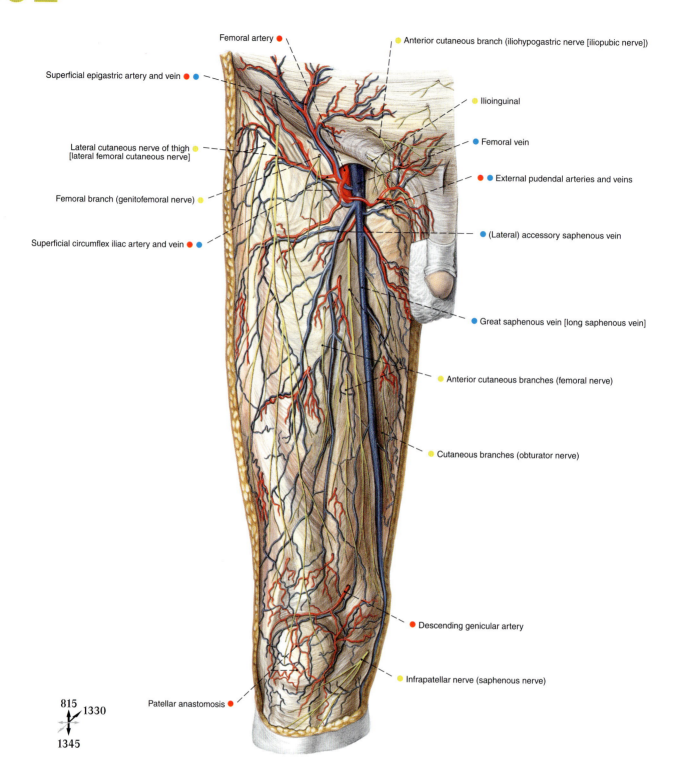

Femoral artery ●

Superficial epigastric artery and vein ● ●

Lateral cutaneous nerve of thigh ●
[lateral femoral cutaneous nerve]

Femoral branch (genitofemoral nerve) ●

Superficial circumflex iliac artery and vein ● ●

Anterior cutaneous branch (iliohypogastric nerve [iliopubic nerve]) ●

Ilioinguinal ●

Femoral vein ●

External pudendal arteries and veins ● ●

(Lateral) accessory saphenous vein ●

Great saphenous vein [long saphenous vein] ●

Anterior cutaneous branches (femoral nerve) ●

Cutaneous branches (obturator nerve) ●

Descending genicular artery ●

Infrapatellar nerve (saphenous nerve) ●

Patellar anastomosis ●

815
1330
1345

Fig. 1327   Epifascial blood vessels and nerves of right groin [inguinal region], anterior regions of thigh and knee; anterior aspect.

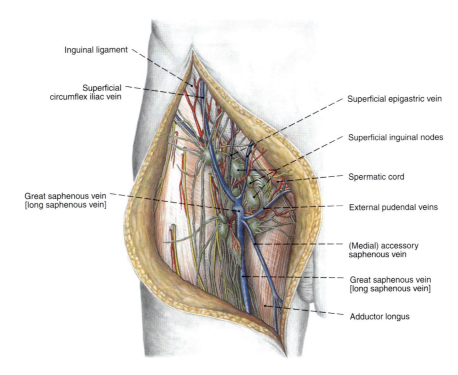

Inguinal ligament

Superficial circumflex iliac vein

Great saphenous vein [long saphenous vein]

Superficial epigastric vein

Superficial inguinal nodes

Spermatic cord

External pudendal veins

(Medial) accessory saphenous vein

Great saphenous vein [long saphenous vein]

Adductor longus

Fig. 1328 Superficial lymphatic vessels and venous trunks of right groin [inguinal region]; anterior aspect.

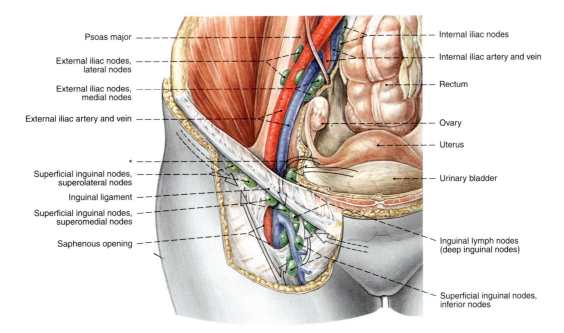

Psoas major

External iliac nodes, lateral nodes

External iliac nodes, medial nodes

External iliac artery and vein

*

Superficial inguinal nodes, superolateral nodes

Inguinal ligament

Superficial inguinal nodes, superomedial nodes

Saphenous opening

Internal iliac nodes

Internal iliac artery and vein

Rectum

Ovary

Uterus

Urinary bladder

Inguinal lymph nodes (deep inguinal nodes)

Superficial inguinal nodes, inferior nodes

Fig. 1329 Tributaries of right inguinal nodes in the female; general survey; anterior aspect.
Arrows indicate possible directions of lymphatic flow.

* The medial part of the uterine tube and the fundus of uterus lymph also may drain into the superficial inguinal nodes via the round ligament of uterus.

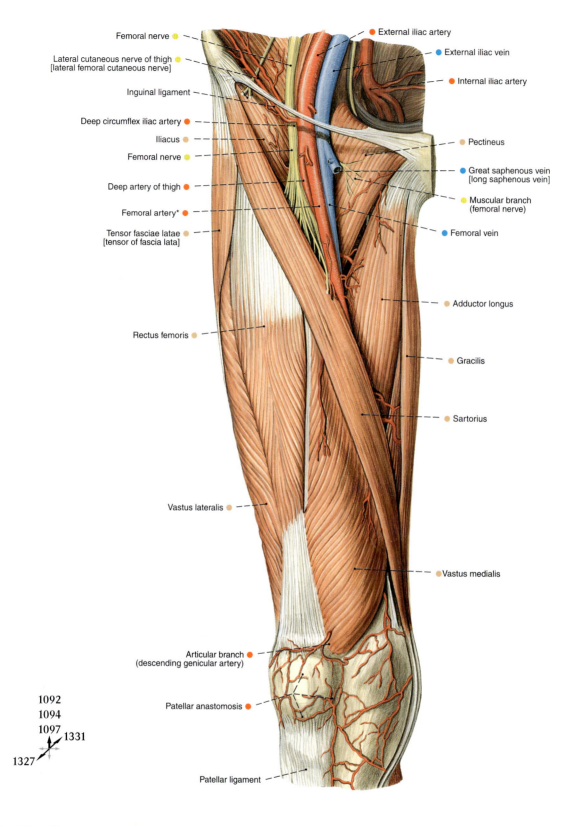

Femoral nerve ●

Lateral cutaneous nerve of thigh ●
[lateral femoral cutaneous nerve]

Inguinal ligament

Deep circumflex iliac artery ●

Iliacus ●

Femoral nerve ●

Deep artery of thigh ●

Femoral artery* ●

Tensor fasciae latae ●
[tensor of fascia lata]

Rectus femoris ●

Vastus lateralis ●

Articular branch ●
(descending genicular artery)

Patellar anastomosis ●

Patellar ligament

External iliac artery ●

External iliac vein ●

Internal iliac artery ●

Pectineus ●

Great saphenous vein ●
[long saphenous vein]

Muscular branch ●
(femoral nerve)

Femoral vein ●

Adductor longus ●

Gracilis ●

Sartorius ●

Vastus medialis ●

1092
1094
1097 1331
1327

Fig. 1330 Blood vessels and nerves of anterior region of right thigh; fascia lata, except iliotibial tract removed; anterior aspect.

*   Clinically, the femoral artery is frequently also known as superficial femoral artery, compared to the deep femoral artery (= deep artery of thigh).

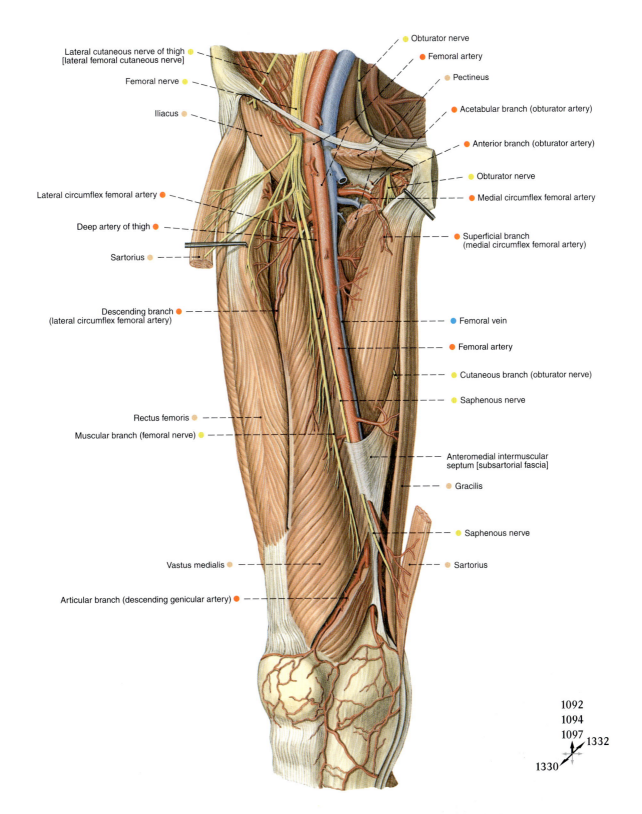

Lateral cutaneous nerve of thigh ●
[lateral femoral cutaneous nerve]

Femoral nerve ●

Iliacus ●

Lateral circumflex femoral artery ●

Deep artery of thigh ●

Sartorius ●

Descending branch ●
(lateral circumflex femoral artery)

Rectus femoris ●

Muscular branch (femoral nerve) ●

Vastus medialis ●

Articular branch (descending genicular artery) ●

● Obturator nerve

● Femoral artery

● Pectineus

● Acetabular branch (obturator artery)

● Anterior branch (obturator artery)

● Obturator nerve

● Medial circumflex femoral artery

● Superficial branch
(medial circumflex femoral artery)

● Femoral vein

● Femoral artery

● Cutaneous branch (obturator nerve)

● Saphenous nerve

Anteromedial intermuscular
septum [subsartorial fascia]

● Gracilis

● Saphenous nerve

● Sartorius

1092
1094
1097
       1332
1330

Fig. 1331 Blood vessels and nerves of anterior region of right thigh; sartorius partially removed and pectineus sectioned; anterior aspect.

* The entrance into the adductor canal is formed by the vastus medialis and the adductor longus, as well as by the anteromedial intermuscular septum [subsartorial fascia], which stretches between them.

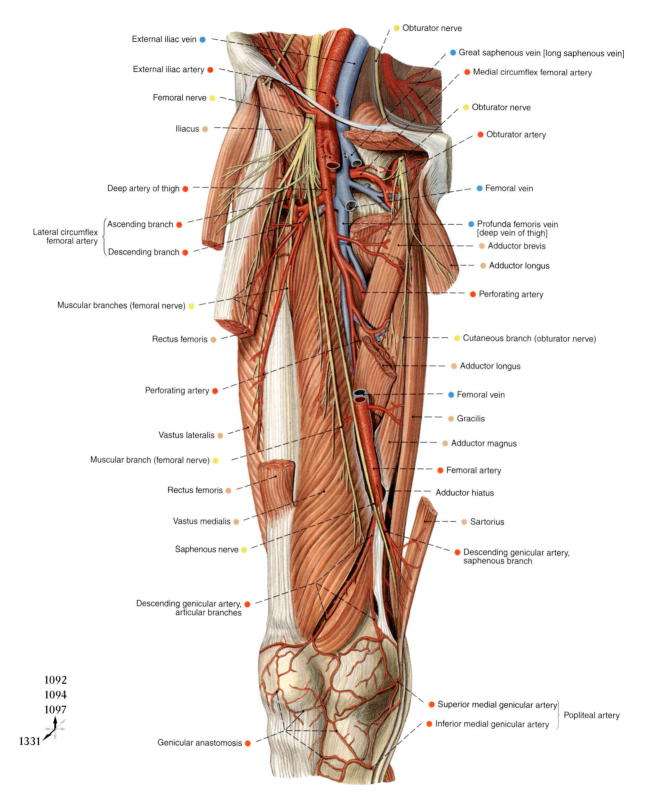

External iliac vein ●
External iliac artery ●
Femoral nerve ●
Iliacus ●
Deep artery of thigh ●
Lateral circumflex femoral artery {
Ascending branch ●
Descending branch ●
}
Muscular branches (femoral nerve) ●
Rectus femoris ●
Perforating artery ●
Vastus lateralis ●
Muscular branch (femoral nerve) ●
Rectus femoris ●
Vastus medialis ●
Saphenous nerve ●
Descending genicular artery, ●
articular branches
Genicular anastomosis ●

Obturator nerve ●
● Great saphenous vein [long saphenous vein]
● Medial circumflex femoral artery
Obturator nerve ●
● Obturator artery
● Femoral vein
● Profunda femoris vein [deep vein of thigh]
Adductor brevis ●
● Adductor longus
● Perforating artery
Cutaneous branch (obturator nerve) ●
Adductor longus ●
● Femoral vein
Gracilis ●
Adductor magnus ●
● Femoral artery
Adductor hiatus
Sartorius ●
● Descending genicular artery, saphenous branch
● Superior medial genicular artery }
Popliteal artery
● Inferior medial genicular artery

1092
1094
1097
1331

Fig. 1332   Blood vessels and nerves of anterior region of right thigh; deep layer after partial removal of sartorius and rectus femoris as well as sectioning pectineus and adductor longus; anteromedial intermuscular septum [subsartorial fascia] cut longitudinally to expose the adductor canal; anterior aspect.

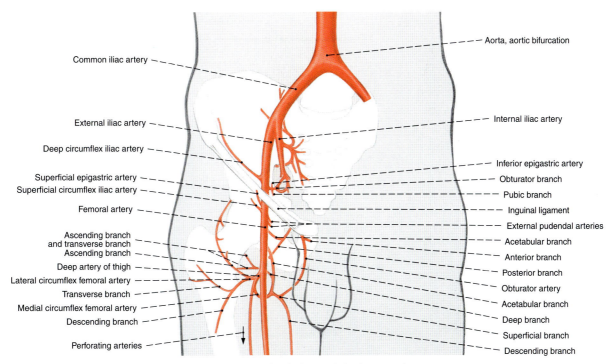

Common iliac artery

External iliac artery

Deep circumflex iliac artery

Superficial epigastric artery
Superficial circumflex iliac artery

Femoral artery

Ascending branch
and transverse branch
Ascending branch
Deep artery of thigh
Lateral circumflex femoral artery
Transverse branch
Medial circumflex femoral artery
Descending branch

Perforating arteries

Aorta, aortic bifurcation

Internal iliac artery

Inferior epigastric artery
Obturator branch
Pubic branch
Inguinal ligament
External pudendal arteries
Acetabular branch
Anterior branch
Posterior branch
Obturator artery
Acetabular branch
Deep branch
Superficial branch
Descending branch

Fig. 1333   Arteries of right hip and thigh; general survey;
anterior aspect.
The shown origin and branching pattern of the deep artery of
thigh can be observed in approximately 58% of cases.

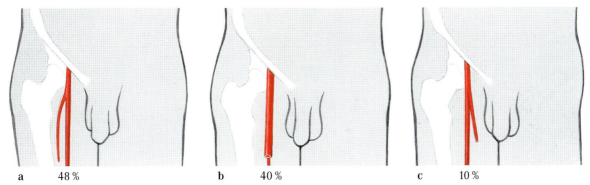

a   48 %   b   40 %   c   10 %

Fig. 1334 a-c   Variations of position of deep artery of thigh.
a   Lateral or laterodorsal to femoral artery
b   Dorsal to femoral artery
c   Medial to femoral artery

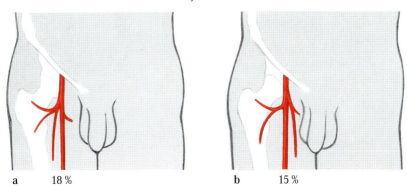

a   18 %   b   15 %

Fig. 1335 a, b   Variations of origin of circumflex femoral arteries.
  a   Separate origin of medial circumflex femoral artery from femoral artery
  b   Separate origin of lateral circumflex femoral artery from femoral artery

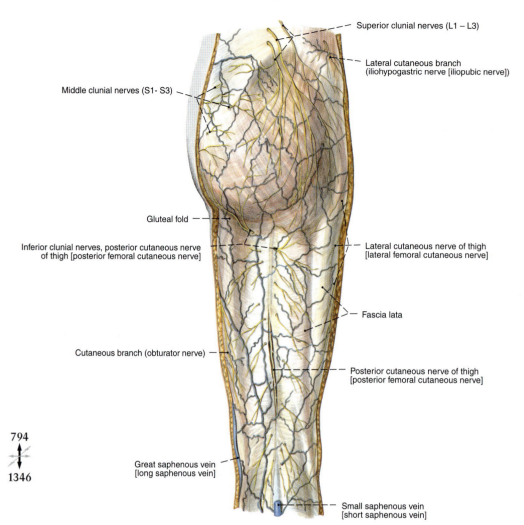

Superior clunial nerves (L1 – L3)

Lateral cutaneous branch
(iliohypogastric nerve [iliopubic nerve])

Middle clunial nerves (S1- S3)

Gluteal fold

Inferior clunial nerves, posterior cutaneous nerve
of thigh [posterior femoral cutaneous nerve]

Lateral cutaneous nerve of thigh
[lateral femoral cutaneous nerve]

Fascia lata

Cutaneous branch (obturator nerve)

Posterior cutaneous nerve of thigh
[posterior femoral cutaneous nerve]

794

1346

Great saphenous vein
[long saphenous vein]

Small saphenous vein
[short saphenous vein]

Fig. 1336   Epifascial blood vessels and nerves of
posterior regions of right thigh, gluteal region, and
popliteal fossa; posterior aspect.

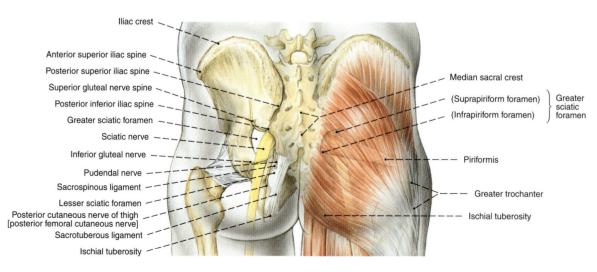

Iliac crest

Anterior superior iliac spine

Posterior superior iliac spine

Superior gluteal nerve spine

Posterior inferior iliac spine

Greater sciatic foramen

Sciatic nerve

Inferior gluteal nerve

Pudendal nerve

Sacrospinous ligament

Lesser sciatic foramen

Posterior cutaneous nerve of thigh
[posterior femoral cutaneous nerve]

Sacrotuberous ligament

Ischial tuberosity

Median sacral crest

(Suprapiriform foramen)

(Infrapiriform foramen)

Greater
sciatic
foramen

Piriformis

Greater trochanter

Ischial tuberosity

Fig. 1337   Projection of skeleton and sciatic
nerve onto the surface of the gluteal region;
posterior aspect.

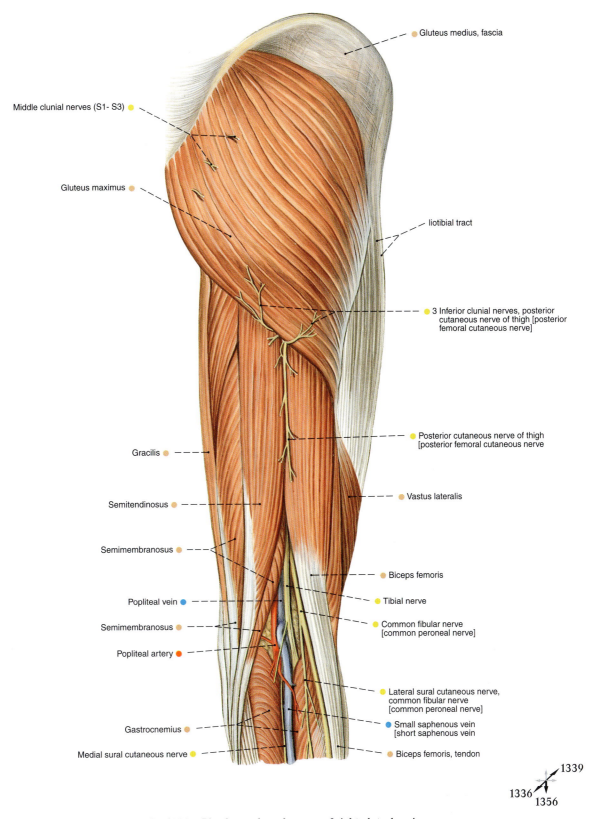

Gluteus medius, fascia

Middle clunial nerves (S1- S3)

Gluteus maximus

Iiotibial tract

3 Inferior clunial nerves, posterior cutaneous nerve of thigh [posterior femoral cutaneous nerve]

Posterior cutaneous nerve of thigh [posterior femoral cutaneous nerve

Gracilis

Semitendinosus

Vastus lateralis

Semimembranosus

Biceps femoris

Popliteal vein

Tibial nerve

Semimembranosus

Common fibular nerve [common peroneal nerve]

Popliteal artery

Lateral sural cutaneous nerve, common fibular nerve [common peroneal nerve]

Small saphenous vein [short saphenous vein

Gastrocnemius

Medial sural cutaneous nerve

Biceps femoris, tendon

1339
1336
1356

Fig. 1338 Blood vessels and nerves of right gluteal region, posterior region of thigh, and popliteal fossa; fascia lata, except iliotibial tract removed; posterior aspect.

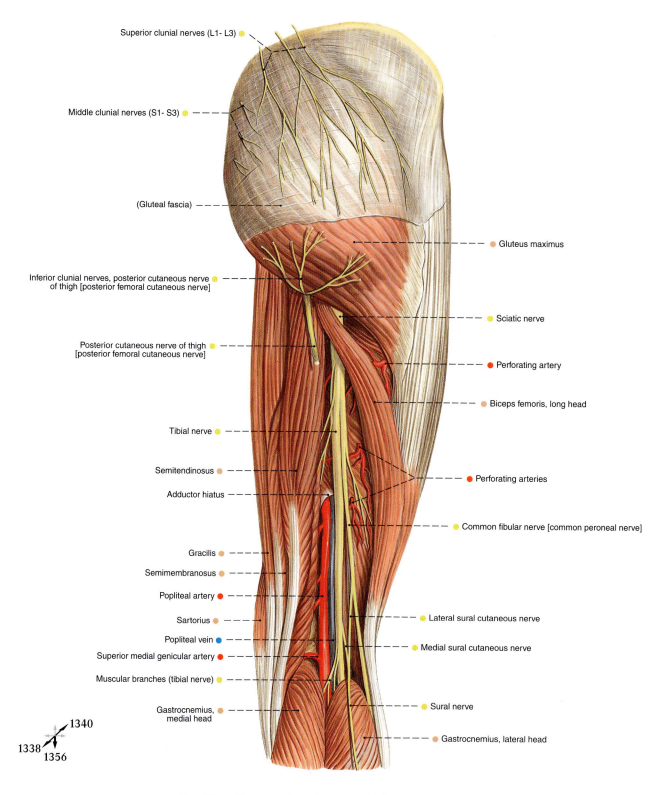

Superior clunial nerves (L1- L3)

Middle clunial nerves (S1- S3)

(Gluteal fascia)

Inferior clunial nerves, posterior cutaneous nerve of thigh [posterior femoral cutaneous nerve]

Posterior cutaneous nerve of thigh [posterior femoral cutaneous nerve]

Tibial nerve

Semitendinosus

Adductor hiatus

Gracilis

Semimembranosus

Popliteal artery

Sartorius

Popliteal vein

Superior medial genicular artery

Muscular branches (tibial nerve)

Gastrocnemius, medial head

Gluteus maximus

Sciatic nerve

Perforating artery

Biceps femoris, long head

Perforating arteries

Common fibular nerve [common peroneal nerve]

Lateral sural cutaneous nerve

Medial sural cutaneous nerve

Sural nerve

Gastrocnemius, lateral head

1340
1338
1356

Fig. 1339 Blood vessels and nerves of right gluteal region, posterior region of thigh, and popliteal fossa; fascia lata removed; long head of biceps femoris retracted laterally; posterior aspect.
In this specimen the medial and lateral sural cutaneous nerves branch off somewhat far proximal.

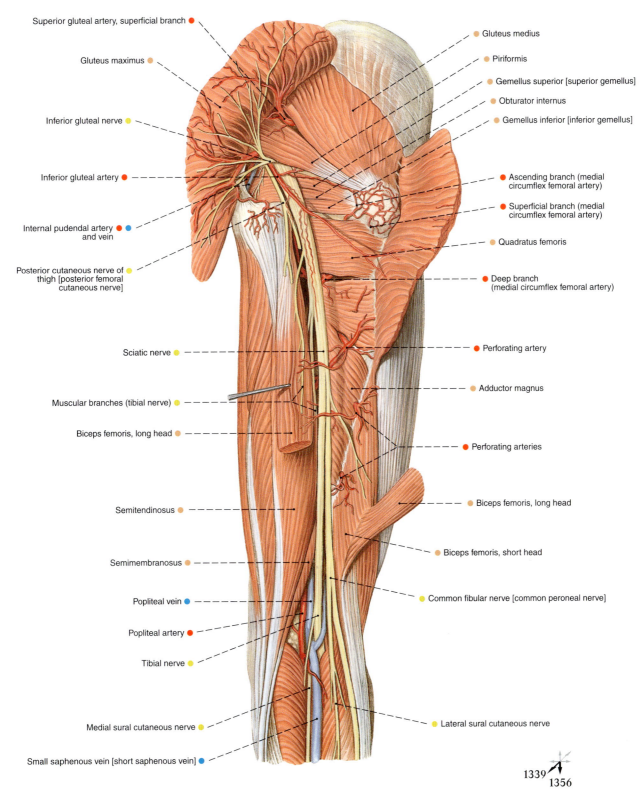

Superior gluteal artery, superficial branch ●

Gluteus maximus ●

Inferior gluteal nerve ●

Inferior gluteal artery ●

Internal pudendal artery ● ● and vein

Posterior cutaneous nerve of ● thigh [posterior femoral cutaneous nerve]

Sciatic nerve ●

Muscular branches (tibial nerve) ●

Biceps femoris, long head ●

Semitendinosus ●

Semimembranosus ●

Popliteal vein ●

Popliteal artery ●

Tibial nerve ●

Medial sural cutaneous nerve ●

Small saphenous vein [short saphenous vein] ●

● Gluteus medius

● Piriformis

● Gemellus superior [superior gemellus]

● Obturator internus

● Gemellus inferior [inferior gemellus]

● Ascending branch (medial circumflex femoral artery)

● Superficial branch (medial circumflex femoral artery)

● Quadratus femoris

● Deep branch (medial circumflex femoral artery)

● Perforating artery

● Adductor magnus

● Perforating arteries

● Biceps femoris, long head

● Biceps femoris, short head

● Common fibular nerve [common peroneal nerve]

● Lateral sural cutaneous nerve

1339
1356

Fig. 1340   Blood vessels and nerves of right gluteal region, posterior region of thigh, and popliteal fossa; gluteus maximus and long head of biceps femoris sectioned; posterior aspect.

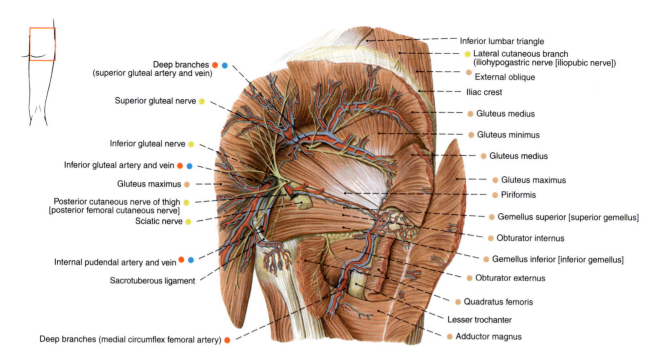

Deep branches ● ●
(superior gluteal artery and vein)

Superior gluteal nerve ●

Inferior gluteal nerve ●

Inferior gluteal artery and vein ● ●

Gluteus maximus ●

Posterior cutaneous nerve of thigh ●
[posterior femoral cutaneous nerve]
Sciatic nerve ●

Internal pudendal artery and vein ● ●

Sacrotuberous ligament

Deep branches (medial circumflex femoral artery) ●

Inferior lumbar triangle
Lateral cutaneous branch
(iliohypogastric nerve [iliopubic nerve])
External oblique
Iliac crest
Gluteus medius
Gluteus minimus
Gluteus medius
Gluteus maximus
Piriformis
Gemellus superior [superior gemellus]
Obturator internus
Gemellus inferior [inferior gemellus]
Obturator externus
Quadratus femoris
Lesser trochanter
Adductor magnus

Fig. 1341   Blood vessels and nerves of right gluteal region; gluteus maximus and medius sectioned and partially removed; sciatic nerve after passage through infrapiriform foramen removed; posterior aspect.

The **greater sciatic foramen** is divided into two passages for blood vessels and nerves by the piriformis.
The **suprapiriform foramen** contains the superior gluteal artery, vein, and nerve; the **infrapiriform foramen** contains the sciatic, inferior gluteal, and pudendal nerves, the posterior cutaneous nerve of thigh [posterior femoral cutaneous nerve] as well as the inferior gluteal and internal pudendal arteries and veins. Through the **lesser sciatic foramen** pass the tendon of obturator internus, the pudendal nerve, and the internal pudendal artery and vein.

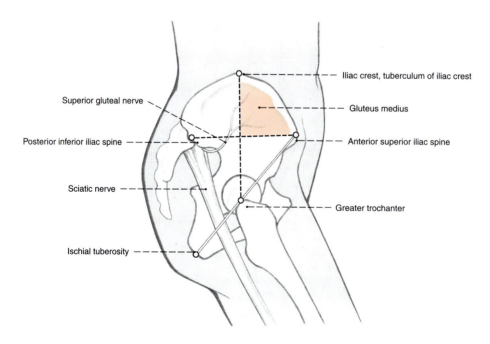

Superior gluteal nerve

Posterior inferior iliac spine

Sciatic nerve

Ischial tuberosity

Iliac crest, tuberculum of iliac crest

Gluteus medius

Anterior superior iliac spine

Greater trochanter

Fig. 1342   Projection of skeletal structures of right hip important for injection into the gluteus medius, lateral aspect.

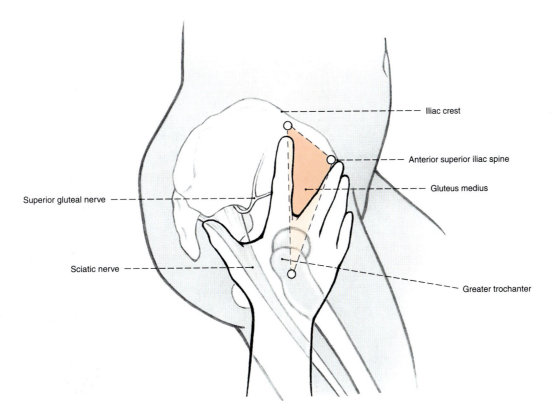

Fig. 1343 Intragluteal injection (according to A. v. HOCHSTETTER). To safely avoid the superior gluteal nerve, and particularly the superior gluteal artery, the injection is made into the triangular area bordered by the two spread fingers and the iliac crest. The middle finger—or when using the left hand the index finger—lies on the anterior superior iliac spine, the palm on the greater trochanter. Because the injected medication should be placed in the belly of the gluteus medius as far as possible from any blood vessels, the direction of the needle must not cross under the fingers. Some risk, however, remains for the branch of the superior gluteal nerve to the tensor fasciae latae [tensor of fascia lata].

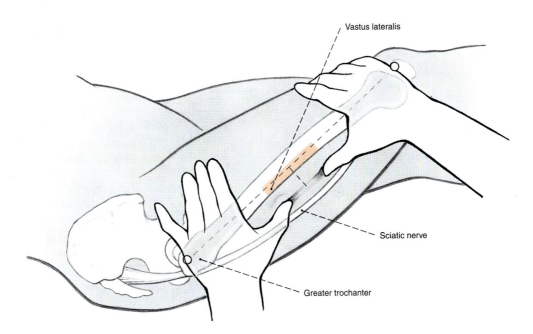

Fig. 1344 Intramuscular injection into the vastus lateralis (according to A. v. HOCHSTETTER). Except for the tiny branches of the lateral cutaneous nerve of thigh [lateral femoral cutaneous nerve] there are no large nerves or blood vessels in the middle of the lateral surface of the thigh. After orientation as to the position of the femur [thigh bone] the needle is inserted transversally directed towards the bone into the belly of the vastus lateralis.

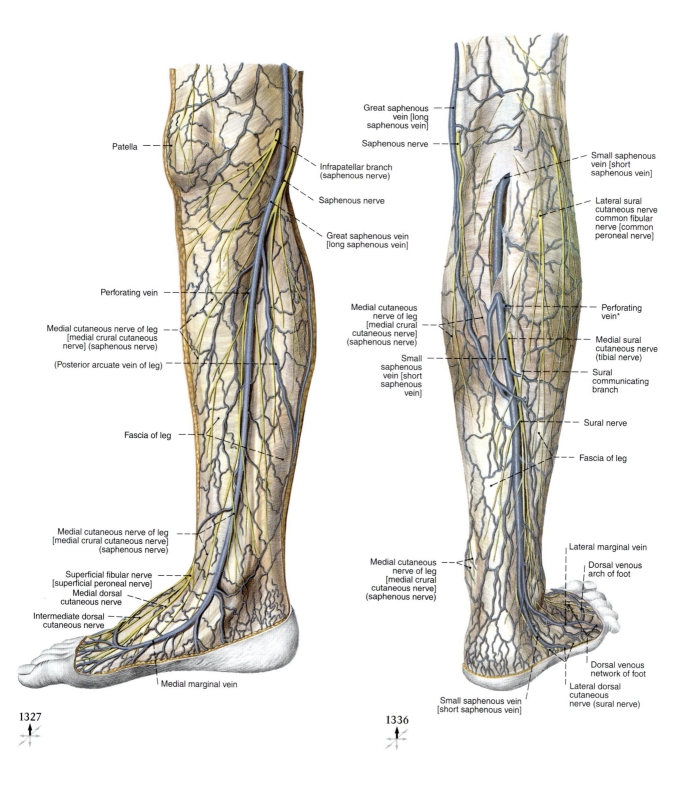

Patella

Infrapatellar branch
(saphenous nerve)

Saphenous nerve

Great saphenous vein
[long saphenous vein]

Perforating vein

Medial cutaneous nerve of leg
[medial crural cutaneous
nerve] (saphenous nerve)

(Posterior arcuate vein of leg)

Fascia of leg

Medial cutaneous nerve of leg
[medial crural cutaneous nerve]
(saphenous nerve)

Superficial fibular nerve
[superficial peroneal nerve]
Medial dorsal
cutaneous nerve

Intermediate dorsal
cutaneous nerve

Medial marginal vein

1327

Great saphenous
vein [long
saphenous vein]

Saphenous nerve

Small saphenous
vein [short
saphenous vein]

Lateral sural
cutaneous nerve
common fibular
nerve [common
peroneal nerve]

Medial cutaneous
nerve of leg
[medial crural
cutaneous nerve]
(saphenous nerve)

Small
saphenous
vein [short
saphenous
vein]

Perforating
vein*

Medial sural
cutaneous nerve
(tibial nerve)

Sural
communicating
branch

Sural nerve

Fascia of leg

Medial cutaneous
nerve of leg
[medial crural
cutaneous nerve]
(saphenous nerve)

Lateral marginal vein

Dorsal venous
arch of foot

Dorsal venous
network of foot

Lateral dorsal
cutaneous
nerve (sural nerve)

Small saphenous vein
[short saphenous vein]

1336

Fig. 1345 Epifascial veins and nerves of right leg
and foot; medial aspect.

Fig. 1346 Epifascial veins and nerves of right leg
and foot; fascia of leg split proximally; posterior aspect.

* Clinically also: MAY's vein.

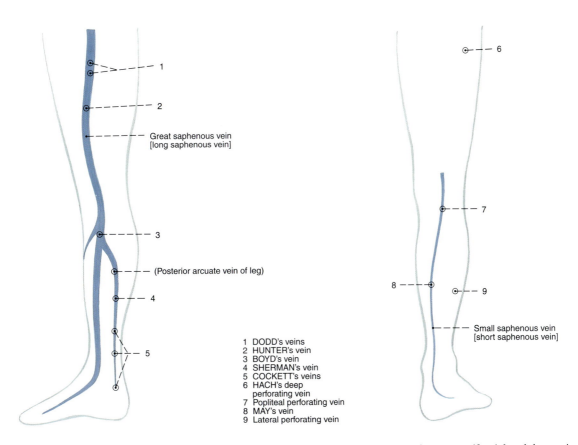

1 DODD's veins
2 HUNTER's vein
3 BOYD's vein
4 SHERMAN's vein
5 COCKETT's veins
6 HACH's deep
  perforating vein
7 Popliteal perforating vein
8 MAY's vein
9 Lateral perforating vein

Great saphenous vein
[long saphenous vein]

(Posterior arcuate vein of leg)

Small saphenous vein
[short saphenous vein]

Fig. 1347 Connections between epifascial and deep veins in the tributary of the right great saphenous vein [long saphenous vein]; general survey (according to HACH, 1986); medial aspect.

Fig. 1348 Connections between epifascial and deep veins in the tributary of the right small saphenous vein [short saphenous vein]; general survey (according to HACH, 1986); posterior aspect.

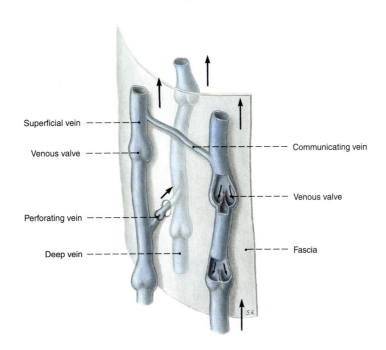

Superficial vein

Venous valve

Perforating vein

Deep vein

Communicating vein

Venous valve

Fascia

Fig. 1349 Veins of lower limb; principles of arrangement.
Disturbances in drainage from veins of the lower limb,

particularly varicosities, are frequent vascular diseases. If one of the venous systems is completely closed, the perforating veins obtain an important role in venous drainage.

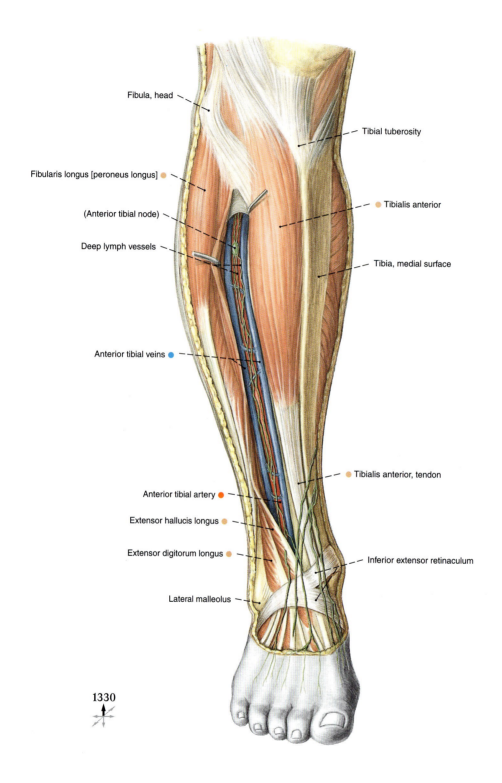

Fibula, head

Tibial tuberosity

Fibularis longus [peroneus longus] ●

● Tibialis anterior

(Anterior tibial node)

Deep lymph vessels

Tibia, medial surface

Anterior tibial veins ●

Tibialis anterior, tendon

Anterior tibial artery ●

Extensor hallucis longus ●

Extensor digitorum longus ●

Inferior extensor retinaculum

Lateral malleolus

1330

Fig. 1350   Blood vessels of anterior region of right leg; fascia of leg removed and extensors spread apart; anterior aspect.
The superficial lymph vessels accompany the epi- fascial veins. They converge along the great saphenous vein [long saphenous vein] on the medial side of the leg. The deep lymph vessels accompany the deep veins and arteries in their connective tissue sheaths.

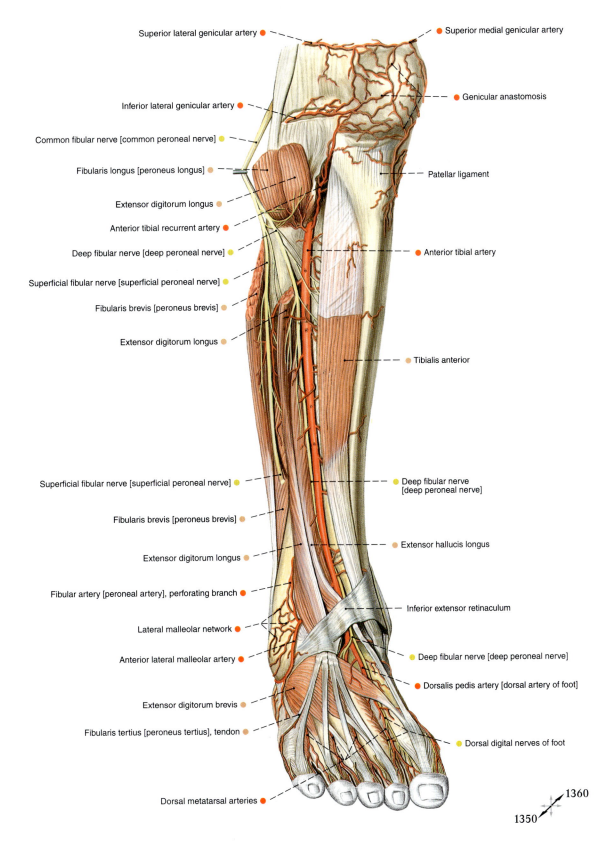

Superior lateral genicular artery ● ---

● Superior medial genicular artery

Inferior lateral genicular artery ● ---

● Genicular anastomosis

Common fibular nerve [common peroneal nerve] ● ---

Fibularis longus [peroneus longus] ● ---

--- Patellar ligament

Extensor digitorum longus ● ---

Anterior tibial recurrent artery ● ---

Deep fibular nerve [deep peroneal nerve] ● ---

● Anterior tibial artery

Superficial fibular nerve [superficial peroneal nerve] ● ---

Fibularis brevis [peroneus brevis] ● ---

Extensor digitorum longus ● ---

● Tibialis anterior

Superficial fibular nerve [superficial peroneal nerve] ● ---

● Deep fibular nerve [deep peroneal nerve]

Fibularis brevis [peroneus brevis] ● ---

Extensor digitorum longus ● ---

● Extensor hallucis longus

Fibular artery [peroneal artery], perforating branch ● ---

--- Inferior extensor retinaculum

Lateral malleolar network ● ---

Anterior lateral malleolar artery ● ---

● Deep fibular nerve [deep peroneal nerve]

● Dorsalis pedis artery [dorsal artery of foot]

Extensor digitorum brevis ● ---

Fibularis tertius [peroneus tertius], tendon ● ---

● Dorsal digital nerves of foot

1360

1350

Dorsal metatarsal arteries ● ---

Fig. 1351 Blood vessels and nerves of anterior region of
right leg and dorsum of foot; fascia of leg removed and
extensor digitorum longus and fibularis longus [peroneus
longus] sectioned; anterior aspect.

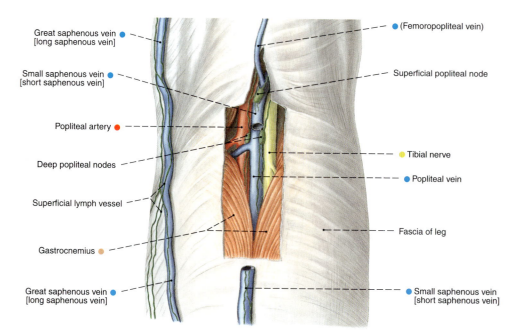

Great saphenous vein [long saphenous vein] ●

Small saphenous vein [short saphenous vein] ●

Popliteal artery ●

Deep popliteal nodes

Superficial lymph vessel

Gastrocnemius ●

Great saphenous vein [long saphenous vein] ●

(Femoropopliteal vein) ●

Superficial popliteal node

Tibial nerve ●

Popliteal vein ●

Fascia of leg

Small saphenous vein [short saphenous vein] ●

Fig. 1352 Blood vessels and nerves of right popliteal fossa; fascia of leg split and small saphenous vein [short saphenous vein] removed; posterior aspect.

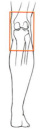

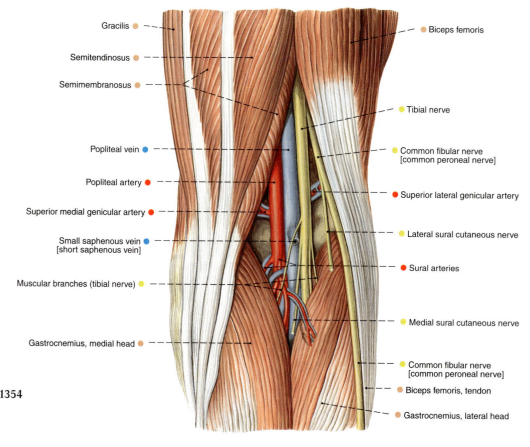

Gracilis ●

Semitendinosus ●

Semimembranosus ●

Popliteal vein ●

Popliteal artery ●

Superior medial genicular artery ●

Small saphenous vein [short saphenous vein] ●

Muscular branches (tibial nerve) ●

Gastrocnemius, medial head ●

Biceps femoris ●

Tibial nerve ●

Common fibular nerve [common peroneal nerve] ●

Superior lateral genicular artery ●

Lateral sural cutaneous nerve ●

Sural arteries ●

Medial sural cutaneous nerve ●

Common fibular nerve [common peroneal nerve] ●

Biceps femoris, tendon ●

Gastrocnemius, lateral head ●

1338
1354
1346
1356

Fig. 1353 Blood vessels and nerves of right popliteal fossa; fascia lata and fascia of leg split removed; posterior aspect.

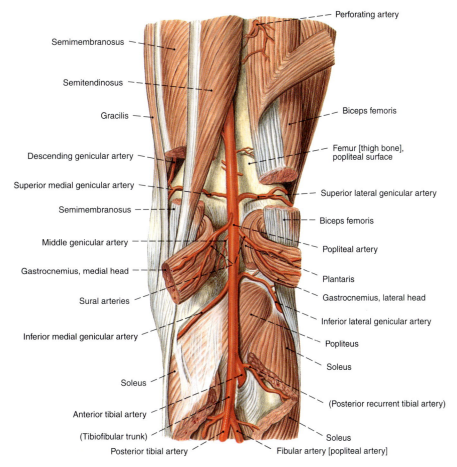

Perforating artery

Semimembranosus

Semitendinosus

Gracilis

Descending genicular artery

Superior medial genicular artery

Semimembranosus

Middle genicular artery

Gastrocnemius, medial head

Sural arteries

Inferior medial genicular artery

Soleus

Anterior tibial artery

(Tibiofibular trunk)

Posterior tibial artery

Biceps femoris

Femur [thigh bone], popliteal surface

Superior lateral genicular artery

Biceps femoris

Popliteal artery

Plantaris

Gastrocnemius, lateral head

Inferior lateral genicular artery

Popliteus

Soleus

(Posterior recurrent tibial artery)

Soleus

Fibular artery [popliteal artery]

1339

1353

1357

Fig. 1354 Arteries of right popliteal fossa;
covering muscles partially removed;
posterior aspect.
This branching pattern can be observed in approximately
90% of cases.

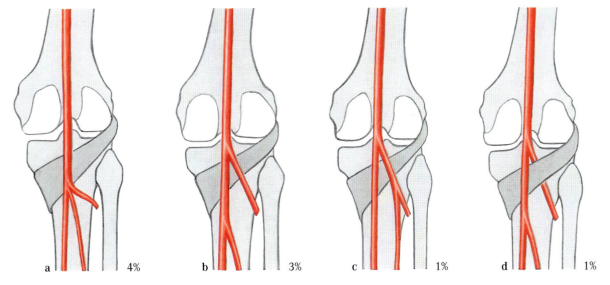

a   4%   b   3%   c   1%   d   1%

Fig. 1355 a-d Variations in the branching pattern of popliteal artery.
a Common trunk of anterior and posterior tibial arteries and fibular [peroneal] artery
b Division of popliteal artery proximal to upper border of popliteus
c Proximal trunk formation of posterior tibial and fibular [peroneal] arteries
d Course of anterior tibial artery ventral to popliteus

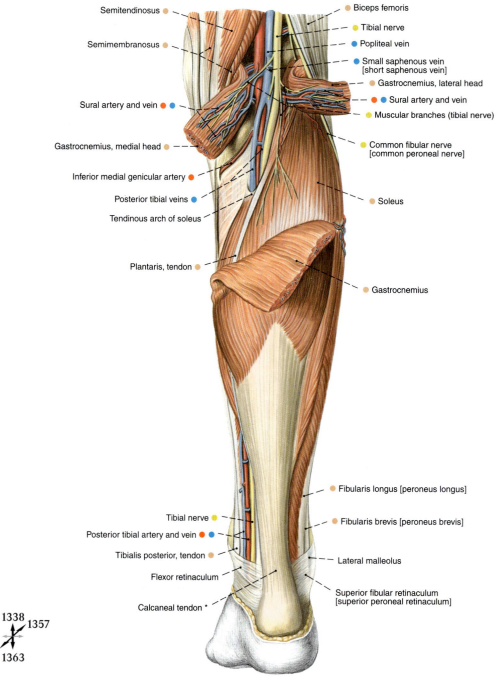

Semitendinosus ●

Semimembranosus ●

Sural artery and vein ● ●

Gastrocnemius, medial head ●

Inferior medial genicular artery ●

Posterior tibial veins ●

Tendinous arch of soleus

Plantaris, tendon ●

Biceps femoris ●

Tibial nerve ●

Popliteal vein ●

Small saphenous vein
[short saphenous vein] ●

Gastrocnemius, lateral head ●

● ● Sural artery and vein

Muscular branches (tibial nerve) ●

Common fibular nerve
[common peroneal nerve] ●

Soleus ●

Gastrocnemius ●

Fibularis longus [peroneus longus] ●

Fibularis brevis [peroneus brevis] ●

Tibial nerve ●

Posterior tibial artery and vein ● ●

Tibialis posterior, tendon ●

Flexor retinaculum

Calcaneal tendon *

Lateral malleolus

Superior fibular retinaculum
[superior peroneal retinaculum]

1338
1357
1346
1363

Fig. 1356   Blood vessels and nerves of popliteal fossa
and posterior region of right leg;
fascia of leg removed and gastrocnemius sectioned;
posterior aspect.

* Also: ACHILLES tendon.

The medial retromalleolar space, covered by the flexor retinaculum, connects the calf to the deep layer of the sole. From anterior to posterior it contains the tendons of tibialis posterior, flexor digitorum longus, tibial blood vessels, tendon of flexor hallucis longus, and the tibial nerve. The distal continuation of this space is known as the tarsal tunnel (see Fig. 1364).

The lateral retromalleolar space is covered by the superior and inferior fibular [peroneal] retinacula. From anterior to posterior it contains the tendons of fibularis [peroneus] brevis and longus.

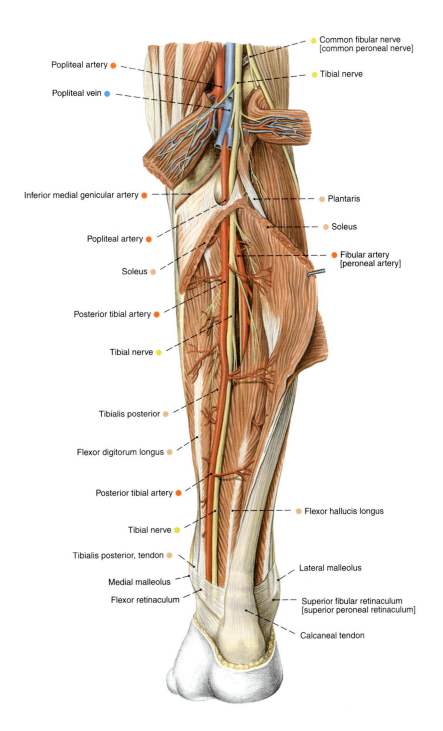

Common fibular nerve [common peroneal nerve]

Popliteal artery

Tibial nerve

Popliteal vein

Inferior medial genicular artery

Plantaris

Soleus

Popliteal artery

Fibular artery [peroneal artery]

Soleus

Posterior tibial artery

Tibial nerve

Tibialis posterior

Flexor digitorum longus

Posterior tibial artery

Flexor hallucis longus

Tibial nerve

Tibialis posterior, tendon

Lateral malleolus

Medial malleolus

Flexor retinaculum

Superior fibular retinaculum [superior peroneal retinaculum]

Calcaneal tendon

1339 1358
1356 1363

Fig. 1357   Blood vessels and nerves of popliteal fossa
and posterior region of right leg;
gastrocnemius extensively removed and soleus split to
expose the deep layer; posterior aspect.

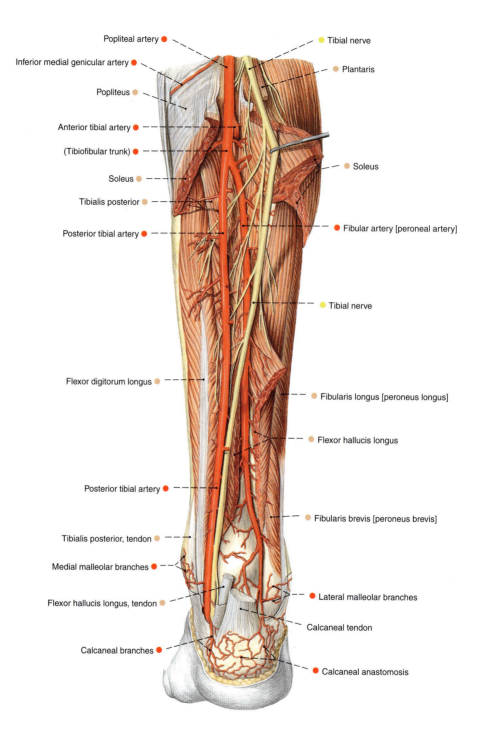

Popliteal artery ●

Inferior medial genicular artery ●

Popliteus ●

Anterior tibial artery ●

(Tibiofibular trunk) ●

Soleus ●

Tibialis posterior ●

Posterior tibial artery ●

Flexor digitorum longus ●

Posterior tibial artery ●

Tibialis posterior, tendon ●

Medial malleolar branches ●

Flexor hallucis longus, tendon ●

Calcaneal branches ●

Tibial nerve ●

Plantaris ●

Soleus ●

Fibular artery [peroneal artery] ●

Tibial nerve ●

Fibularis longus [peroneus longus] ●

Flexor hallucis longus ●

Fibularis brevis [peroneus brevis] ●

Lateral malleolar branches ●

Calcaneal tendon

Calcaneal anastomosis ●

1340
1357
1363

Fig. 1358 Arteries and nerves of popliteal fossa and posterior region of right leg; triceps surae and extensor hallucis longus extensively removed; posterior aspect.

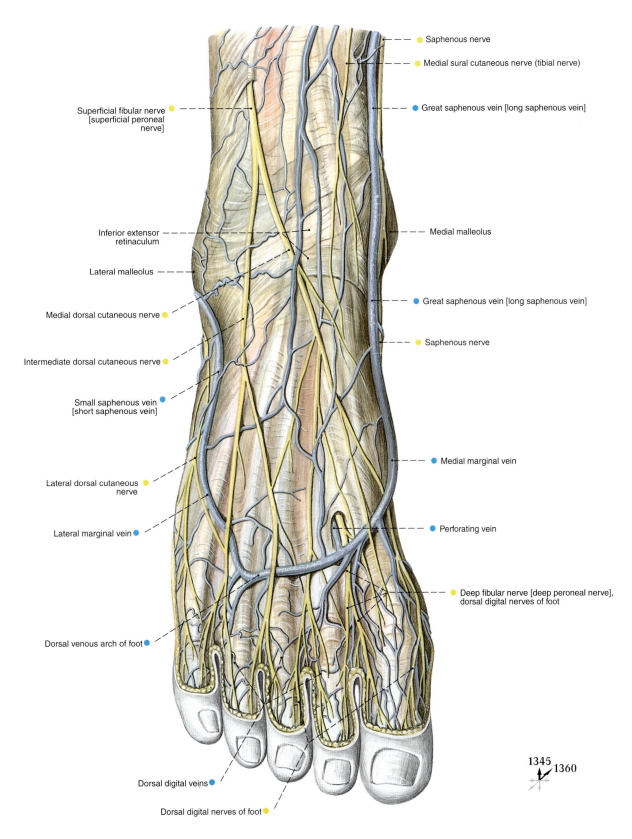

Saphenous nerve

Medial sural cutaneous nerve (tibial nerve)

Great saphenous vein [long saphenous vein]

Superficial fibular nerve [superficial peroneal nerve]

Inferior extensor retinaculum

Medial malleolus

Lateral malleolus

Great saphenous vein [long saphenous vein]

Medial dorsal cutaneous nerve

Saphenous nerve

Intermediate dorsal cutaneous nerve

Small saphenous vein [short saphenous vein]

Medial marginal vein

Lateral dorsal cutaneous nerve

Perforating vein

Lateral marginal vein

Deep fibular nerve [deep peroneal nerve], dorsal digital nerves of foot

Dorsal venous arch of foot

1345 1360

Dorsal digital veins

Dorsal digital nerves of foot

Fig. 1359 Epifascial veins and nerves of right dorsum of foot [dorsal region of foot]; dorsal aspect.

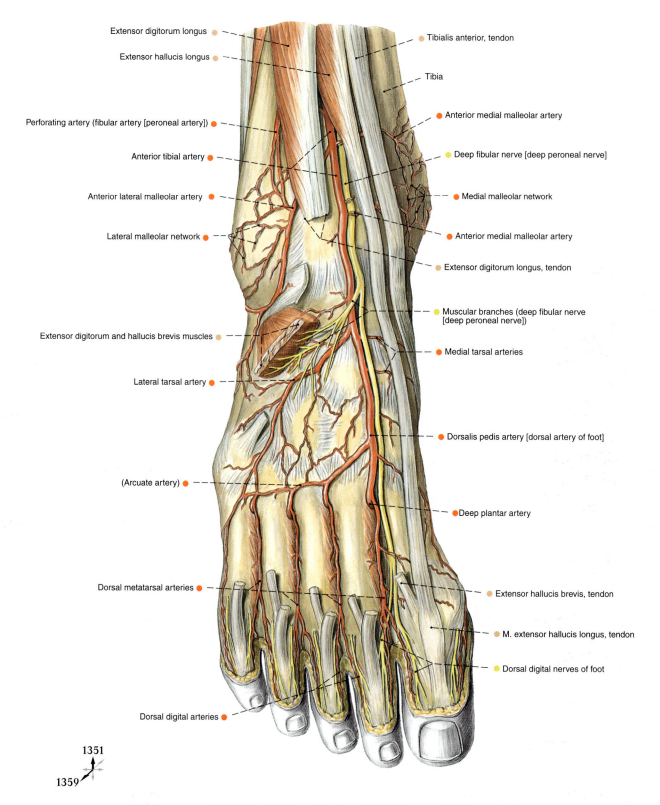

Extensor digitorum longus

Extensor hallucis longus

Perforating artery (fibular artery [peroneal artery])

Anterior tibial artery

Anterior lateral malleolar artery

Lateral malleolar network

Extensor digitorum and hallucis brevis muscles

Lateral tarsal artery

(Arcuate artery)

Dorsal metatarsal arteries

Dorsal digital arteries

Tibialis anterior, tendon

Tibia

Anterior medial malleolar artery

Deep fibular nerve [deep peroneal nerve]

Medial malleolar network

Anterior medial malleolar artery

Extensor digitorum longus, tendon

Muscular branches (deep fibular nerve [deep peroneal nerve])

Medial tarsal arteries

Dorsalis pedis artery [dorsal artery of foot]

Deep plantar artery

Extensor hallucis brevis, tendon

M. extensor hallucis longus, tendon

Dorsal digital nerves of foot

1351

1359

Fig. 1360   Arteries and nerves of right dorsum of foot [dorsal region of foot]; dorsal fascia of foot and extensor digitorum and hallucis muscles partially removed; dorsal aspect.

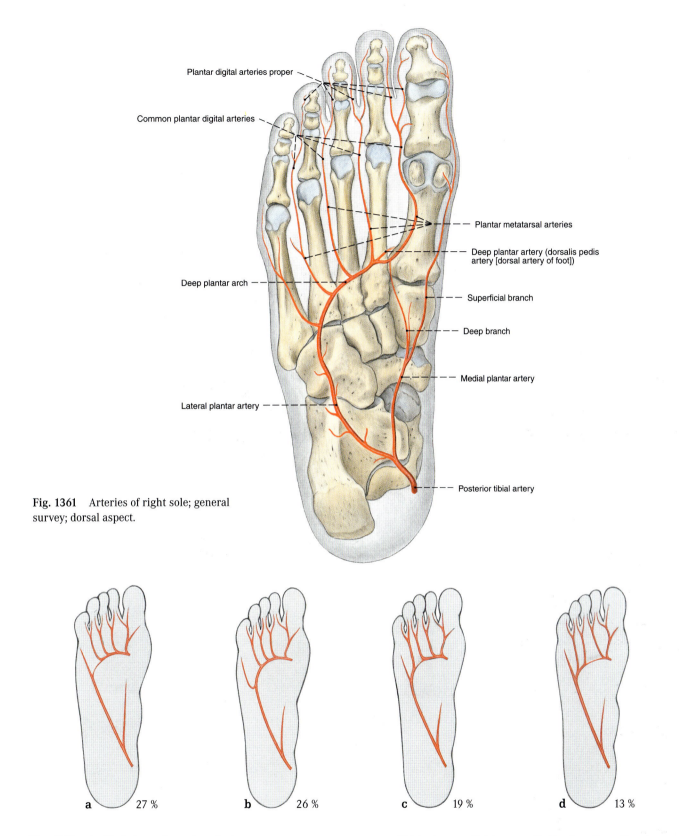

Plantar digital arteries proper

Common plantar digital arteries

Plantar metatarsal arteries

Deep plantar artery (dorsalis pedis artery [dorsal artery of foot])

Deep plantar arch

Superficial branch

Deep branch

Medial plantar artery

Lateral plantar artery

Posterior tibial artery

Fig. 1361   Arteries of right sole; general survey; dorsal aspect.

a   27 %   b   26 %   c   19 %   d   13 %

Fig. 1362 a-d   Variations of arteries of sole.
  a Deep plantar arch supplied mainly by the dorsalis pedis artery [dorsal artery of foot]
  b Deep plantar arch supplied mainly by the tibialis posterior artery
  c 5th and lateral part of 4th toe supplied by the posterior tibial artery, medial toes supplied by dorsalis pedis artery [dorsal artery of foot]
  d 5th, 4th, and lateral part of 3rd toe supplied by the posterior tibial artery, medial toes supplied by dorsalis pedis artery [dorsal artery of foot]

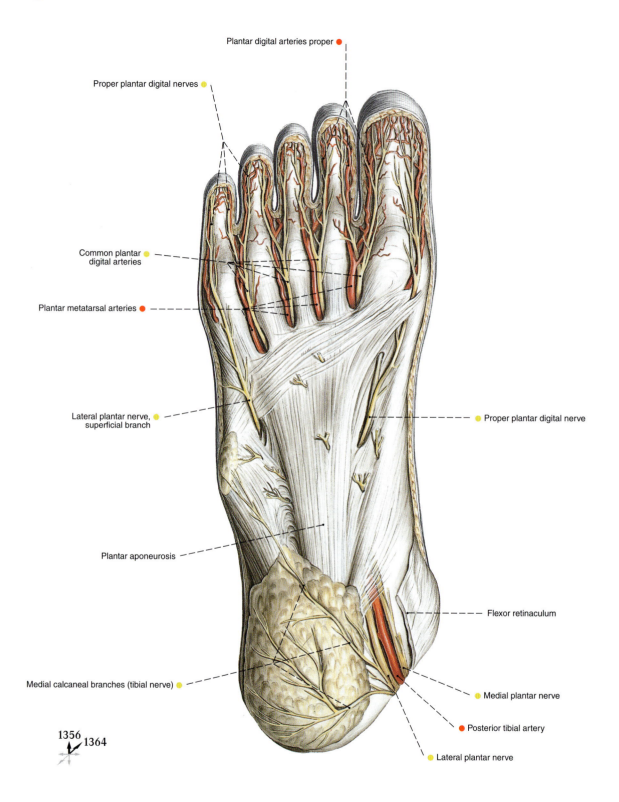

Plantar digital arteries proper ●

Proper plantar digital nerves ●

Common plantar ●
digital arteries

Plantar metatarsal arteries ●

Lateral plantar nerve, ●
superficial branch

Proper plantar digital nerve ●

Plantar aponeurosis

Flexor retinaculum

Medial calcaneal branches (tibial nerve) ●

Medial plantar nerve ●

Posterior tibial artery ●

Lateral plantar nerve ●

1356
1364

Fig. 1363   Arteries and nerves of right sole;
flexor retinaculum split; plantar aspect.

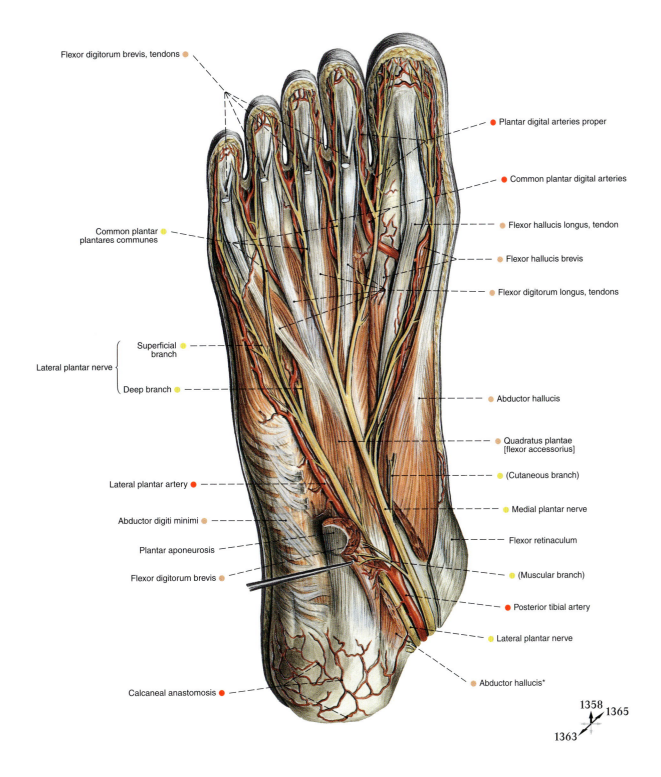

Flexor digitorum brevis, tendons ●

Plantar digital arteries proper ●

Common plantar digital arteries ●

Common plantar plantares communes ●

Flexor hallucis longus, tendon ●

Flexor hallucis brevis ●

Flexor digitorum longus, tendons ●

Superficial branch ●

Lateral plantar nerve {

Deep branch ●

Abductor hallucis ●

Quadratus plantae [flexor accessorius] ●

(Cutaneous branch) ●

Lateral plantar artery ●

Medial plantar nerve ●

Abductor digiti minimi ●

Flexor retinaculum

Plantar aponeurosis ●

(Muscular branch) ●

Flexor digitorum brevis ●

Posterior tibial artery ●

Lateral plantar nerve ●

Abductor hallucis* ●

Calcaneal anastomosis ●

1358
1365
1363

Fig. 1364 Arteries and nerves of right sole; plantar aponeurosis and flexor digitorum brevis extensively removed and abductor hallucis split; plantar aspect.

* The distal continuation of the medial retromalleolar space beneath the abductor hallucis is also known as tarsal tunnel (see also page 370).

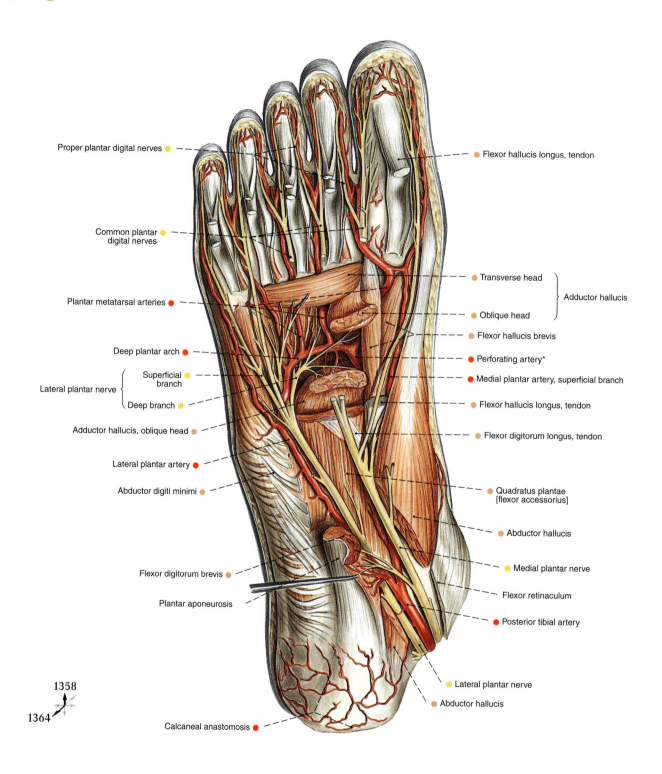

Proper plantar digital nerves

Common plantar digital nerves

Plantar metatarsal arteries

Deep plantar arch

Lateral plantar nerve
  Superficial branch
  Deep branch

Adductor hallucis, oblique head

Lateral plantar artery

Abductor digiti minimi

Flexor digitorum brevis

Plantar aponeurosis

1358
1364

Calcaneal anastomosis

Flexor hallucis longus, tendon

Transverse head
Oblique head
  } Adductor hallucis

Flexor hallucis brevis

Perforating artery*

Medial plantar artery, superficial branch

Flexor hallucis longus, tendon

Flexor digitorum longus, tendon

Quadratus plantae [flexor accessorius]

Abductor hallucis

Medial plantar nerve

Flexor retinaculum

Posterior tibial artery

Lateral plantar nerve

Abductor hallucis

Fig. 1365   Arteries and nerves of right sole;
flexor digitorum brevis and longus and flexor hallucis
longus extensively removed; abductor hallucis and oblique
head of adductor hallucis split; plantar aspect.

* Anastomosis with dorsalis pedis artery [dorsal artery of foot].

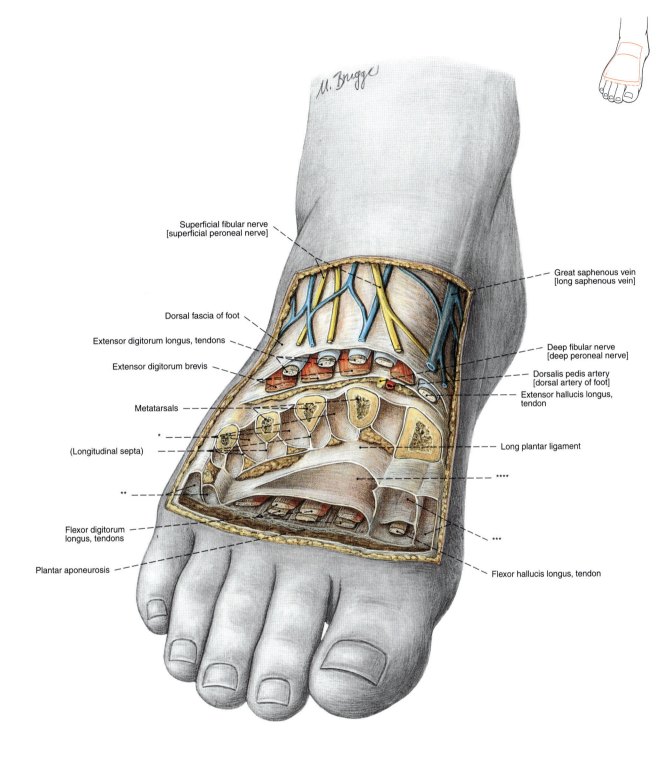

M. Brugge

Superficial fibular nerve
[superficial peroneal nerve]

Great saphenous vein
[long saphenous vein]

Dorsal fascia of foot

Extensor digitorum longus, tendons

Extensor digitorum brevis

Deep fibular nerve
[deep peroneal nerve]

Dorsalis pedis artery
[dorsal artery of foot]

Extensor hallucis longus,
tendon

Metatarsals

*

(Longitudinal septa)

Long plantar ligament

****

**

***

Flexor digitorum
longus, tendons

Plantar aponeurosis

Flexor hallucis longus, tendon

Fig. 1366 Compartments of right foot
opened layer by layer; anterior dorsal
aspect (30%).

*   Spaces for interossei.
**   Lateral compartment.
***   Medial compartment.
****   Intermediate [middle] compartment.

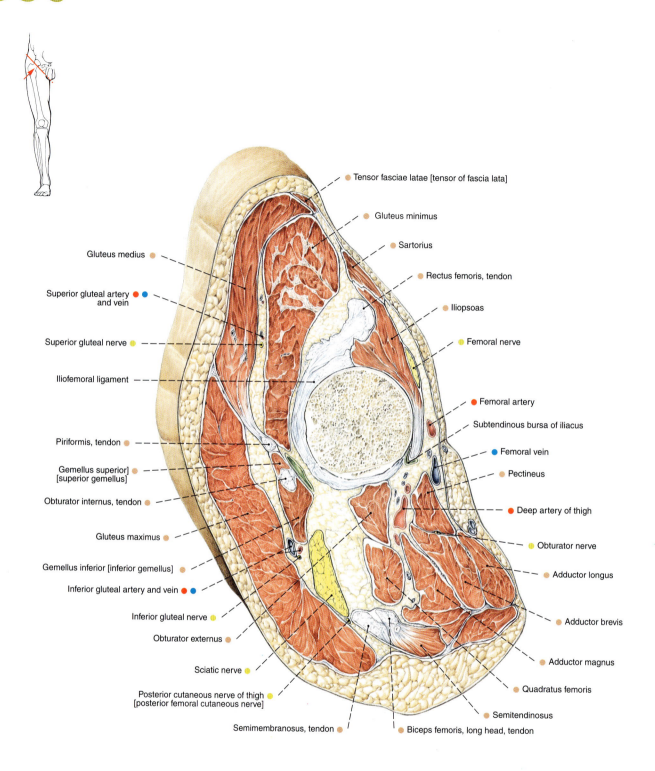

Tensor fasciae latae [tensor of fascia lata]

Gluteus minimus

Sartorius

Rectus femoris, tendon

Iliopsoas

Femoral nerve

Femoral artery

Subtendinous bursa of iliacus

Femoral vein

Pectineus

Deep artery of thigh

Obturator nerve

Adductor longus

Adductor brevis

Adductor magnus

Quadratus femoris

Semitendinosus

Biceps femoris, long head, tendon

Semimembranosus, tendon

Posterior cutaneous nerve of thigh [posterior femoral cutaneous nerve]

Sciatic nerve

Obturator externus

Inferior gluteal nerve

Inferior gluteal artery and vein

Gemellus inferior [inferior gemellus]

Gluteus maximus

Obturator internus, tendon

Gemellus superior] [superior gemellus]

Piriformis, tendon

Iliofemoral ligament

Superior gluteal nerve

Superior gluteal artery and vein

Gluteus medius

Fig. 1367　Right thigh; oblique section through hip joint; distal aspect.

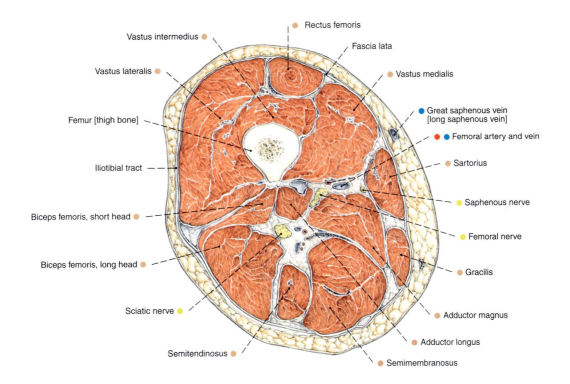

Vastus intermedius

Vastus lateralis

Femur [thigh bone]

Iliotibial tract

Biceps femoris, short head

Biceps femoris, long head

Sciatic nerve

Semitendinosus

Rectus femoris

Fascia lata

Vastus medialis

Great saphenous vein [long saphenous vein]

Femoral artery and vein

Sartorius

Saphenous nerve

Femoral nerve

Gracilis

Adductor magnus

Adductor longus

Semimembranosus

Fig. 1368 Right thigh; cross-section through middle of thigh; distal aspect.

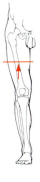

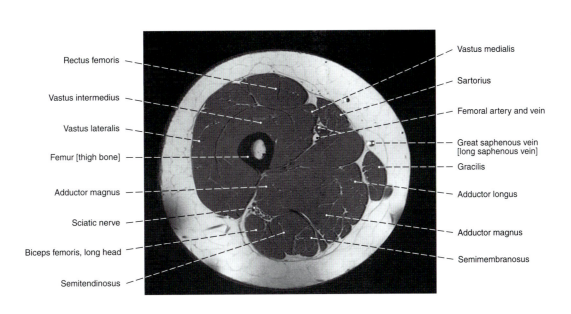

Rectus femoris

Vastus intermedius

Vastus lateralis

Femur [thigh bone]

Adductor magnus

Sciatic nerve

Biceps femoris, long head

Semitendinosus

Vastus medialis

Sartorius

Femoral artery and vein

Great saphenous vein [long saphenous vein]

Gracilis

Adductor longus

Adductor magnus

Semimembranosus

Fig. 1369 Right thigh; magnetic resonance image (MRI); cross-section slightly above middle of thigh; distal aspect.

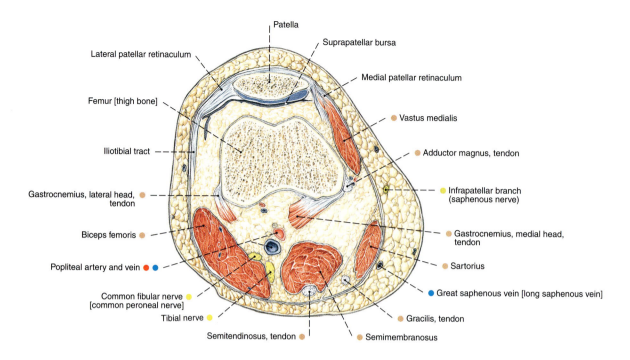

Patella

Lateral patellar retinaculum

Suprapatellar bursa

Medial patellar retinaculum

Femur [thigh bone]

Vastus medialis

Iliotibial tract

Adductor magnus, tendon

Gastrocnemius, lateral head, tendon

Infrapatellar branch (saphenous nerve)

Biceps femoris

Gastrocnemius, medial head, tendon

Popliteal artery and vein

Sartorius

Common fibular nerve [common peroneal nerve]

Great saphenous vein [long saphenous vein]

Tibial nerve

Gracilis, tendon

Semitendinosus, tendon

Semimembranosus

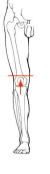

Fig. 1370   Right thigh; cross section through distal extremity of femur [thigh bone] and patella; distal aspect.

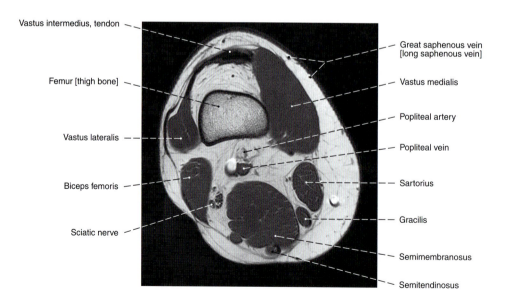

Vastus intermedius, tendon

Great saphenous vein [long saphenous vein]

Femur [thigh bone]

Vastus medialis

Popliteal artery

Vastus lateralis

Popliteal vein

Biceps femoris

Sartorius

Sciatic nerve

Gracilis

Semimembranosus

Semitendinosus

Fig. 1371   Right thigh; magnetic resonance image (MRI); cross-section through lower third of thigh slightly above patella; distal aspect.

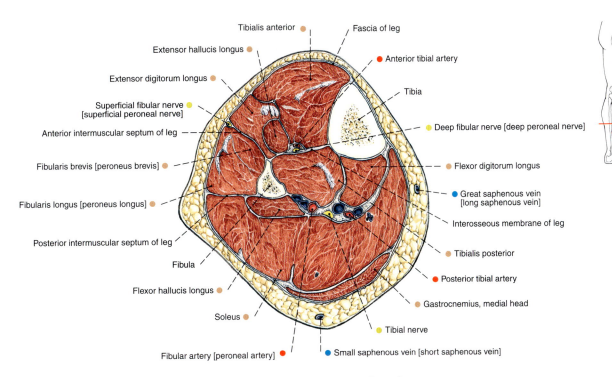

Tibialis anterior
Fascia of leg
Extensor hallucis longus
Extensor digitorum longus
Superficial fibular nerve [superficial peroneal nerve]
Anterior intermuscular septum of leg
Fibularis brevis [peroneus brevis]
Fibularis longus [peroneus longus]
Posterior intermuscular septum of leg
Fibula
Flexor hallucis longus
Soleus
Fibular artery [peroneal artery]

Anterior tibial artery
Tibia
Deep fibular nerve [deep peroneal nerve]
Flexor digitorum longus
Great saphenous vein [long saphenous vein]
Interosseous membrane of leg
Tibialis posterior
Posterior tibial artery
Gastrocnemius, medial head
Tibial nerve
Small saphenous vein [short saphenous vein]

Fig. 1372 Right leg; cross-section through middle of leg; distal aspect.

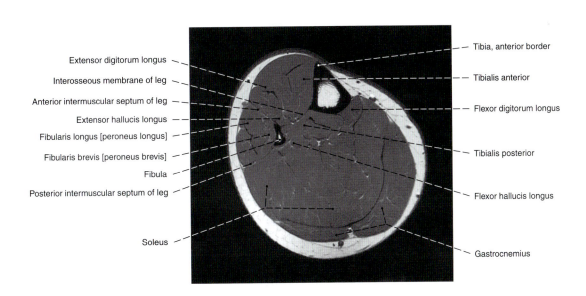

Extensor digitorum longus
Interosseous membrane of leg
Anterior intermuscular septum of leg
Extensor hallucis longus
Fibularis longus [peroneus longus]
Fibularis brevis [peroneus brevis]
Fibula
Posterior intermuscular septum of leg
Soleus

Tibia, anterior border
Tibialis anterior
Flexor digitorum longus
Tibialis posterior
Flexor hallucis longus
Gastrocnemius

Fig. 1373 Right leg; magnetic resonance image (MRI); cross-section through middle of leg; distal aspect.

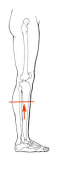

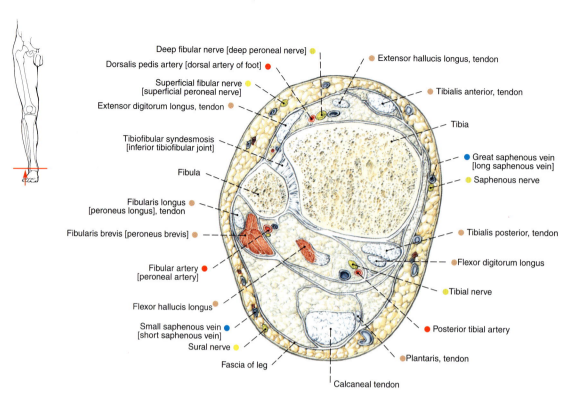

Deep fibular nerve [deep peroneal nerve]
Dorsalis pedis artery [dorsal artery of foot]
Superficial fibular nerve [superficial peroneal nerve]
Extensor digitorum longus, tendon
Tibiofibular syndesmosis [inferior tibiofibular joint]
Fibula
Fibularis longus [peroneus longus], tendon
Fibularis brevis [peroneus brevis]
Fibular artery [peroneal artery]
Flexor hallucis longus
Small saphenous vein [short saphenous vein]
Sural nerve
Fascia of leg
Calcaneal tendon

Extensor hallucis longus, tendon
Tibialis anterior, tendon
Tibia
Great saphenous vein [long saphenous vein]
Saphenous nerve
Tibialis posterior, tendon
Flexor digitorum longus
Tibial nerve
Posterior tibial artery
Plantaris, tendon

Fig. 1374   Right leg;
cross-section slightly above ankle joint;
distal aspect.

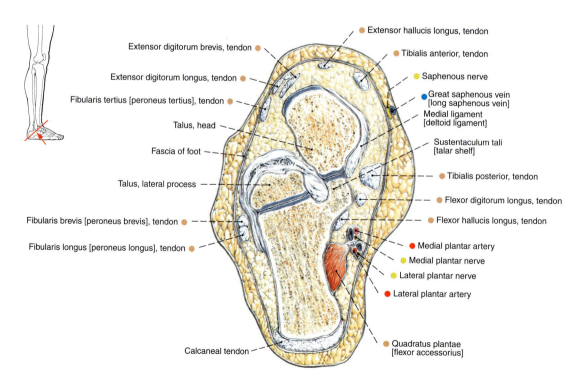

Extensor digitorum brevis, tendon
Extensor digitorum longus, tendon
Fibularis tertius [peroneus tertius], tendon
Talus, head
Fascia of foot
Talus, lateral process
Fibularis brevis [peroneus brevis], tendon
Fibularis longus [peroneus longus], tendon
Calcaneal tendon

Extensor hallucis longus, tendon
Tibialis anterior, tendon
Saphenous nerve
Great saphenous vein [long saphenous vein]
Medial ligament [deltoid ligament]
Sustentaculum tali [talar shelf]
Tibialis posterior, tendon
Flexor digitorum longus, tendon
Flexor hallucis longus, tendon
Medial plantar artery
Medial plantar nerve
Lateral plantar nerve
Lateral plantar artery
Quadratus plantae [flexor accessorius]

Fig. 1375   Right foot;
oblique section through calcaneus and head of talus;
distal aspect.

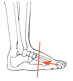

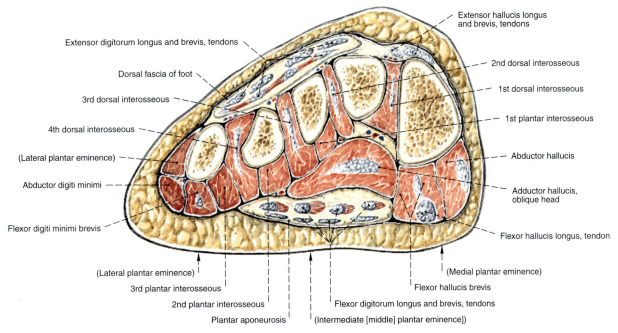

Extensor hallucis longus and brevis, tendons

Extensor digitorum longus and brevis, tendons

2nd dorsal interosseous

Dorsal fascia of foot

1st dorsal interosseous

3rd dorsal interosseous

1st plantar interosseous

4th dorsal interosseous

(Lateral plantar eminence)

Abductor hallucis

Abductor digiti minimi

Adductor hallucis, oblique head

Flexor digiti minimi brevis

Flexor hallucis longus, tendon

(Lateral plantar eminence)

(Medial plantar eminence)

3rd plantar interosseous

Flexor hallucis brevis

2nd plantar interosseous

Flexor digitorum longus and brevis, tendons

Plantar aponeurosis

(Intermediate [middle] plantar eminence])

Fig. 1376   Right foot;
frontal section through metatarsus;
distal aspect.

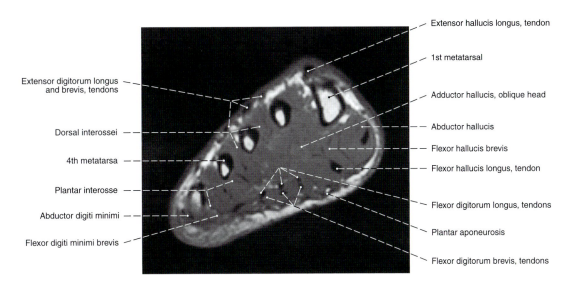

Extensor hallucis longus, tendon

1st metatarsal

Extensor digitorum longus and brevis, tendons

Adductor hallucis, oblique head

Dorsal interossei

Abductor hallucis

4th metatarsa

Flexor hallucis brevis

Plantar interosse

Flexor hallucis longus, tendon

Abductor digiti minimi

Flexor digitorum longus, tendons

Flexor digiti minimi brevis

Plantar aponeurosis

Flexor digitorum brevis, tendons

Fig. 1377   Right foot;
magnetic resonance image (MRI);
frontal section through metatarsus;
distal aspect.

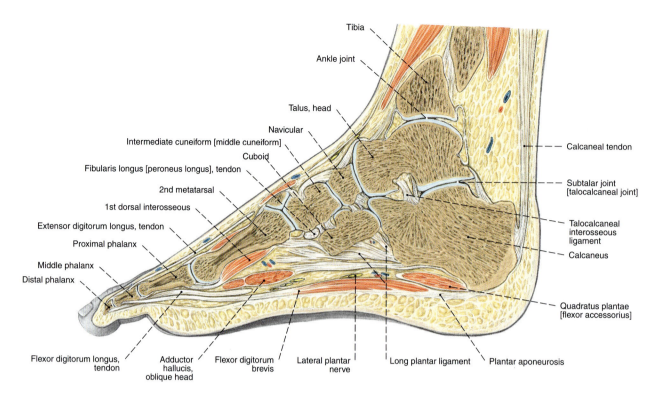

Tibia

Ankle joint

Talus, head

Navicular

Intermediate cuneiform [middle cuneiform]

Cuboid

Fibularis longus [peroneus longus], tendon

2nd metatarsal

1st dorsal interosseous

Extensor digitorum longus, tendon

Proximal phalanx

Middle phalanx

Distal phalanx

Calcaneal tendon

Subtalar joint [talocalcaneal joint]

Talocalcaneal interosseous ligament

Calcaneus

Quadratus plantae [flexor accessorius]

Flexor digitorum longus, tendon

Adductor hallucis, oblique head

Flexor digitorum brevis

Lateral plantar nerve

Long plantar ligament

Plantar aponeurosis

Fig. 1378   Foot; sagittal section through 2nd toe; medial aspect.

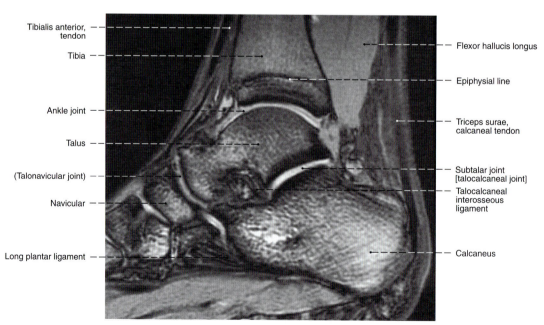

Tibialis anterior, tendon

Tibia

Ankle joint

Talus

(Talonavicular joint)

Navicular

Long plantar ligament

Flexor hallucis longus

Epiphysial line

Triceps surae, calcaneal tendon

Subtalar joint [talocalcaneal joint]

Talocalcaneal interosseous ligament

Calcaneus

Fig. 1379   Foot; magnetic resonance image (MRI); sagittal slightly medial to longitudinal axis of neck of talus; medial aspect.

	Motor	Sensory
Lumbar plexus (T 12) L 1–L 3 (L 4)		
Iliohypogastric nerve [iliopubic nerve] T 12, L 1	Rectus abdominis, external oblique, internal oblique, transversus abdominis [transverse abdominal]	
Lateral cutaneous branch		Skin of hip
Anterior cutaneous branch		Skin of external inguinal ring and mons pubis
Ilio-inguinal nerve (T 12) L 1 (L 2)	Rectus abdominis, external oblique, internal oblique, transversus abdominis [transverse abdominal]	
Anterior scrotal nerves/ anterior labial nerves		Skin of inguinal region, root of penis, and scrotum Skin of inguinal region and labia majora
Genitofemoral nerve L 1, L 2	Cremaster	
Genital branch		
Femoral branch		Layers of testis (including dartos fascia)
Lateral cutaneous nerve of thigh [lateral femoral cutaneous nerve] L 2, L 3		Skin over saphenous opening Skin of lateral and anterior side of thigh proximal to knee
Obturator nerve L 2- L 4 Anterior branch	Obturator externus, pectineus, adductor brevis, adductor longus, gracilis	Joint capsule of hip joint
Cutaneous branch	Adductor magnus, (adductor brevis), adductor minimus	Skin of medial side of thigh proximal to knee
Posterior branch Muscular branches		Joint capsule of hip joint, periosteum of posterior surface of femur [thigh bone]
Accessory obturator nerve L 3, L 4	Pectineus	Joint capsule of hip joint
Femoral nerve L 2 - L 4 Muscular branches	Iliopsoas, pectineus, sartorius, quadriceps femoris	Joint capsule of hip joint
Anterior cutaneous branches Saphenous nerve Infrapatellar branch Medial cutaneous nerve of leg		Skin of anterior and medial side of thigh proximal to knee, periosteum of anterior surface of femur [thigh bone] Skin of medial and anterior side of knee and medial side of leg and foot
Sacral plexus (L 4) L 5- S 3 (S 4)		
Nerve to obturator internus L 5- S 2	Obturator internus	
Nerve to piriformis S 1, S 2	Piriformis	
Nerve to quadratus femoris L 5 - S 1 (S 2)	Quadratus femoris	
Superior gluteal nerve L 4 - S 1	Gluteus medius and minimus, tensor fasciae latae [tensor of fascia lata]	
Inferior gluteal nerve L 5 - S 2	Gluteus maximus	
Posterior cutaneous nerve of thigh [posterior femoral cutaneous nerve] S 1- S 3		Skin of posterior side of thigh and proximal leg
Inferior clunial nerves Perineal nerves		Skin of gluteal region Perineum, skin of scrotum resp. skin of labia majora
Sciatic nerve L 4 - S 3	Flexors of thigh, all muscles of leg and foot	
Common fibular nerve L 4- S 2	Biceps femoris, short head	Joint capsule of knee joint Skin of calf up proximal to lateral malleolus Communicating branch with sural nerve
Lateral sural cutaneous nerve Sural communicating branch		
Superficial fibular nerve Muscular branches	Fibularis [peroneus] longus and brevis	
Medial dorsal cutaneous nerve Intermediate dorsal cutaneous nerve		Skin of leg and dorsum of foot down to 1st- 3rd toe Skin of lateral border of foot
Dorsal digital nerves of foot		Skin of dorsum of toes except 1st interdigital space and lateral border of 5th toe

Continued → 388

	Motor	Sensory
Deep fibular nerve Muscular branches	Tibialis anterior, extensor digitorum longus, extensor hallucis longus, extensor digitorum brevis, and extensor hallucis brevis	Periosteum of tibia and fibula and joint capsule of ankle joint
Dorsal digital nerves of foot		Skin of 1st interdigital space
Tibial nerve L 4 - S 3 Muscular branches	Triceps surae, plantaris, popliteus, tibialis posterior, flexor digitorum longus, flexor hallucis longus	Joint capsule of knee joint
Interosseous nerve of leg [crural interosseous nerve]		Periosteum of tibia and fibula and joint capsule of ankle joint
Medial sural cutaneous nerve		Merges with lateral sural cutaneous nerve to form the sural nerve
Sural nerve Lateral dorsal cutaneous nerve		Skin of lateral border of foot up to lateral border of little toe
Lateral calcaneal branches		Lateral skin of heel
Medial calcaneal branches		Medial skin of heel
Medial plantar nerve	Abductor hallucis, flexor digitorum brevis, flexor hallucis brevis (medial head), 1st and 2nd lumbricals	Medial skin of sole
Common plantar digital nerves		Skin of plantar side of medial 3 1/2 toes and nail area
Proper plantar digital nerves		
Lateral plantar nerve Superficial branch	Abductor digiti minimi, quadratus plantae [flexor accessorius], flexor digiti minimi brevis, opponens digiti minimi, interossei of 4th interdigital space	
Common plantar digital nerves	2nd - 4th lumbricals, adductor hallucis (transverse head), interossei of 1st - 4th interdigital space	Skin of plantar side of lateral 1 1/2 toes and nail area
Proper plantar digital nerves		
Deep branch		
Pudendal nerve (S 1) S 2 - S 4 Inferior anal [rectal] nerves S 3, S 4		Skin of anal triangle and perineum
Perineal nerves Posterior scrotal nerves/ posterior labial nerves Muscular branches	Superficial and deep transverse perineal muscles, bulbospongiosus and ischiocavernosus, external anal sphincter	Dorsal skin of scrotum resp. labia majora and minora, mucosa of urethra, vestibule of vagina
Dorsal nerve of penis/ dorsal nerve of clitoris	Deep transverse perineal muscle	Skin of penis, glans penis/ clitoris, prepuce
Coccygeal nerve S 4, S 5 (Co 1) Coccygeal plexus S 4, S 5, (Co 1) Anococcygeal nerve	Ischiococcygeus [coccygeus], levator ani	Skin over coccyx and between coccyx and anus

Muscles used in clinical diagnosis of segmental innervation of lower limb

Spinal segment resp. segmental spinal nerve	Resp. muscle(s) / tendon(s) reflex
L 3	Quadriceps femoris (paralysis and loss of patellar tendon reflex)
L 4	Quadriceps femoris and tibialis anterior (weakening of patellar tendon reflex)
L 5	Extensor hallucis longus, possibly also brevis (paralysis and atrophy)
S 1	Fibular [peroneal] muscles, possibly also triceps surae and glutei (loss of Achilles tenodn reflex)

Index

Bold numbers indicate pages in which terms occur also in legends or tables.